Drug Reference Guide to Brand Names and Active Ingredients

OTHER MOSBY PUBLICATIONS BY THE PAGLIAROS

Pharmacologic Aspects of Nursing, 1986.

Pharmacologic Aspects of Aging, 1983.

Drug Reference Guide to Brand Names and Active Ingredients

LOUIS A. PAGLIARO, M.S., Pharm.D., Ph.D.

Associate Professor
Faculty of Pharmacy and Pharmaceutical Sciences
University of Alberta
Edmonton, Alberta

ANN M. PAGLIARO, R.N., B.S.N., M.S.N.

Associate Professor
Faculty of Nursing
University of Alberta
Edmonton, Alberta

The C.V. Mosby Company

St. Louis • Toronto • Princeton • 1986

PRINTED IN THE UNITED STATES OF AMERICA

The C.V. Mosby Company
11830 Westline Industrial Drive
St. Louis, Missouri 63146

Library of Congress Cataloging in Publication Data

Pagliaro, Louis A.
Drug reference guide to brand names and active ingredients.

1. Drugs--Dictionaries. 2. Drugs--Trade-marks--Dictionaries. I. Pagliaro, Ann M. II. Title.
[DNLM: 1. Drug Interactions--handbooks. 2. Drugs--handbooks. 3. Nomenclature--handbooks. 4. Therapeutic Equivalency--handbooks. QV 39 P138d]
RS51.P24 1986 615'.1 85-21486
ISBN 0-8016-3773-2

VH/VH 9 8 7 6 5 4 3 2 1 05/C/617

To Abigail, Bernadette, and P.D.B.
Semper fidelis

Preface

The purpose of this reference guide is to provide the clinician with a comprehensive list of brand (trade) names and the corresponding active ingredients for prescription and non-prescription products commonly available in North America.

In addition, in order to keep the list as current, up-to-date, and useful as possible, drugs that are undergoing experimental use in North America for which brand names have been tentatively assigned are included. Likewise, selected newer drugs that are used clinically in Britain and Europe and that are likely to be marketed in North America have also been included. Since this guide is primarily concerned with products used in human therapeutics, veterinary products and diagnostic agents are omitted unless their inclusion is warranted by clinical reports of toxicity in humans. This reference guide contains complete information on both single- and multiple-ingredient products that are available for human use. Over 8,000 different brand names and over 1,600 different active ingredients are listed in this reference guide. Each entry is fully cross-referenced to facilitate retrieval of information, so that this guide contains in total over 21,000 entries.

Products are generally maintained in this listing for a minimum of five years after they have been taken off the market. This provides the clinician with information that is typically missing from most *current* references. The reason for maintaining these listings for a minimum of five years is demonstrated in clinical examples of the usefulness of such "dated" information, which includes (1) the clinician treating a patient who has not been seen for two years and who now wants a refill for a product no longer on the market; (2) a clinician treating a child who has accidentally ingested the contents of a prescription bottle of a product taken off the market several years ago but which nevertheless remained in the bathroom cabinet; and (3) the clinician involved in chart review who wants to know what the active ingredient was in a prescription product the patient was receiving, but which is now no longer available.

This reference is divided into two fully cross-referenced lists. The first list contains in alphabetical order drug brand names and their corresponding active ingredient(s). For the sake of clarity and uniformity, all active ingredients are referred to by their generic United States Adopted Names. The second list contains in alphabetical order generic names of active ingredients with a corresponding alphabetized list of brand names. An asterisk after a brand name, in either list, indicates that the product contains more than one active ingredient. Inactive ingredients, such as binders, fillers, preservatives, suspending agents, and the like, are *not* included in the listings. Omission of these inactive ingredients, as well as of other data which may be related to drug products (but which are extraneous to the stated purpose of this reference guide), has been done to facilitate clarity and usability.

The first list, which presents brand names and their corresponding active ingredient(s), should be of particular assistance to:

1. Clinicians working in an emergency department when, for example, an overdose patient is brought in with a number of different prescription or nonprescription drug vials, which list brand names, but not the generic active ingredients.
2. Clinicians involved in public health, who, for example, may in their assessment of the home situation be presented with a variety of drugs identified by brand name only.
3. Clinicians involved in taking drug and other histories (e.g., medical, nursing, social, etc.), who may elicit drug names from their patients, but may not be aware of the generic names of the active ingredients.
4. Clinicians involved in providing drug information to patients or other health care providers, who, for example, may need to know what active ingredients are contained in the various proprietary preparations.

The second list, which presents the generic names of the active ingredients together with a corresponding alphabetized list of brand names, should be of particular assistance to:

1. Clinicians involved in prescribing who want to check, for example, what brand names are associated with a particular active ingredient or if perhaps the same active ingredient, but under a different brand name, is available.

2. Clinicians involved with therapeutic or toxicologic assessment who may want to know, for example, if the patient is receiving any other products which contain a specific ingredient. For example, if the patient is allergic to aspirin, the clinician can look at the second list and under aspirin find all of the various single ingredient *and* combination products which should be avoided. Likewise, if a patient is taking a drug with a relatively narrow therapeutic index, a quick check of the second list may prevent inadvertent duplication and resultant overdose. This last example is particularly relevant when a drug with a narrow therapeutic index is found in combination- as well as single-ingredient products (e.g., theophylline).

This reference guide has been carefully constructed and checked in order to ensure that it is both accurate and up-to-date. However, because manufacturers may change formulations from time to time, it is imperative that the user check the current package insert or contact the manufacturer directly whenever in doubt or whenever further information about product formulation is required. For information regarding the pharmacology of the listed ingredients, the user is referred to one of the texts listed opposite the title page of this reference guide.

We trust that this reference guide will be of practical use to both the clinician who is directly involved in patient care and to the student who is assimilating clinical knowledge and skills, and that its use will assist health care professionals in optimizing patient care.

We wish to extend special thanks to Darin Brox and Dominant Chung for their assistance.

LOUIS A. PAGLIARO
ANN M. PAGLIARO

Contents

Part I

Brand Names and Corresponding Active Ingredients

A

AARANE
  Cromolyn Sodium
AAS*
  Allantoin
  Aminacrine
  Sulfanilamide
ABBOKINASE
  Urokinase
ABSORBINE ARTHRITIC
    PAIN*
  Cetyl Alcohol
  Isopropyl Alcohol
  Menthol
  Methylnicotinate
  Methyl Salicylate
ACCUTANE
  Isotretinoin
ACENOL
  Acetaminophen
ACETA-GESIC*
  Acetaminophen
  Phenyltoloxamine
ACET-AM
  Theophylline
ACET-AM EXPECTORANT*
  Guaifenesin
  Theophylline
ACETAMIN
  Acetaminophen
ACETAMINOPHEN WITH
    CODEINE ELIXIR*
  Acetaminophen
  Codeine
ACETATE-AS
  Hydrocortisone
ACETAZOLAM
  Acetazolamide
ACETEST
  Sodium Nitroprusside
    Reagent
ACETEXA
  Nortriptyline
ACETONYL
  Aspirin
ACETOPHEN
  Aspirin
ACETOXYL
  Benzoyl Peroxide
ACETYL ADALIN
  Acecarbromal
ACETYL-SAL
  Aspirin
ACHROMYCIN
  Tetracycline
ACHROMYCIN OPHTHALMIC
  Tetracycline
ACHROMYCIN V
  Tetracycline
ACHROSTATIN V*
  Nystatin
  Tetracycline
ACIDFLUD
  Fluoride
ACID MANTLE
  Aluminum Acetate
ACIDOGEN
  Glutamic Acid
ACIDORIDE
  Glutamic Acid
ACIDULIN
  Glutamic Acid
ACI-JEL*
  Acetic Acid
  Boric Acid
  Oxyquinoline
  Ricinoleic Acid
ACILLIN
  Ampicillin
A.C.N.*
  Ascorbic Acid
  Niacin
  Vitamin A

ACNAVEEN*
  Salicylic Acid
  Sulfur
ACNE-AID*
  Resorcinol
  Sulfur
ACNEDERM LOTION*
  Isopropyl Alcohol
  Sulfur
  Zinc Oxide
  Zinc Sulfate
ACNE-DOME CREME & LOTION*
  Resorcinol
  Sulfur
ACNE-DOME MEDICATED CLEANSER*
  Salicylic Acid
  Sulfur
ACNESARB
  Salicylic Acid
ACNO*
  Salicylic Acid
  Sulfur
ACNOMEL*
  Resorcinol
  Sulfur
ACNOTEX*
  Salicylic Acid
  Sulfur
ACNYCIN*
  Resorcinol
  Sulfur
ACON
  Vitamin A
ACRIDIL
  Triprolidine
ACRIFLEX
  Aminacrine
ACTACIN*
  Pseudoephedrine
  Triprolidine
ACTAGEN*
  Pseudoephedrine
  Triprolidine
ACTAMER
  Bithionol
ACTAMIN
  Acetaminophen
ACTAMINE*
  Pseudoephedrine
  Triprolidine
ACTASE
  Fibrinolysin, Human
ACTAZINE
  Piperacetazine
ACTEST
  Corticotropin
ACTH
  Corticotropin
ACTHAR
  Corticotropin
ACTICORT-100
  Hydrocortisone
ACTIDIL
  Triprolidine
ACTIDILON
  Triprolidine
ACTIFED*
  Pseudoephedrine
  Triprolidine
ACTIFED-C*
  Codeine
  Guaifenesin
  Pseudoephedrine
  Triprolidine
ACTIFED EXPECTORANT*
  Guaifenesin
  Pseudoephedrine
  Triprolidine
ACTIFED WITH CODEINE COUGH SYRUP*
  Codeine
  Pseudoephedrine
  Triprolidine
ACTIF VIII
  Antihemophilic Factor
ACTIHIST*
  Pseudoephedrine
  Triprolidine
ACTI-PREM*
  Pseudoephedrine
  Triprolidine
ACTOL EXPECTORANT*
  Guaifenesin
  Noscapine
ACTOSPAR
  Sparteine
ACTOZINE

Benactyzine
ACTRAPID, HUMAN
Insulin Regular, Human
ACTRAPID MC
Insulin Regular
ACU-DYNE
Povidone-Iodine
ACUPAN
Nefopam
ACUTRAN
Amphecloral
ACUTRIM
Phenylpropanolamine
ACUTUSS EXPECTORANT WITH CODEINE*
Codeine
Guaifenesin
Phenylephrine
ACYLANID
Acetyldigitoxin
ADABEE
Vitamins, Multiple
ADABEE WITH MINERALS*
Minerals, Multiple
Vitamins, Multiple
ADALAT
Nifedipine
ADALIN
Carbromal
ADANON
Methadone
ADAPETTES*
Edetic Acid
Povidone
Thimerosal
ADAPIN
Doxepin
ADASEPT CLEANSER
Triclosan
ADATUSS D.C. EXPECTORANT*
Guaifenesin
Hydrocodone
ADEFLOR CHEWABLE*
Sodium Fluoride
Vitamins, Multiple
ADEFLOR DROPS*
Sodium Fluoride
Vitamins, Multiple
ADEMIL
Flumethiazide
ADEMOL
Flumethiazide
ADENEX
Ascorbic Acid
ADENO
Adenosine
ADENOTRIPHOS
Adenosine
ADIPEX
Phentermine
ADIPEX-P
Phentermine
ADLERIKA
Magnesium Sulfate
ADPHEN
Phendimetrazine
A-D-R
Racemethionine
ADRENALEX
Adrenal Cortex Extract
ADRENALIN
Epinephrine
ADRENALINE CHLORIDE SOLUTION, INJECTABLE
Epinephrine
ADRENALIN IN OIL
Epinephrine
ADRENATRATE
Epinephrine
ADRENOSEM SALICYLATE
Carbazochrome Salicylate
ADRENOXYL
Carbazochrome Salicylate
ADRESTAT F
Carbazochrome Salicylate
ADRIAMYCIN
Doxorubicin
ADRIBLASTINA
Doxorubicin
ADROYD
Oxymetholone
ADRUCIL
Fluorouracil

ADSORBOCARPINE
  Pilocarpine
ADSORBONAC
  Sodium Chloride
ADSORBOTEAR
  Methylcellulose
ADUMBRAN
  Oxazepam
ADVANCED FORMULA
    DRISTAN*
  Acetaminophen
  Chlorpheniramine
  Phenylephrine
ADVIL
  Ibuprofen
AEROBID
  Flunisolide
AERO CAINE
  Benzocaine
AERODINE
  Povidone-Iodine
AEROLATE III
  Theophylline
AEROLATE JR.
  Theophylline
AEROLATE LIQUID
  Theophylline
AEROLATE SR.
  Theophylline
AEROLONE*
  Cyclopentamine
  Isoproterenol
AEROPHYLLINE
  Dyphylline
AEROSEB-DEX
  Dexamethasone
AEROSEB-HC
  Hydrocortisone
AEROSOL OT
  Docusate Sodium
AEROSPORIN
  Polymyxin B
AERO THERM
  Benzocaine
AFAXIN
  Vitamin A
A-FIL*
  Menthyl anthranilate
  Titanium Dioxide
AFKO-LUBE
  Docusate Sodium
AFKO-LUBE LAX*
  Casanthranol
  Docusate Sodium
AFRIN
  Oxymetazoline
AFRINOL
  Pseudoephedrine
AFRIN PEDIATRIC
  Oxymetazoline
AFTATE
  Tolnaftate
AGESTIN
  Norethindrone
AGORAL*
  Glycerin
  Mineral Oil
  Phenolphthalein
AGORAL PLAIN*
  Glycerin
  Mineral Oil
AGRIBON
  Sulfadimethoxine
A-H GEL
  Aluminum Hydroxide
A-HYDROCORT
  Hydrocortisone
AID-TUSS*
  Atropine
  Caramiphen
  Chlorpheniramine
  Phenylpropanolamine
AIRBRON
  Acetylcysteine
AIRET
  Dyphylline
AIRHEUMAT
  Ketoprofen
AKARPINE
  Pilocarpine
AK-CON OPHTHALMIC
  Naphazoline
AK-DEX
  Dexamethasone
AK-DILATE OPHTHALMIC
  Phenylephrine
AKES-N-PAIN*
  Acetaminophen
  Caffeine
  Calcium Gluconate

Salicylamide
AK-FLUOR
  Fluorescein
AKINETON
  Biperiden
AKNE DRYING*
  Benzalkonium
    Chloride
  Isopropyl Alcohol
  Salicyclic Acid
  Sulfur
  Urea
  Zinc Oxide
AK-NEFRIN OPHTHALMIC
  Phenylephrine
AK-PENTOLATE
  Cyclopentolate
AKRINOL
  Acrisorcin
AK-TAINE
  Proparacaine
AKWA TEARS*
  Chlorobutanol
  Polyvinyl Alcohol
AK-ZOL
  Acetazolamide
ALAMINE*
  Chlorpheniramine
  Phenylephrine
ALAMINE-C*
  Chlorpheniramine
  Codeine
  Phenylephrine
ALAMINE EXPECTORANT*
  Chlorpheniramine
  Codeine
  Guaifenesin
  Phenylephrine
ALAMINO
  Dihydroxyaluminum
    Aminoacetate
ALAXIN
  Poloxamer
AL-AY*
  Acetaminophen
  Caffeine
  Chlorpheniramine
  Phenylephrine
ALBA-CE
  Ascorbic Acid
ALBA-DOME
  Monobenzone
ALBAFORT INJECTABLE*
  Iron
  Vitamin B Complex
ALBALON
  Naphazoline
ALBALON-A*
  Antazoline
  Naphazoline
ALBALON LIQUIFILM
  Naphazoline
ALBA-LYBE*
  Calcium Pantothenate
  Cyanocobalamin
  Lysine
  Niacinamide
  Pyridoxine
  Riboflavin
  Thiamine
ALBAMYCIN
  Novobiocin
ALBA-TEMP
    SUPPOSITORIES
  Acetaminophen
ALBATUSSIN*
  Citric Acid
  Dextromethorphan
  Guaifenesin
  Phenylephrine
  Pyrilamine
  Sodium Citrate
ALBA-3 OINTMENT*
  Bacitracin
  Neomycin
  Polymyxin B
ALBICON*
  Aluminum Hydroxide
  Calcium Carbonate
  Magnesium Carbonate
  Magnesium Oxide
ALBON
  Sulfadimethoxine
ALCAINE
  Proparacaine
ALCID
  Aluminum Hydroxide
ALCOJEL
  Isopropyl Alcohol
ALCONEFRIN

Phenylephrine
ALCOPARA
Bephenium
ALCORUB
Isopropyl Alcohol
ALDACTAZIDE*
Hydrochlorothiazide
Spironolactone
ALDACTONE
Spironolactone
ALDECIN INHALER
Beclomethasone
ALDINAMIDE
Pyrazinamide
ALDOCLOR*
Chlorothiazide
Methyldopa
ALDOCORTIN
Aldosterone
ALDOMET
Methyldopa
ALDOMET ESTER
Methyldopate
ALDORIL*
Hydrochlorothiazide
Methyldopa
ALDROX
Aluminum Hydroxide
ALERMINE
Chlorpheniramine
ALERSULE*
Chlorpheniramine
Methscopolamine
Phenylephrine
ALFATHESIN*
Alfadolone
Alfaxalone
ALFICETYN
Chloramphenicol
ALFLORONE
Fludrocortisone
ALGAFAN
Propoxyphene
ALGEMOL*
Alginic Acid
Aluminum Hydroxide
Magnesium Hydroxide
Sodium Bicarbonate
ALGENIC ALKA IMPROVED TABLETS*
Aluminum Hydroxide
Magnesium Hydroxide
ALGESAL CREAM
Diethylamine Salicylate
ALGLYN
Dihydroxyaluminum Aminoacetate
ALGODEX
Propoxyphene
ALGOVERINE
Phenylbutazone
ALIDASE
Hyaluronidase
ALISED*
Atropine
Phenobarbital
ALKA BUTAZOLIDIN
Phenylbutazone
ALKABUTAZONE
Phenylbutazone
ALKA-MINTS
Calcium Carbonate
ALKARAU
Reserpine
ALKA-SELTZER EFFERVESCENT ANTACID*
Citric Acid
Potassium Bicarbonate
Sodium Bicarbonate
ALKA-SELTZER EFFERVESCENT PAIN RELIEVER AND ANTACID*
Aspirin
Citric Acid
Sodium Bicarbonate
ALKA-SELTZER PLUS*
Aspirin
Chlorpheniramine
Phenylpropanolamine
ALKA-TANDEARIL
Oxyphenbutazone
ALKA-2 CHEWABLE ANTACID
Calcium Carbonate
ALKERAN
Melphalan

ALKETS*
Calcium Carbonate
Magnesium Carbonate
Magnesium Oxide
ALKOISOL
Isopropyl Alcohol
ALKO-LUBE LAX*
Casanthranol
Docusate Sodium
ALLBEE-T
Vitamins, Multiple
ALLBEE WITH C
Vitamins, Multiple
ALLEGRON
Nortriptyline
ALLERBID
Chlorpheniramine
ALLER-CHLOR
Chlorpheniramine
ALLERCUR
Clemizole
ALLERDRYL
Diphenhydramine
ALLEREST*
Methapyrilene
Phenylpropanolamine
Pyrilamine
ALLEREST EYE DROPS
Naphazoline
ALLEREST NASAL
Phenylephrine
ALLEREST REGULAR AND CHILDREN'S*
Chlorpheniramine
Phenylpropanolamine
ALLEREST SINUS PAIN FORMULA*
Acetaminophen
Chlorpheniramine
Phenylpropanolamine
ALLERFORM*
Chlorpheniramine
Phenylpropanolamine
ALLERFRIN*
Pseudoephedrine
Triprolidine
ALLERGEFON
Carbinoxamine
ALLERGESIC*
Chlorpheniramine
Phenylpropanolamine
ALLERGIN*
Chlorpheniramine
Phenylpropanolamine
ALLERGY RELIEF MEDICINE*
Chlorpheniramine
Phenylpropanolamine
ALLERID
Chlorpheniramine
ALLERID-D.C.*
Chlorpheniramine
Pseudoephedrine
ALLERPROP*
Belladonna
Chlorpheniramine
Phenylpropanolamine
ALLERSONE*
Diperodon
Hydrocortisone
Zinc Oxide
ALLERTOC
Pyrilamine
ALLOPRIN
Allopurinol
ALMACONE*
Aluminum Hydroxide
Magnesium Trisilicate
ALMINATE
Dihydroxyaluminum Aminoacetate
ALMOCARPINE*
Benzalkonium Chloride
Pilocarpine
ALONDRA
Paramethasone
ALONDRA-F
Flurandrenolide
ALOPHEN
Phenolphthalein
ALPEN
Ampicillin
ALPHA CHYMAR
Chymotrypsin
ALPHA CHYMOLEAN
Chymotrypsin
ALPHADERM
Hydrocortisone

ALPHADROL
  Fluprednisolone
ALPHA KERI*
  Lanolin
  Mineral Oil
ALPHA KERI SOAP*
  Lanolin
  Mineral Oil
ALPHALIN
  Vitamin A
ALPHAMETTES*
  Cholecalciferol
  Vitamin A
ALPHAMUL
  Castor Oil
ALPHAONE*
  Resorcinol
  Salicylic Acid
ALPHAREDISOL
  Hydroxocobalamin
ALPHA-RUVITE
  Hydroxocobalamin
ALPHOSYL-HC LOTION & CREAM*
  Allantoin
  Crude Coal Tar Extract
  Hydrocortisone
ALPHOSYL LOTION & CREAM*
  Allantoin
  Crude Coal Tar Extract
AL-R
  Chlorpheniramine
ALSERIN
  Reserpine
ALTAFUR
  Furaltadone
ALTERNAGEL
  Aluminum Hydroxide
ALTHOSE
  Methadone
ALTILEV
  Nortriptyline
ALU-CAP
  Aluminum Hydroxide
AL-U-CREME
  Aluminum Hydroxide
ALUDRIN
  Isoproterenol
ALUDROX*
  Aluminum Hydroxide
  Magnesium Oxide
ALUMADRINE*
  Acetaminophen
  Chlorpheniramine
  Phenylpropanolamine
ALUMID SUSPENSION*
  Aluminum Hydroxide
  Magnesium Hydroxide
ALUPENT
  Metaproterenol
ALURATE
  Aprobarbital
ALUREX*
  Aluminum Hydroxide
  Magnesium Hydroxide
ALUREX NO.2
  Aluminum Hydroxide
  Magnesium Hydroxide
ALUSCOP*
  Aluminum Hydroxide
  Dihydroxyaluminum Acetate
  Magnesium Hydroxide
  Magnesium Oxide
ALU-TAB
  Aluminum Hydroxide
AL-VITE*
  Intrinsic Factor
  Vitamins, Multiple
ALVODINE
  Piminodine
ALYSINE
  Sodium Salicylate
ALZINOX
  Dihydroxyaluminum Aminoacetate
AMAPHEN*
  Acetaminophen
  Butalbital
  Caffeine
AMARIL D*
  Chlorpheniramine
  Phenylephrine
  Phenylpropanolamine
  Phenyltoloxamine
AMBENYL-D DECONGESTANT COUGH FORMULA*
  Dextromethorphan
  Guaifenesin

Pseudoephedrine
AMBENYL EXPECTORANT*
Ammonium Chloride
Bromodiphenhydramine
Codeine
Diphenhydramine
Guaifenesin
Menthol
AMBILHAR
Niridazole
AMBODRYL
Bromodiphenhydramine
AMCAP
Ampicillin
AMCHLOR
Ammonium Chloride
AMCILL
Ampicillin
AMEN
Medroxyprogesterone
AMERICAINE
Benzocaine
AMERICAINE-OTIC*
Benzocaine
Glycerin
AMERICAN MCGAW
Sorbitol
AMERSOL
Ibuprofen
AMERTAN
Tannic Acid
AMESEC*
Aminophylline
Amobarbital
Ephedrine
A-METHAPRED
Methylprednisolone
AMETHONE
Amolanone
AMETYCIN
Mitomycin
AMICAR
Aminocaproic Acid
AMIDATE
Etomidate
AMIDE-VC*
Allantoin
Aminacrine
Sulfanilamide
AMIDONE
Methadone
AMIKIN
Amikacin
AMILINE
Amitriptyline
AMINO-CERV
Urea
AMINODUR DURA-TABS
Aminophylline
AMINOPHYL
Aminophylline
AMIPAQUE
Metrizamide
AMITID
Amitriptyline
AMITONE
Calcium Carbonate
AMITRIL
Amitriptyline
AMLAX*
Bile Salts
Cascara Sagrada
Phenolphthalein
AMMIVIN
Khellin
AMMONERIC
Ammonium Chloride
AMNESTROGEN
Estrogens,
Esterified
AMOBELL*
Belladonna Extract
Phenobarbital
AMODRINE*
Aminophylline
Ephedrine
Phenobarbital
AMOGEL*
Bismuth Subgallate
Kaolin
Opium
Pectin
Zinc Phenolsulfonate
AMOGEL PG*
Belladonna Alkaloids
Kaolin
Paregoric
Pectin
AMOLINE
Aminophylline
AMONIDRIN*
Ammonium Chloride

Guaifenesin
AMOSAN
Carbamide Peroxide
AMOSTAT
Caffeine
AMOTRIL
Clofibrate
AMOXICAN
Amoxicillin
AMOXIL
Amoxicillin
AMPEN
Ampicillin
AMPHENOL
Acetaminophen
AMPHICHLOR
Chloramphenicol
AMPHICOL
Chloramphenicol
AMPHISOL
Amiphenazole
AMPHOJEL
Aluminum Hydroxide
AMPHOJEL 65*
Aluminum Hydroxide
Simethicone
AMPHYLLINE
Aminophylline
AMPICIN
Ampicillin
AMPICIN-PRB*
Ampicillin
Probenecid
AMPILEAN
Ampicillin
AMPLIN
Ampicillin
A.M.T.*
Aluminum Hydroxide
Magnesium
Trisilicate
AMUNO
Indomethacin
AMYTAL
Amobarbital
AMYTAL & ASPIRIN*
Amobarbital
Aspirin
AMYTALILY
Amobarbital
ANABACTYL
Carbenicillin
ANACARDONE
Nikethamide
ANACEL
Tetracaine
ANACIN*
Aspirin
Caffeine
ANACIN-3
Acetaminophen
ANACOBIN
Cyanocobalamin
ANADROL
Oxymetholone
ANAFED*
Chlorpheniramine
Pseudoephedrine
ANAFRANIL
Clomipramine
ANAHIST
Thonzylamine
ANALATE
Magesium Salicylate
ANALBALM*
Camphor
Menthol
Methyl Salicylate
ANALEXIN
Phenyramidol
ANALGESIC BALM*
Menthol
Methyl Salicylate
ANAMINE*
Chlorpheniramine
Pseudoephedrine
ANAMINE T.D. CAPS*
Chlorpheniramine
Pseudoephedrine
ANANASE
Proteolytic Enzymes
ANANASE-50
Bromelains
ANAPHEN*
Acetaminophen
Butalbital
Caffeine
ANAPOLON 50
Oxymetholone
ANAPREL-500

Rescinnamine
ANAPROX
Naproxen
ANASPAZ
Hyoscyamine
ANASPAZ PB*
Hyoscyamine
Phenobarbital
ANATOLA
Vitamin A
ANATUSS*
Acetaminophen
Chlorpheniramine
Dextromethorphan
Guaifenesin
Phenylephrine
Phenylpropanolamine
ANAVAR
Oxandrolone
ANBESOL ANTISEPTIC ANESTHETIC*
Benzocaine
Phenol
Povidone-Iodine
ANCASAL
Aspirin
ANCASAL COMPOUND NO.1*
Aspirin
Codeine
ANCASAL COMPOUND NO.2*
Aspirin
Codeine
ANCASAL COMPOUND NO.3*
Aspirin
Codeine
ANCAZINE
Piperazine
ANCEF
Cefazolin
ANCOBON
Flucytosine
ANCOLAN
Meclizine
ANCOTIL
Flucytosine
ANDOIN*
Allantoin
Cholecalciferol
Vitamin A
ANDRO-CYP 100
Testosterone
ANDRO-CYP 200
Testosterone
ANDROID
Methyltestosterone
ANDROID-T
Testosterone
ANDROLONE
Stanolone
ANDROSTALONE
Mestanolone
ANDROYD
Oxymetholone
ANDRO 100
Testosterone
ANDRUSOL
Testosterone
ANDURACAINE
Procaine
ANECTINE
Succinylcholine
ANERGEN 25
Promethazine
ANESTACON
Lidocaine
ANESTHESIN
Benzocaine
ANETHAINE
Tetracaine
ANEURAL
Meprobamate
ANEVRAL
Phenylbutazone
ANEXSIA WITH CODEINE*
Aspirin
Caffeine
Codeine
ANGIOAMIN
Xanthinol Niacinate
ANGIO-CONRAY
Iothalamate Sodium
ANGIOGRAFIN
Meglumine
ANGISED
Nitroglycerin
ANGITRATE
Pentaerythritol Tetranitrate
ANGITRIT
Trolnitrate

ANGLOVIST 370
  Diatrizoate
    Meglumine
ANG-O-SPAN
  Nitroglycerin
ANHYDRON
  Cyclothiazide
ANODYNOS*
  Acetaminophen
  Aspirin
  Caffeine
  Salicylamide
ANODYNOS FORTE*
  Acetaminophen
  Chlorpheniramine
  Phenylephrine
  Salicylamide
ANOQUAN*
  Acetaminophen
  Butalbital
  Caffeine
ANOREX
  Phendimetrazine
ANOREXIN*
  Carboxymethyl-
    cellulose
  Phenylpropanolamine
ANOREXIN ONE-SPAN*
  Caffeine
  Phenylpropanolamine
ANSAID
  Flurbiprofen
ANSEMCO #2*
  Aspirin
  Caffeine
ANSOLYSEN
  Pentolinium
ANSPOR
  Cephradine
ANTABUSE
  Disulfiram
ANTACID POWDER*
  Aluminum Hydroxide
  Magnesium Carbonate
  Magnesium
    Trisilicate
  Sodium Bicarbonate
ANTALKA
  Glutamic Acid
ANTASTAN
  Antazoline
ANTEPAR
  Piperazine
ANTERON
  Gonadotropin
ANTHATEST
  Testosterone
ANTHERA
  Anthralin
ANTHIPHEN
  Dichlorophen
ANTHISAN
  Pyrilamine
ANTHRA-DERM
  Anthralin
ANTHRA-DERM OIL
  Anthralin
ANTI-ACID NO.1*
  Bismuth Subnitrate
  Calcium Carbonate
  Magnesium Carbonate
ANTIBIOPTO OPHTHALMIC*
  Boric Acid
  Chloramphenicol
  Sodium Borate
ANTILIRIUM
  Physostigmine
ANTIMINTH
  Pyrantel Pamoate
ANTIPRESS
  Imipramine
ANTISPAS
  Dicyclomine
ANTISTINE
  Antazoline
ANTISTINE-PRIVINE*
  Antazoline
  Naphazoline
ANTITREM
  Trihexyphenidyl
ANTI-TUSS
  Guaifenesin
ANTI-TUSS DM*
  Dextromethorphan
  Guaifenesin
ANTIVERT
  Meclizine
ANTIVERT/25
  Meclizine
ANTORA

Pentaerythritol
Tetranitrate
ANTRENYL
Oxyphenonium
ANTROCOL*
Atropine
Phenobarbital
ANTRYPOL
Suramin
ANTUITRIN-S
Gonadotropin,
Chorionic
ANTURAN
Sulfinpyrazone
ANTURANE
Sulfinpyrazone
ANTURIDIN
Sulfinpyrazone
ANUGARD-HC*
Benzyl Benzoate
Bismuth Resorcinol
Bismuth Subgallate
Hydrocortisone
Peruvian Balsam
ANUJECT
Procaine
ANUPHEN SUPPOSITORIES
Acetaminophen
ANUSOL*
Benzyl Benzoate
Bismuth Resorcinol
Bismuth Subgallate
Peruvian Balsam
Zinc Sulfate
ANUSOL-HC*
Benzyl Benzoate
Bismuth Resorcinol
Bismuth Subgallate
Hydrocortisone
Peruvian Balsam
Zinc Sulfate
ANUSOL OINTMENT*
Benzyl Benzoate
Peruvian Balsam
Zinc Sulfate
ANUSOL SUPPOSITORIES*
Bismuth Resorcinol
Bismuth Subgallate
Peruvian Balsam
Zinc Sulfate
AOLEPT
Periciazine
APAC*
Aspirin
Caffeine
Phenacetin
APA-DEINE*
Aspirin
Caffeine
Codeine
APAMIDE
Acetaminophen
APAP*
Acetaminophen
Aspirin
Caffeine
APARKANE
Trihexyphenidyl
APAURIN
Diazepam
APC*
Aspirin
Caffeine
APCOHIST ALLERGY*
Methapyrilene
Phenylpropanolamine
APC WITH CODEINE*
Aspirin
Caffeine
Codeine
APECTOL*
Aspirin
Butalbital
Caffeine
APF
Aspirin
A.P.L.
Gonadotropin,
Chorionic
APLISOL
Tuberculin
APLITEST
Tuberculin
APO-DIAZEPAM
Diazepam
APODOL
Anileridine
APOGEN
Gentamicin
APO-IMIPRAMINE

Imipramine
APO-INDOMETHACIN
Indomethacin
APOMITERAL
Cinnarizine
APONAL
Doxepin
APO-TRIAZIDE*
Hydrochlorothiazide
Triamterene
A-POXIDE
Chlordiazepoxide
APPEDRINE*
Carboxymethyl-cellulose
Phenylpropanolamine
APPRESS
Phenylpropanolamine
APRESAZIDE*
Hydralazine
Hydrochlorothiazide
APRESOLINE
Hydralazine
APRINOX
Bendroflumethiazide
APRISAC*
Minerals, Multiple
Vitamin E
APTROL
Phendimetrazine
AQUACARE
Urea
AQUACHLORAL
Chloral Hydrate
AQUADIOL
Estradiol
AQUA-FLOW*
Benzalkonium Chloride
Edetic Acid
Hydroxyethyl-cellulose
Polyvinyl Alcohol
Potassium Chloride
Sodium Bicarbonate
AQUA IVY
Poison Ivy Extract
AQUALIN SUPRETTES
Theophylline
AQUAMEPHYTON
Phytonadione
AQUAMOX
Quinethazone
AQUAPHYLLIN
Theophylline
AQUARIUS
Hydrochlorothiazide
AQUASOL A
Vitamin A
AQUASOL A CREAM
Tretinoin
AQUASOL A & D*
Cholecalciferol
Vitamin A
AQUASOL E
Vitamin E
AQUASTAT
Benzthiazide
AQUATAG
Benzthiazide
AQUATENSEN
Methyclothiazide
AQUEX
Trichlormethiazide
ARA-A
Vidarabine
ARALEN*
Chloroquine
Primaquine
ARAMINE
Metaraminol
ARCO-LASE*
Lipase
Trizyme
ARCO-LASE PLUS*
Atropine
Hyoscyamine
Lipase
Phenobarbital
Trizyme
ARCYLATE
Salsalate
ARET-A
Vitamin A
ARFONAD
Trimethaphan Camsylate
ARGESIC*
Magnesium Salicylate
Phenyltoloxamine

ARGYROL
  Silver Protein
ARISTAMID
  Sulfisomidine
ARISTFORM*
  Clioquinol
  Triamcinolone
ARISTFORM D*
  Clioquinol
  Triamcinolone
ARISTFORM R*
  Clioquinol
  Triamcinolone
ARISTOCORT
  Triamcinolone
ARISTODERM
  Triamcinolone
ARISTOGEL
  Triamcinolone
ARISTOSOL
  Triamcinolone
ARISTOSPAN
  Triamcinolone
ARLIDIN
  Nylidrin
ARMAZIDE
  Isoniazid
ARMOUR THYROID*
  Liothyronine
  Thyroxine
ARNE TIMESULES
  Ferrous Sulfate
AROVIT
  Vitamin A
ARS
  Antirabies Serum
    Equine
ARSOBAL
  Melarsoprol
ARTANE
  Trihexyphenidyl
ARTHRALGEN*
  Acetaminophen
  Salicylamide
ARTHRIN
  Magnesium Salicylate
ARTHRITIS PAIN FORMULA*
  Aluminum Hydroxide
  Aspirin
  Magnesium Hydroxide
ARTHRITIS STRENGTH
    BUFFERIN*
  Aspirin
  Dihydroxyaluminum
    Aminoacetate
  Magnesium Carbonate
ARTHROGESIC*
  Magnesium Salicylate
  Phenyltoloxamine
ARTHROLATE
  Sodium Thiosalicylate
ARTHROPAN
  Choline Salicylate
ARTRA
  Hydroquinone
ARVYNOL
  Ethchlorvynol
ASA
  Aspirin
A.S.A. AND CODEINE
    COMPOUND*
  Aspirin
  Caffeine
  Codeine
A.S.A. COMPOUND*
  Aspirin
  Caffeine
A.S.A. ENSEALS
  Aspirin
ASBRON G INLAY*
  Guaifenesin
  Theophylline
ASCODEEN-30*
  Aspirin
  Codeine
ASCOFER
  Ferrous Ascorbate
ASCORBICAP
  Ascorbic Acid
ASCORBIN
  Sodium Ascorbate
ASCORIL
  Ascorbic Acid
ASCRIPTIN*
  Aluminum Hydroxide
  Aspirin
  Codeine
  Magnesium Hydroxide
ASCRIPTIN A/D*
  Aluminum Hydroxide

Aspirin
Magnesium Hydroxide
ASELLACRIN
Somatropin
ASENDIN
Amoxapine
ASMA-LIEF*
Ephedrine
Phenobarbital
Theophylline
ASMALIX
Theophylline
ASMATANE MIST
Epinephrine
ASMINORL IMPROVED*
Ephedrine
Hydroxyzine
Theophylline
ASMINYL*
Ephedrine
Phenobarbital
Theophylline
ASMOLIN
Epinephrine
A-SOL
Vitamin A
ASPERBUF
Aspirin
ASPERCREME
Triethanolamine
Trolamine
Salicylate
ASPERGUM
Aspirin
ASPHAC-G*
Aspirin
Caffeine
Phenacetin
ASPHAL-G*
Aspirin
Caffeine
ASPIRIN FREE ANACIN-3*
Acetaminophen
Caffeine
ASPIRIN FREE DRISTAN*
Acetaminophen
Chlorpheniramine
Phenylephrine
ASPOGEN
Dihydroxyaluminum
Aminoacetate
ASPROJECT
Sodium
Thiosalicylate
ASTHMACON*
Aminophylline
Amobarbital
Ephedrine
ASTHMAGYL*
Ephedrine
Phenobarbital
Theophylline
ASTHMAHALER
Epinephrine
ASTHMANEFRIN
Epinephrine
ASTHMOPHYLLINE
Theophylline
ASTRAFER
Dextriferron
ASTRIN
Aspirin
ATABRINE
Quinacrine
ATARAX
Hydroxyzine
ATARAXOID*
Hydroxyzine
Prednisolone
ATARZINE
Promazine
ATASOL
Acetaminophen
ATASOL FORTE
Acetaminophen
ATASOL-15*
Acetaminophen
Caffeine
Codeine
ATASOL-30*
Acetaminophen
Caffeine
Codeine
ATASOL-8*
Acetaminophen
Caffeine
Codeine
ATEMPOL
Meparfynol
ATENSINE
Diazepam
ATHEMOL

Theobromine
Magnesium Oleate
ATHEMOL-N*
Magnesium Nicotinate
Theobromine
Magnesium Oleate
ATHROMBIN-K
Warfarin
ATIVAN
Lorazepam
ATLACHLOR
Chlorpheniramine
ATLANSIL
Amiodarone
ATOPHAN
Cinchophen
ATOSIL
Promethazine
ATROBARB*
Atropine
Phenobarbital
ATROBARBITAL*
Atropine
Phenobarbital
ATROMIDIN
Clofibrate
ATROMID-S
Clofibrate
ATROPINE WITH DEMEROL*
Atropine
Meperidine
ATROPISOL
Atropine
ATROSED*
Atropine
Phenobarbital
ATROVENT
Ipratropium
A.T.S.*
Allantoin
Coal Tar
ATTENUVAX
Measles Virus
Vaccine
ATUSSIN D.M.
EXPECTORANT*
Chlorpheniramine
Dextromethorphan
Guaifenesin
Phenylephrine
Phenylpropanolamine
ATUSSIN EXPECTORANT*
Chlorpheniramine
Guaifenesin
Phenylephrine
Phenylpropanolamine
A.T.V.
Diethylstilbestrol
A.T.10
Dihydrotachysterol
AUBASON
Desoximetasone
AUGMENTIN*
Amoxicillin
Clavulanic Acid
AURALGAN*
Antipyrine
Benzocaine
AURASOL*
Antipyrine
Benzocaine
AUREOMYCIN
Chlortetracycline
AURICRINE*
Antipyrine
Benzocaine
AURO
Boric Acid
AUROCAINE*
Boric Acid
Isopropyl Alcohol
AURO-DRI*
Boric Acid
Isopropyl Alcohol
AURO EAR DROPS
Carbamide Peroxide
AUROMID*
Antipyrine
Benzocaine
AUTOPLEX
Anti-inhibitor
coagulant complex
AVANTYL
Nortriptyline
AVAZYME
Chymotrypsin
AVC CREAM*
Allantoin
Aminacrine
Sulfanilamide
AVC SUPPOSITORIES*
Allantoin

Aminacrine
Sulfanilamide
AVC WITH DIENESTROL*
Dienestrol
Sulfanilamide
AVEENO PREPARATIONS
Oatmeal Compound
AVENTYL
Nortriptyline
A-VITAN
Vitamin A
AVLOCARDYL
Propranolol
AVLOCHLOR
Chloroquine
AVP NATAL*
Ascorbic Acid
Iron
Pyridoxine
Vitamin A
AXMACORT
Triamcinolone
AXON*
Benzocaine
Cetylpyridinium
AXOTAL*
Aspirin
Butalbital
AYDS APPETITE SUPPRESSANT
Benzocaine
AYDS WEIGHT SUPPRESSANT
Phenylpropanolamine
AYERCILLIN
Penicillin G Procaine
AYGESTIN
Norethindrone
AYR
Saline Solution
AZACTAM
Aztreonam
AZAPEN
Methicillin
AZENE
Clorazepate
AZIONYL
Clofibrate
AZLIN
Azlocillin
AZMA AID*
Ephedrine
Phenobarbital
Theophylline
AZMACORT
Triamcinolone
AZODINE
Phenazopyridine
AZO GANTANOL*
Phenazopyridine
Sulfamethoxazole
AZO GANTRISIN*
Phenazopyridine
Sulfisoxazole
AZOLID
Phenylbutazone
AZOLID-A*
Aluminum Hydroxide
Magnesium Trisilicate
Phenylbutazone
AZO-MANDELAMINE*
Methenamine Mandelate
Phenazopyridine
AZOMINE
Phenazopyridine
AZOPYRIN
Sulfasalazine
AZO-SOXAZOLE*
Phenazopyridine
Sulfisoxazole
AZO-STANDARD
Phenazopyridine
AZOSUL*
Phenazopyridine
Sulfisoxazole
AZO-SULFISOXAZOLE*
Phenazopyridine
Sulfisoxazole
AZO-SULFSTAT*
Phenazopyridine
Sulfamethizole
AZOTREX*
Phenazopyridine
Sulfamethizole
Tetracycline
AZULFIDINE
Sulfasalazine

AZULFIDINE EN-TABS
  Sulfasalazine
A-200 PYRINATE*
  Piperonyl Butoxide
  Pyrethrins

B

B-A*
  Aluminum Hydroxide
  Aspirin
  Magnesium Hydroxide
BABY COUGH
  Ammonium Chloride
BABY ORAJEL
  Benzocaine
BABY TEETHING LOTION
  Benzocaine
BACARATE
  Phendimetrazine
BACID*
  Carboxymethyl-
    cellulose
  Lactobacillus
    acidophilus
BACIGUENT OINTMENT
  Bacitracin
BACIGUENT OPHTHALMIC*
  Bacitracin
  Chlorobutanol
BACIMYCIN*
  Bacitracin
  Neomycin
BACITIN
  Bacitracin
BACTALIN*
  Alcohol
  Cetylpyridinium
BACTIGRAS
  Chlorhexidine
BACTINE*
  Benzalkonium
    Chloride
  Methylbenzethonium
BACTINE ANTISEPTIC
    ANESTHETIC*
  Benzalkonium
    Chloride
  Lidocaine
BACTINE HYDROCORTISONE
  Hydrocortisone
BACTOCILL
  Oxacillin
BACTOPEN
  Cloxacillin
BACTRATYCIN
  Tyrothricin
BACTRIM
  Trimethoprim
BACTRIM DS
  Co-Trimoxazole
BACTRIM IV
  Co-Trimoxazole
BAL IN OIL
  Dimercaprol
BALMEX*
  Lanolin
  Peruvian Balsam
BALMINIL DM
  Dextromethorphan
BALMINIL EXPECTORANT
  Guaifenesin
BALNEOL*
  Lanolin
  Mineral Oil
BALNETAR*
  Coal Tar
  Lanolin
  Mineral Oil
BANACID*
  Aluminum Hydroxide
  Magnesium Hydroxide
  Magnesium
    Trisilicate
BANALG LINIMENT*
  Camphor
  Eucalyptus Oil
  Menthol
  Methyl Salicylate
BANCAP*
  Acetaminophen
  Salicylamide
BANCAP HC*
  Acetaminophen
  Hydrocodone
BANCAP WITH CODEINE*
  Acetaminophen
  Codeine
  Salicylamide

BANESIN*
  Acetaminophen
  Salicylamide
BANFLEX
  Orphenadrine
BANISTYL
  Fonazine
BANLIN
  Propantheline
BANOCIDE
  Diethylcarbamazine
BANTHINE
  Methantheline
BARATOL
  Indoramin
BARBENYL
  Phenobarbital
BARBIDONNA*
  Atropine
  Hyoscyamine
  Phenobarbital
BARBITA
  Phenobarbital
BARBIVIS
  Phenobarbital
BARBOSEC
  Secobarbital
BARBSEB*
  Hydrocortisone
  Isopropyl Alcohol
  Salicylic Acid
BARC
  Pyrethrins
BARCONE
  Benzoxiquine
BARIDIUM
  Phenazopyridine
BARIUM ENEMA PREP KIT*
  Bisacodyl
  Sodium Biphosphate
  Sodium Phosphate
BARODENSE
  Barium
BAROFLAVE
  Barium
BAROLOID
  Barium
BAROSPERSE
  Barium
BAROTRAST
  Barium
BARRIERE
  Simethicone
BARSEB HC
  Hydrocortisone
BARSED THERA-SPRAY*
  Hydrocortisone
  Isopropyl Alcohol
  Isopropyl Myristate
  Propylene Glycol
  Salicylic Acid
BASALJEL*
  Aluminum Carbonate
  Aluminum Hydroxide
BASALJEL EXTRA STRENGTH
  Aluminum Hydroxide
BAUMODYNE*
  Menthol
  Methyl Salicylate
  Oil of Eucalyptus
BAYAMINIC EXTRACT*
  Guaifenesin
  Phenylpropanolamine
BAYAMINICOL*
  Ammonium Chloride
  Dextromethorphan
  Pheniramine
  Phenylpropanolamine
  Pyrilamine
BAYAMINIC SYRUP*
  Chlorpheniramine
  Phenylpropanolamine
BAYAPAP
  Acetaminophen
BAYDEC*
  Carbinoxamine
  Dextromethorphan
  Pseudoephedrine
BAYER ASPIRIN
  Aspirin
BAYER CHILDREN'S ASPIRIN
  Aspirin
BAYER CHILDREN'S COLD*
  Aspirin
  Phenylpropanolamine
BAYER COUGH FOR CHILDREN*
  Dextromethorphan

Phenylpropanolamine
BAYER DECONGESTANT*
Aspirin
Chlorpheniramine
Phenylpropanolamine
BAYER TIMED-RELEASE ARTHRITIC PAIN
Aspirin
BAYER TIMED-RELEASE ASPIRIN
Aspirin
BAYER 205
Suramin
BAYHISTINE*
Chlorpheniramine
Phenylpropanolamine
BAYMETHAZINE
Promethazine
BAY-ORNADE*
Caramiphen
Doxylamine
Phenylpropanolamine
BAYTUSSIN
Guaifenesin
BAYTUSSIN DM*
Dextromethorphan
Guaifenesin
BC*
Aspirin
Potassium Chloride
B-C-BID
Vitamins, Multiple
B COMPLEX
Vitamins, Multiple
B-COMPLEX
Vitamins, Multiple
B COMPLEX WITH VITAMIN C
Vitamins, Multiple
BC POWDER*
Aspirin
Caffeine
Salicylamide
BC TABLETS*
Aspirin
Caffeine
Salicylamide
BEBEN
Betamethasone
BECAUSE
Nonoxynol
BECLOVENT INHALER
Beclomethasone
BECONASE
Beclomethasone
BECOTIDE INHALER
Beclomethasone
BECOTIN
Vitamin B Complex
BECOTIN-T*
Ascorbic Acid
Vitamin B Complex
BECOTIN WITH VITAMIN C*
Ascorbic Acid
Vitamin B Complex
BECRINOL
Thiamine
BEDOZ
Cyanocobalamin
BEELITH*
Magnesium Oxide
Pyridoxine
BEEPEN-VK
Penicillin V Potassium
BEESIX
Pyridoxine
BEJECTAL
Vitamin B Complex
BEJECTAL WITH VITAMIN C*
Ascorbic Acid
Vitamin B Complex
BEJEX*
Ascorbic Acid
Vitamin B Complex
BEKUNIS HERBAL TEA
Senna
BELAP
Belladonna Extract
BELIX
Diphenhydramine
BELLADENAL*
Belladonna
Phenobarbital
BELLADENAL-S*
Belladonna
Phenobarbital
BELL-ANS

Sodium Bicarbonate
BELLAPHEN*
Atropine
Hyoscyamine
Phenobarbital
Scopolamine
BELLASTAL*
Atropine
Hyoscyamine
Phenobarbital
Scopolamine
BELLERGAL*
Belladonna
Ergotamine
Phenobarbital
BELLERGAL-S*
Belladonna
Ergotamine
Phenobarbital
BELLERMINE-O.D.*
Belladonna
Ergotamine
Phenobarbital
BELLKATAL*
Belladonna Extract
Kaolin
Phenobarbital
BELLOPHEN*
Belladonna Extract
Phenobarbital
BEMINAL FORTE WITH VITAMIN C
Vitamins, Multiple
BEMINAL 500
Vitamins, Multiple
BENA-D
Diphenhydramine
BENADRYL
Diphenhydramine
BENADRYL WITH EPHEDRINE*
Diphenhydramine
Ephedrine
BENADYNE EAR DROPS
Carbamide Peroxide
BENAHIST
Diphenhydramine
BEN-AQUA-5
Benzoyl Peroxide
BENDECTIN*
Doxylamine
Pyridoxine
BENDOPA
Levodopa
BENDYLATE
Diphenhydramine
BENEGYN*
Allantoin
Aminacrine
Sulfanilamide
BENEMID
Probenecid
BEN-GAY EXTERNAL ANALGESIC*
Menthol
Methyl Salicylate
BEN-GAY OINTMENT*
Menthol
Methyl Salicylate
BENISONE
Betamethasone
BENOJECT
Diphenhydramine
BENOQUIN
Monobenzone
BENOXYL
Benzoyl Peroxide
BEN-P
Penicillin G
BENSULFOID*
Resorcinol
Sulfur
BENSYLATE
Benztropine
BENTYL
Dicyclomine
BENTYLOL
Dicyclomine
BENTYLOL WITH PHENOBARBITAL*
Dicyclomine
Phenobarbital
BENTYL WITH PHENOBARB*
Dicyclomine
Phenobarbital
BENURON
Bendroflumethiazide
BENURYL
Probenecid
BENVIL

Tybamate
BENYLATE
Benzyl Benzoate
BENYLIN
Diphenhydramine
BENYLIN DECONGESTANT*
Diphenhydramine
Pseudoephedrine
BENYLIN DM*
Ammonium Chloride
Dextromethorphan
Diphenhydramine
BENYLIN PEDIATRIC COUGH
Diphenhydramine
BENZAC
Benzoyl Peroxide
BENZACHLOR-50
Benzalkonium Chloride
BENZAGEL
Benzoyl Peroxide
BENZAMYCIN*
Benzoyl Peroxide
Erythromycin
BENZEDREX
Propylhexedrine
BENZEDRINE
Amphetamine
BENZIDE
Benzthiazide
BENZOCOL
Benzocaine
BENZODENT*
Benzocaine
Eugenol
Hydroxyquinoline
BENZODYNE DROPS*
Acetic Acid
Benzalkonium Chloride
Chloroxylenol
Glycerin
BENZOXAL
Tripelennamine
BEPLETE
Vitamin B Complex
BERKOMINE
Imipramine
BERKOZIDE
Bendroflumethiazide
BEROCCA*
Ascorbic Acid
Folic Acid
Vitamin B Complex
BEROCCA-C*
Ascorbic Acid
Vitamin B Complex
BEROTEC
Fenoterol
BEROTEC INHALER
Fenoterol
BERUBIGEN
Cyanocobalamin
BESAN
Pseudoephedrine
BEST C CAPS
Ascorbic Acid
BESTRONE
Estrone
BETA-CHLOR
Chloral Betaine
BETACORT
Betamethasone
BETACREST
Vitamins, Multiple
BETADERM
Betamethasone
BETADINE
Povidone-Iodine
BETALIN
Vitamin B Complex
BETALIN-S
Thiamine
BETALIN 12 CRYSTALLINE
Cyanocobalamin
BETALOC
Metoprolol
BETAPAR
Meprednisone
BETAPEN-VK
Penicillin V Potassium
BETAPRED
Meprednisone
BETATREX
Betamethasone
BETA-VAL
Betamethasone
BETA-VITE LIQUID

Vitamins, Multiple
BETA-VITE WITH IRON LIQUID
Vitamins, Multiple
BETAXIN
Thiamine
BETA-2
Isoetharine
BETHANID
Bethanidine
BETIM
Timolol
BETNELAN
Betamethasone
BETNESOL
Betamethasone
BETNOVATE
Betamethasone
BETONAL CAP
Vitamins, Multiple
BETULINE*
Camphor
Menthol
Methyl Salicylate
Peppermint oil
BEVIDOX
Cyanocobalamin
BEVILL'S LOTION
Salicylic Acid
BEWON
Thiamine
BEWON ELIXIR
Vitamins, Multiple
BFL
Methylcellulose
BHI
Insulin,Human
BICHLORACETIC ACID
Dichloroacetic Acid
BICILLIN
Penicillin G Benzathine
BICILLIN L-A
Penicillin G Benzathine
BICITRA
Potassium Citrate
BICITRA-SUGAR FREE*
Citric Acid
Sodium Citrate
BICNU
Carmustine
BICOL
Bisacodyl
BICOZENE CREME*
Benzocaine
Resorcinol
BILAGOG*
Atropine
Magnesium Sulfate
Ox Bile
BILAMIDE*
Homatropine
Ox Bile
Phenobarbital
BILAX*
Dehydrocholic Acid
Docusate Sodium
BILEZYME*
Amylase
Dehydrocholic Acid
Desoxycholic Acid
Protease
BILIGRAFIN
Meglumine
BILIODYL
Phenobutiodil
BILIVIST
Ipodate
BILOGEN*
Desoxycholic Acid
Ox Bile Extract
Pancreatin
BILOMBRINE
Iodoalphionic Acid
BILOPAQUE
Tyropanoate Sodium
BILOSTAT
Dehydrocholic Acid
BILRON*
Bile Salts
Iron
BILTRICIDE
Praziquantel
BINOTAL
Ampicillin
BIO-CHOLIN
Dehydrocholic Acid
BIOCIDIN
Mephentermine

BIOGASTRONE
Carbenoxolone
BIOLAX
Cascara Sagrada
BIOLAX SP
Cascara Sagrada
BIOMYDRIN
Phenylephrine
BIO-PHYLLINE
Etofylline
BIOREX
Carbenoxolone
BIOSAN
Ampicillin
BIO SLIM T*
Caffeine
Phenylpropanolamine
BIOSONE
Enoxolone
BIO-TAB
Cascara Sagrada
BIO-TETRA
Tetracycline
BIOTUSSIN
Guaifenesin
BIOZYME*
Chymotrypsin
Neomycin
Trypsin
BIOZYME-C
Collagenase
BIO-12
Cyanocobalamin
BIPHETAMINE*
Amphetamine
Dextroamphetamine
BIQUIN DURULES
Quinidine
BISCOLAX
Bisacodyl
BISCO-LAX
Bisacodyl
BI-SECOGEN*
Amobarbital
Secobarbital
BISILAD*
Bismuth Subgallate
Kaolin
BISMOL
Bismuth Subsalicylate
BISODOL*
Calcium Carbonate
Magnesium Carbonate
Magnesium Oxide
Sodium Bicarbonate
BISOLVON
Bromhexine
BISTREPTASE
Streptokinase
BISTRIMATE
Bismuth Sodium
Triglycollamate
BISTRIUM
Hexamethonium
BI-SUB-SAL
Bismuth
Subsalicylate
BITIN
Bithionol
BLACK AND WHITE
BLEACHING CREAM
Hydroquinone
BLACK DRAUGHT
Senna
BLAINTRATE
Pentaerythritol
Tetranitrate
BLANDLUBE
Mineral Oil
BLENOXANE
Bleomycin
BLEPH
Sulfacetamide
BLEPHAMIDE LIQUIFILM*
Phenylephrine
Prednisolone
Sulfacetamide
BLEPHAMIDE OINTMENT*
Prednisolone
Sulfacetamide
BLEPHAMIDE OPHTHALMIC*
Prednisolone
Sulfacetamide
BLEPHAMIDE S.O.P.*
Prednisolone
Sulfacetamide
BLEPH-10 LIQUIFILM
Sulfacetamide
BLINX*
Boric Acid

Phenylmercuric
Acetate
Sodium Borate
BLISTEX*
Ammonia
Beeswax
Camphor
Glycerin
Peppermint Oil
Sodium Borate
BLIS-TO-SOL*
Benzoic Acid
Salicylic Acid
Undecylenic Acid
Zinc Stearate
BLISTR KLEAR
Camphor
BLOCADREN
Timolol
BLOCK-AID*
Aminobenzoic Acid
Oxybenzone
BLOCK OUT*
Oxybenzone
Padimate O
BLOXANTH
Allopurinol
BLUBORO*
Aluminum Acetate
Boric Acid
BLUTENE
Tolonium
B NUTRON
Vitamins, Multiple
BO-CAR-AL
Boric Acid
BOIL-EASE*
Benzocaine
Camphor
Ichthammol
Juniper tar
Phenol
Sulfur
BOIL N SOAK*
Boric Acid
Edetic Acid
Sodium Borate
Sodium Chloride
Thimerosal
BOLVIDON
Mianserin
BONAMINE
Meclizine
BONINE
Meclizine
BONTRIL PDM
Phendimetrazine
BORNATE
Isobornyl
Thiocyanoacetate
BOROFAX
Boric Acid
BOROSORB
Boric Acid
BOROWAS
Boric Acid
BOWMAN COLD TABLETS*
Acetaminophen
Caffeine
Phenylpropanolamine
BOYOL*
Benzocaine
Ichthammol
Lanolin
BPN OINTMENT*
Bacitracin
Neomycin
Polymyxin B
BPS
Povidone-Iodine
BP-5
Benzoyl Peroxide
BRADOSOL
Domiphen
BRASIVOL
Aluminum Oxide
BREACOL*
Chlorpheniramine
Dextromethorphan
Phenylpropanolamine
BREATHEASY
Epinephrine
BREOKINASE
Urokinase
BREONESIN
Guaifenesin
BRETHINE
Terbutaline
BRETYLATE
Bretylium
BRETYLIN
Bretylium

BRETYLOL
  Bretylium
BREVATINE-12
  Cyanocobalamin
BREVICON*
  Ethinyl Estradiol
  Norethindrone
BREVICON-28*
  Ethinyl Estradiol
  Norethindrone
BREVIDIL 'M'
  Succinylcholine
BREVIMYTAL NATRIUM
  Methohexital
BREVITAL
  Methohexital
BREWER'S YEAST
  Vitamins, Multiple
BREXIN*
  Carbinoxamine
  Guaifenesin
  Pseudoephedrine
BRICANYL
  Terbutaline
BRIDINE
  Povidone-Iodine
BRIETAL
  Methohexital
BRIOSCHI
  Sodium Bicarbonate
BRISTACYCLINE
  Tetracycline
BRISTAGEN
  Gentamicin
BRISTAMIN
  Phenyltoloxamine
BRISTAMYCIN
  Erythromycin Stearate
BRISTOPEN
  Oxacillin
BRISTURON
  Bendroflumethiazide
BROCASIPAL
  Orphenadrine
BROCON CHEWABLE*
  Brompheniramine
  Phenylephrine
  Phenylpropanolamine
BROCON C.R.*
  Brompheniramine
  Phenylephrine
  Phenylpropanolamine
BRO-LAC
  Methylcellulose
BROMALATE
  Magnesium Glutamate
    Hydrobromide
BROMFED*
  Brompheniramine
  Pseudoephedrine
BROMOPHEN*
  Brompheniramine
  Phenylephrine
BROMO-SELTZER*
  Acetaminophen
  Caffeine
  Citric Acid
  Sodium Bicarbonate
BROMPHEN*
  Brompheniramine
  Phenylpropanolamine
BROMSULPHALEIN
  Sulfobromophthalein
BROMURAL
  Bromisovalum
BRONCHIAL CAPSULES*
  Guaifenesin
  Theophylline
BRONCHICIDE
  Guaifenesin
BRONCHO-GRIPPEX
  Guaifenesin
BRONCHO-GRIPPOL-DM
  Dextromethorphan
BRONCHOLATE*
  Guaifenesin
  Pseudoephedrine
BRONCHO-TUSSIN*
  Codeine
  Terpin Hydrate
BRONDECON*
  Guaifenesin
  Oxtriphylline
BRONITIN*
  Ephedrine
  Guaifenesin
  Pyrilamine
  Theophylline
BRONITIN MIST
  Epinephrine
BRONKAID*
  Ephedrine

Guaifenesin
Magnesium
Trisilicate
Theophylline
BRONKAID MIST
Epinephrine
BRONKAID MISTOMETER
Epinephrine
BRONKEPHRINE
Ethylnorepinephrine
BRONKODYL
Theophylline
BRONKODYL S-R
Theophylline
BRONKOLIXIR*
Ephedrine
Guaifenesin
Phenobarbital
Theophylline
BRONKOMETER
Isoetharine
BRONKOSOL
Isoetharine
BRONKOTABS*
Ephedrine
Guaifenesin
Phenobarbital
Theophylline
BRONSECUR
Carbuterol
BROXIL
Phenethicillin
BROXOLIN
Glycobiarsol
BRUFEN
Ibuprofen
BRYREL
Piperazine
B-TWELV-ORA
Cyanocobalamin
BUBARTAL TT
Butabarbital
BUCLADIN-S
Buclizine
BUF ACNE-CLEANSING
BAR*
Bentonite
Salicylic Acid
BUFF-A COMP*
Aspirin
Butalbital
Caffeine
BUFFADYNE*
Aspirin
Caffeine
BUFFADYNE-LEMMON*
Aspirin
Caffeine
BUFFAPRIN*
Aspirin
Magnesium Oxide
BUFFAZONE
Phenylbutazone
BUFFERGEL*
Aluminum
Magnesium
BUFFERIN*
Aspirin
Dihydroxyaluminum
Aminoacetate
Magnesium Carbonate
BUFFERIN WITH CODEINE
NO. 3*
Aspirin
Codeine
Dihydroxyaluminum
Aminoacetate
Magnesium Carbonate
BUFFETS*
Aluminum Hydroxide
Aspirin
Caffeine
Phenacetin
BUFFEX
Aspirin
BUFFINOL*
Aspirin
Magnesium Oxide
BUF FOOT-CARE LOTION*
Propylene Glycol
Trolamine
BUF FOOT-CARE SOAP*
Glycerin
Petrolatum
Titanium Dioxide
Tolyl Biguanide
BUFOPTO ATROPINE
SOLUTION
Atropine
BUF-OXAL

Benzoyl Peroxide
BUF-TABS
Aspirin
BU-LAX
Docusate Sodium
BU-LAX PLUS*
Casanthranol
Docusate Sodium
BUMEX
Bumetanide
BUPRENEX
Buprenorphine
BURDEO*
Aluminum Acetate
Boric Acid
Hexachlorophene
BURNTAME
Benzocaine
BURO-SOL
Aluminum Acetate
BUSCOPAN
Hyoscine
Butylbromide
BUSONE
Phenylbutazone
BUSPAR
Buspirone
BUTA-BARB
Butabarbital
BUTABELL HMB*
Atropine
Butabarbital
Hyoscyamine
Scopolamine
BUTAGESIC
Phenylbutazone
BUTAGESIC-B
Phenylbutazone
BUTALGAN
Phenylbutazone
BUTAPHYLLAMINE
Ambuphylline
BUTAZOLIDIN
Phenylbutazone
BUTAZOLIDIN ALKA
Phenylbutazone
BUTESIN
Butamben
BUTHOID
Ambuphylline
BUTIBEL*
Belladonna Extract
Butabarbital
BUTICAPS
Butabarbital
BUTIGETIC*
Acetaminophen
Butabarbital
Caffeine
BUTISERPAZIDE*
Butabarbital
Hydrochlorothiazide
Reserpine
BUTISOL
Butabarbital
BUTONE
Phenylbutazone
BUTYLONE
Pentobarbital
BUTYN
Butacaine

C

CABADON M
Cyanocobalamin
CAFACETIN*
Aspirin
Caffeine
Gelseminium
Phenacetin
CAFAMINE T.D.*
Caffeine
Phenylpropanolamine
CAFERGOT*
Caffeine
Ergotamine
CAFERMINE*
Caffeine
Ergotamine
CAFERTABS*
Caffeine
Ergotamine
CAFERTRATE*
Caffeine
Ergotamine
CAFFEDRINE
Caffeine
CAFFEINE AND SODIUM BENZOATE*

Caffeine
Sodium Benzoate
CALADRYL*
Calamine
Diphenhydramine
CALADRYL HYDROCORTISONE*
Calamine
Diphenhydramine
Hydrocortisone
CALAMATUM*
Benzocaine
Calamine
Camphor
Phenol
Zinc Oxide
CALAMINE*
Bentonite
Calamine
Glycerin
Zinc Oxide
CALAMOX
Calamine
CALAN
Verapamil
CALCET*
Calcium Carbonate
Calcium Gluconate
Calcium Lactate
Ergocalciferol
CALCIBIND
Sodium Cellulose Phosphate
CALCIBRONAT
Calcium Bromidolactobionate
CALCICAPS
Vitamins, Multiple
CALCICAPS WITH IRON*
Iron
Vitamins, Multiple
CALCIDRINE*
Calcium Iodide
Codeine
CALCIFEROL
Ergocalciferol
CALCILAC*
Aminoacetic Acid
Calcium Carbonate
CALCIMAR
Calcitonin
CALCIPARINE
Heparin
CALCISORB
Sodium Cellulose
CALCIUM DISODIUM VERSENATE
Edetate Calcium Disodium
CALCIVITAM
Calcium
CALCIWAFERS
Vitamins, Multiple
CALDECORT
Hydrocortisone
CALDEROL
Calcifediol
CALDESENE
Calcium Undecylenate
CALDESENE MEDICATED OINTMENT
Zinc Oxide
CALDESENE MEDICATED POWDER
Calcium Undecylenate
CALGLYCINE*
Calcium Carbonate
Glycerin
CALICYLIC
Salicylic Acid
CALINATE-FA
Vitamins, Multiple
CAL-M*
Calcium
Cholecalciferol
Magnesium
Niacin
Pyridoxine
Thiamine
CALMEX
Diphenhydramine
CALMURID
Urea
CALM-X
Phosphorated Carbohydrate
CALORA
Calcium
CAL-PAN
Calcium Pantothenate

CALPHOSAN
Calcium Lactate
CALPHOSAN B-12*
Calcium
Glycerophosphate
Calcium Lactate
Cyanocobalamin
CALPOL
Acetaminophen
CAL-PRENAL
Vitamins, Multiple
CALTRATE 600 + D*
Calcium Carbonate
Vitamin D
CALURIN
Carbaspirin Calcium
CAL-ZO DRESSING*
Calamine
Camphor
Phenol
Zinc Oxide
CAMA*
Aluminum Hydroxide
Aspirin
Magnesium Hydroxide
CAMALOX*
Aluminum Hydroxide
Calcium Carbonate
Magnesium Oxide
CAMCOLIT
Lithium Carbonate
CAMOFORM
Bialamicol
CAMOQUIN
Amodiaquine
CAMPAIN
Acetaminophen
CAMPHO-PHENIQUE*
Camphor
Phenol
CANDEPTIN
Candicidin
CANDEX
Nystatin
CANDIMON
Candicidin
CANESTEN
Clotrimazole
CANESTEN-1
Clotrimazole
CANK-AID
Carbamide Peroxide
CANTAXIN FORTE
Ascorbic Acid
CANTET
Tetracycline
CANTHACUR
Cantharidin
CANTHARONE
Cantharidin
CANTIL
Mepenzolate
CANTRI VAGINAL CREAM*
Allantoin
Aminacrine
Sulfisoxazole
CAPASTAT
Capreomycin
CAPITAL
Acetaminophen
CAPITAL WITH CODEINE*
Acetaminophen
Codeine
CAPITROL CREAM SHAMPOO
Chloroxine
CAPITUS
Ethosuximide
CAPLA
Mebutamate
CA-PLUS
Calcium
CAPOTEN
Captopril
CAPOZIDE*
Captopril
Hydrochlorothiazide
CAPROCIN
Capreomycin
CAPROKOL
Hexylresorcinol
CAPROMOL
Aminocaproic Acid
CAPRON*
Acetaminophen
Aspirin
Caffeine
CAQUIN CREAM*
Clioquinol
Hydrocortisone
CARAFATE

Sucralfate
CARAMIPHEN EDISYLATE*
Caramiphen
Phenylpropanolamine
CARBACEL OPH
Carbachol
CARBENOLINE
Carbenoxolone
CARBOCAINE
Mepivacaine
CARBOCAINE HYDROCHLORIDE 2% WITH NEO-COBEFRIN INJECTION*
Levonordefrin
Mepivacaine
CARBODEC*
Carbinoxamine
Dextromethorphan
Pseudoephedrine
CARBOLITH
Lithium Carbonate
CARBRITAL*
Carbromal
Pentobarbital
CARCHOLIN
Carbachol
CARDABID
Nitroglycerin
CARDELMYCIN
Novobiocin
CARDENZ
Vitamins, Multiple
CARDIALINE
Vitamin E
CARDIAZOL
Pentylenetetrazol
CARDIDIGIN
Digitoxin
CARDILATE
Erythrityl Tetranitrate
CARDILATE-P*
Erythrityl Tetranitrate
Phenobarbital
CARDIOGRAFIN
Diatrizoate Meglumine
CARDIO-GREEN
Indocyanine Green
CARDIOQUIN
Quinidine
CARDIZEM
Diltiazem
CARDRASE
Ethoxzolamide
CARDUI*
Acetaminophen
Pamabrom
Pyrilamine
CARISOMA
Carisoprodol
CARISOPODOL*
Caffeine
Phenacetin
CARI-TAB SOFTAB*
Fluoride
Vitamins, Multiple
CARMETHOSE
Carboxymethyl-cellulose
CARMOL
Urea
CARMOL HC CREAM
Hydrocortisone
CARMOL 10 LOTION
Urea
CAROID
Papain
CAROID LAXATIVE*
Cascara Sagrada
Phenolphthalein
CARTOSE
Dextrose
CARTRAX*
Hydroxyzine
Pentaerythritol Tetranitrate
CARVASIN
Isosorbide Dinitrate
CASAFRU
Senna
CASEC
Calcium Caseinate
CAS-EVAC
Cascara Sagrada
CASILAN
Calcium Caseinate
CASSA-LAUD*

Casanthranol
Docusate Sodium
CASTELLANIS PAINT*
Alcohol
Basic Fuchsin
Phenol
Resorcinol
CASTORIA
Sennosides A and B
CASTOR OIL
Bisacodyl
CASYLLIUM*
Cascara Sagrada
Plantago Seed
Prune Powder
CATAPRES
Clonidine
CATAPRES-TTS
Clonidine
CATARASE
Chymotrypsin
CATASAL
Aspirin
CATAZOL
Acetaminophen
CATHOMYCIN
Novobiocin
CATRON
Pheniprazine
CAVODIL
Pheniprazine
CAYTINE
Protokylol
C-B VONE
Vitamins, Multiple
CEBEFORTIS
Vitamins, Multiple
CEBETINIC
Vitamins, Multiple
CEBIONE
Ascorbic Acid
CEBRAL
Ethaverine
CECLOR
Cefaclor
CECON
Ascorbic Acid
CECON SOLUTION
Vitamins, Multiple
CEDILANID-D
Deslanoside
CEDILANID INJECTION
Deslanoside
CEEBATE
Ascorbic Acid
CEEBEC
Vitamins, Multiple
CEENU
Lomustine
CEENU
Lomustine
CEEPRYN
Cetylpyridinium
CEE-500
Sodium Ascorbate
CEE-500 T.D.
Ascorbic Acid
CEFADYL
Cephapirin
CEFERA*
Ascorbic Acid
Ferrous Fumarate
CEFIZOX
Ceftizoxime
CEFOBID
Cefoperazone
CEFOL
Vitamins, Multiple
CEFRACYCLINE
Tetracycline
CELBENIN
Methicillin
CELESTAN
Betamethasone
CELESTODERM
Betamethasone
CELESTODERM-V
Betamethasone
CELESTONE
Betamethasone
CELLOGRAN
Methylcellulose
CELLOTHYL
Methylcellulose
CELLUMETH
Methylcellulose
CELONTIN
Methsuximide
CEL-U-JEC
Betamethasone

CEMILL
  Ascorbic Acid
CENAC*
  Resorcinol
  Sulfur
CENADEX
  Phenylpropanolamine
CENAFED
  Pseudoephedrine
CENAGESIC*
  Phenylephrine
  Pyrilamine
  Salicylamide
CENAID*
  Acetaminophen
  Caffeine
  Chlorpheniramine
  Phenylephrine
CENALAX
  Bisacodyl
CENALENE*
  Cyanocobalamin
  Niacinamide
  Pentylenetetrazol
  Thiamine
CENOLATE
  Ascorbic Acid
CENTEDRIN
  Methylphenidate
CENTRAX
  Prazepam
CENTRINE
  Aminopentamide
CENTRUM
  Vitamins, Multiple
CENTYL
  Bendroflumethiazide
CEO-TWO SUPPOSITORIES*
  Potassium Bitartrate
  Sodium Bicarbonate
CEPACOL
  Cetylpyridinium
CEPACOL TROCHES*
  Benzocaine
  Cetylpyridinium
CEPASTAT
  Phenol
CEPHALOMYCIN
  Cephaloridine
CEPHOREX
  Cephalexin
CEPHULAC
  Lactulose
CEPOR
  Cephalexin
CEPORACIN
  Cephalothin
CEPORAN
  Cephaloridine
CEPOREX
  Cephalexin
CEPOREXINE
  Cephalexin
CEPORIN
  Cephaloridine
CEREBID
  Papaverine
CEREBRO-NICIN*
  Ascorbic Acid
  Glutamic Acid
  Niacin
  Niacinamide
  Pentylenetetrazol
  Pyridoxine
  Riboflavin
  Thiamine
CERESPAN
  Papaverine
CEREVON
  Ferrous Succinate
CEROSE*
  Codeine
  Ipecac Fluidextract
  Phenindamine
  Phenylephrine
  Potassium
    Guaiacolsulfonate
CEROSE DM*
  Dextromethorphan
  Ipecac Fluidextract
  Phenindamine
  Phenylephrine
  Potassium
    Guaiacolsulfonate
CERUBIDINE
  Daunorubicin
CERUCAL
  Metoclopramide
CERVEX VAGINAL CREAM*
  Allantoin

Aminacrine
Sulfanilamide
CERVOXAN
Deanol
Acetamidobenzoate
C.E.S.
Conjugated Estrogens
CESAMET
Nabilone
CETACAINE TOPICAL ANESTHETIC*
Benzocaine
Tetracaine
CETACORT
Hydrocortisone
CETAMIDE
Sulfacetamide
CETANE
Ascorbic Acid
CETANE-CAPS TD
Ascorbic Acid
CETANE TIMED
Ascorbic Acid
CETAPHIL*
Cetyl Alcohol
Propylene Glycol
CETAPRED*
Prednisolone
Sulfacetamide
CETAVLON
Cetrimide
CETRIL
Cetrimide
CETRO-CIROSE*
Codeine
Ipecac Fluidextract
Potassium
Guaiacolsulfonate
CEVALIN
Ascorbic Acid
CEVEX
Ascorbic Acid
CEVI-BID
Vitamins, Multiple
CE-VI-SOL
Ascorbic Acid
CE-VI-SOL DROPS
Ascorbic Acid
CHAPSTICK SUNBLOCK*
Oxybenzone
Padimate
CHARCOCAPS
Charcoal
CHARDONNA-2*
Belladonna
Phenobarbital
CHEALAMIDE
Edetate Calcium
Disodium
CHEL-IRON
Ferrocholinate
CHEL-IRON LIQUID
Ferrocholinate
CHEL-IRON PEDIATRIC DROPS
Ferrocholinate
CHEMDROX*
Aluminum
Magnesium
CHEMFEDRAL*
Ephedrine
Phenobarbital
Theophylline
CHEM-FLURAZINE
Trifluoperazine
CHEMGASTRIC*
Aluminum
Magnesium
Simethicone
CHEMGEL ANTACID
Aluminum Hydroxide
CHEMIOFURAN
Nitrofurantoin
CHEMIPEN
Phenethicillin
CHEMLOX*
Aluminum
Magnesium
CHEMPHYL*
Aminophylline
Amobarbital
Ephedrine
CHENATAL*
Minerals, Multiple
Vitamins, Multiple
CHENDOL
Chenodiol
CHENIX
Chenodiol
CHENO

Chenodiol
CHERACOL*
Codeine
Guaifenesin
CHERACOL D*
Dextromethorphan
Guaifenesin
CHERACOL PLUS*
Chlorpheniramine
Dextromethorphan
Phenylpropanolamine
CHERRI-B LIQUID
Vitamins, Multiple
CHERRY CHLORASEPTIC*
Phenol
Sodium Phenolate
CHEW-E
Vitamins, Multiple
CHEW-VITE
Vitamins, Multiple
CHEXIT*
Acetaminophen
Dextromethorphan
Pheniramine
Phenylpropanolamine
Pyrilamine
Terpin Hydrate
CHIGGEREX
Benzocaine
CHILDREN'S CHLORASEPTIC LOZENGES
Benzocaine
CHILDREN'S HOLD 4 HOUR COUGH SUPPRESSANT*
Dextromethorphan
Phenylpropanolamine
CHILDREN'S 217*
Aspirin
Caffeine
CHILDRENS CO TYLENOL*
Acetaminophen
Alcohol
Chlorpheniramine
Phenylpropanolamine
CHILDRENS PANADOL
Acetaminophen
CHLOMIN
Chloramphenicol
CHLORAFED TIMECELLES*
Chlorpheniramine
Pseudoephedrine
CHLORALEX
Chloral Hydrate
CHLORALOL
Dichloralphenazone
CHLORALONE
Chloramine-T
CHLORALVAN
Chloral Hydrate
CHLORAMATE UNICELLES
Chlorpheniramine Maleate
CHLORAMEAD
Chlorpromazine
CHLORAMINOPHENE
Chlorambucil
CHLORASEPTIC DM COUGH CONTROL LOZENGES*
Dextromethorphan
Phenol
Sodium Phenolate
CHLORASEPTIC GEL*
Phenol
Sodium Phenolate
CHLORASEPTIC LOZENGES*
Phenol
Sodium Phenolate
CHLORASEPTIC SPRAY*
Phenol
Sodium Phenolate
CHLORATED ADULT TIMECELLS*
Chlorpheniramine
Pseudoephedrine
CHLORDINIUM SEALETS*
Chlordiazepoxide
Clidinium
CHLORESIUM
Chlorophyllin
CHLORETONE
Chlorobutanol
CHLOROFED INJECTION*
Atropine
Chlorpheniramine
CHLOROFON-F*
Acetaminophen
Chlorzoxazone
CHLOROMIDE
Chlorpropamide

CHLOROMYCETIN
Chloramphenicol
CHLOROMYCETIN HYDROCORTISONE*
Chloramphenicol
Hydrocortisone
CHLOROMYXIN*
Chloramphenicol
Polymyxin B
CHLORONASE
Chlorpropamide
CHLOROPHEN
Chlorphentermine
CHLORO-PRO
Chlorpheniramine
CHLOROPTIC
Chloramphenicol
CHLOROPTIC S.O.P.
Chloramphenicol
CHLOROSERPINE*
Chlorothiazide
Reserpine
CHLORO-100
Chlorpheniramine
CHLORPACTIN XCB
Oxychlorosene
CHLORPHEN
Chlorpheniramine
CHLORPROM
Chlorpromazine
CHLOR-PROMANYL
Chlorpromazine
CHLOR-PZ
Chlorpromazine
CHLOR-REST*
Chlorpheniramine
Phenylpropanolamine
CHLORTAB
Chlorpheniramine
CHLOR-TRIMETON
Chlorpheniramine
CHLOR-TRIMETON DECONGESTANT*
Chlorpheniramine
Pseudoephedrine
CHLOR-TRIMETON EXPECTORANT*
Ammonium Chloride
Chlorpheniramine
Guaifenesin
Phenylephrine
CHLOR-TRIMETON EXPECTORANT WITH CODEINE*
Ammonium Chloride
Chlorpheniramine
Codeine
Guaifenesin
Phenylephrine
CHLOR-TRIPOLON
Chlorpheniramine
CHLORYLEN
Trichloroethylene
CHLORZIDE
Hydrochlorothiazide
CHLORZOXAZONE W/APAP*
Acetaminophen
Chlorzoxazone
CHLOTRIDE
Chlorothiazide
CHOCKS
Vitamins, Multiple
CHOCKS-BUGS BUNNY
Vitamins, Multiple
CHOCKS-BUGS BUNNY PLUS IRON*
Iron
Vitamins, Multiple
CHOCKS PLUS IRON*
Iron
Vitamins, Multiple
CHOLAN DH
Dehydrocholic Acid
CHOLEDBRINE
Iocetamic Acid
CHOLEDYL
Oxtriphylline
CHOLEDYL EXPECTORANT*
Guaifenesin
Oxtriphylline
CHOLOGRAFIN
Iodipamide Meglumine
CHOLOGRAFIN MEGLUMINE
Iodipamide Meglumine
CHOLOVUE
Iodoxamate Meglumine
CHOLOXIN
Dextrothyroxine
CHOLYPYL
Dehydrocholic Acid

CHOOZ*
  Calcium Carbonate
  Magnesium
    Trisilicate
CHORANID
  Gonadotropin
CHROMAGEN*
  Ascorbic Acid
  Cyanocobalamin
  Ferrous Fumarate
CHROMPHOSPHOTOPE
  Chromic Phosphate
CHRONULAC
  Lactulose
CHRYSOMYSIN
  Chlortetracycline
CHYMAR
  Chymotrypsin
CHYMASE
  Chymotrypsin
CHYMETIN
  Chymotrypsin
CHYMEX
  Bentiromide
CHYMODIACTIN
  Chymopapain
CHYMOLASE
  Chymotrypsin
CHYMORAL
  Chymotrypsin
CHYMOTEST
  Chymotrypsin
CIBALITH-S
  Lithium Carbonate
CIDALON
  Isobornyl
    Thiocyanoacetate
CIDEX
  Glutaral
CIDOMYCIN
  Gentamicin
CIGNOLIN
  Anthralin
CILLIMYCIN
  Lincomycin
CIMADON
  Piminodine
CINALONE 40
  Triamcinolone
CINNASIL
  Rescinnamine
CINOBAC
  Cinoxacin
CINOLONE-T
  Triamcinolone
CIN-QUIN
  Quinidine
CIRCANOL
  Ergoloid Mesylates
CIRCLADIN
  Bromindione
CIRCLIDRIN
  Nylidrin
CIRCUBID
  Ethaverine
CITANEST
  Prilocaine
CITRA*
  Ascorbic Acid
  Caffeine
  Chlorpheniramine
  Pheniramine
  Phenylephrine
  Pyrilamine
  Salicylamide
CITRATE DE BETAINE
  Betaine Citrate
CITROCARBONATE*
  Sodium Bicarbonate
  Sodium Citrate
CITROLITH
  Potassium Citrate
CITRO-MAG
  Magnesium Citrate
CITROTEIN*
  Minerals, Multiple
  Vitamins, Multiple
CLAFORAN
  Cefotaxime
CLARIPEX
  Clofibrate
CLAVITON
  Tridihexethyl
CLEANING & SOAKING*
  Benzalkonium
    Chloride
  Edetic Acid
CLEAN-N-SOAK
  Phenylmercuric
    Nitrate

CLEARASIL*
Resorcinol
Sulfur
CLEARASIL BP
Benzoyl Peroxide
CLEARASIL MEDICATED CLEANSER
Salicylic Acid
CLEARASIL MEDICATED SOAP
Triclosan
CLEARASIL VANISHING FORMULA*
Resorcinol
Sulfur
CLEAR&BRIGHT
Tetrahydrozoline
CLEAR BY DESIGN
Benzoyl Peroxide
CLEAR EYES
Naphazoline
CLEOCIN
Clindamycin
C-LEVEL
Ascorbic Acid
CLIMESTRONE
Estrogens, Esterified
CLINAZINE
Trifluoperazine
CLINDEX*
Chlordiazepoxide
Clidinium
CLINICAINE
Lidocaine
CLINICORT
Hydrocortisone
CLINICYDIN*
Bacitracin
Neomycin
Polymyxin B
CLINISTIX
Glucose Oxidase Reagent
CLINORIL
Sulindac
CLIOXIDE*
Chlordiazepoxide
Clidinium
CLIPOXIDE*
Chlordiazepoxide
Clidinium
CLISTIN
Carbinoxamine
CLISTIN-D*
Acetaminophen
Carbinoxamine
Phenylephrine
CLODERM
Clocortolone
CLOMID
Clomiphene
C-LONG
Ascorbic Acid
CLONOPIN
Clonazepam
CLONT
Metronidazole
CLOREVAN
Chlorphenoxamine
CLORILAX
Chlormezanone
CLORPACTIN WCS-90
Sodium Oxychlorosene
CLOSINA
Cycloserine
CLOXAPEN
Cloxacillin
CLOXILEAN
Cloxacillin
CLUSIVOL
Vitamins, Multiple
CLUSIVOL 130
Vitamins, Multiple
COACTIN
Amdinocillin
COASTALDYNE*
Acetaminophen
Codeine
COBADOCE FORTE
Cyanocobalamin
COBALASINE
Adenosine
COBIONE
Cyanocobalamin
COCILLIN V-K
Penicillin V Potassium
COCO-QUININE
Quinine

CODALAN*
  Acetaminophen
  Caffeine
  Codeine
  Salicylamide
CODASA*
  Aspirin
  Codeine
CODIAZINE
  Sulfadiazine
CODIMAL*
  Acetaminophen
  Chlorpheniramine
  Pseudoephedrine
  Salicylamide
CODIMAL DM*
  Dextromethorphan
  Phenylephrine
  Potassium
    Guaiacolsulfonate
  Pyrilamine
CODIMAL EXPECTORANT*
  Phenylpropanolamine
  Potassium
    Guaiacolsulfonate
CODIMAL-L.A. CENULES*
  Chlorpheniramine
  Pseudoephedrine
CODIMAL PH*
  Codeine
  Phenylephrine
  Potassium
    Guaiacolsulfonate
  Pyrilamine
CODISTAN*
  Dextromethorphan
  Guaifenesin
COD LIVER OIL
    CONCENTRATE
  Vitamins, Multiple
COD LIVER OIL WITH
    VITAMIN C
  Vitamins, Multiple
CODONE
  Hydrocodone
CODOPHEN-R*
  Aspirin
  Caffeine
  Codeine
CODRIN L.A*
  Chlorpheniramine
  Phenylpropanolamine
CODROXOMIN
  Hydroxocobalamin
CODYLIN
  Pholcodine
COFFEE, TEA & A NEW ME
  Phenylpropanolamine
COFFEE BREAK CUBES
    WEIGHT REDUCTION
    PLAN
  Phenylpropanolamine
CO-GEL LIQUITABS*
  Aminoacetic Acid
  Calcium Carbonate
  Trizyme
COGENTIN
  Benztropine
COGESIC
  Prodilidine
COHIDRATE
  Chloral Hydrate
COLACE
  Docusate Sodium
COLBENEMID*
  Colchicine
  Probenecid
COLDECON
  Phenylpropanolamine
COLDRINE*
  Acetaminophen
  Pseudoephedrine
COLESTID GRANULES
  Colestipol
COL-EVAC*
  Potassium Bitartrate
  Sodium Bicarbonate
COLISONE
  Prednisone
COLLYRIUM*
  Antipyrine
  Boric Acid
COLLYRIUM DROPS*
  Antipyrine
  Boric Acid
  Ephedrine
COLOCTYL
  Docusate Sodium
COLOGEL
  Methylcellulose
COLONATRAST
  Barium

COLPRO
Medrogestone
COLPRONE
Medrogestone
COLPROSTERONE
Progesterone
COLREX*
Acetaminophen
Chlorpheniramine
Phenylephrine
COLREX ANTITUSSIVE*
Chlorpheniramine
Dextromethorphan
Phenylephrine
COLREX COUGH SYRUP*
Chlorpheniramine
Dextromethorphan
Phenylephrine
COLREX EXPECTORANT*
Ammonium Chloride
Guaifenesin
COLREX TROCHES
Benzocaine
COLSALIDE
Colchicine
COLTAB*
Chlorpheniramine
Phenylephrine
COL-VI-NOL
Benzocaine
COLY-MYCIN
Colistin
COLY-MYCIN M PARENTERAL
Colistimethate
COLY-MYCIN S OTIC*
Colistin
Hydrocortisone
Neomycin
COMBANTRIN
Pyrantel Pamoate
COMBEX KAPSEALS
Vitamins, Multiple
COMBEX KAPSEALS WITH VITAMIN C
Vitamins, Multiple
COMBID*
Isopropamide
Prochlorperazine
COMBID SPANSULE*
Isopropamide
Prochlorperazine
COMBIPRES*
Chlorthalidone
Clonidine
COMFOLAX
Docusate Sodium
COMFOLAX PLUS*
Casanthranol
Docusate Sodium
COMFORT DROPS*
Benzalkonium Chloride
Edetic Acid
COMHIST*
Atropine
Chlorpheniramine
Hyoscyamine
Phenindamine
Phenylephrine
Scopolamine
COMPAZINE
Prochlorperazine
COMPAZINE SPANSULES
Prochlorperazine
COMPLAMIN
Xanthinol Niacinate
COMPLOMENT
Pyridoxine
COMPOCILLIN V
Penicillin V Potassium
COMPOCILLIN-VK
Penicillin V Potassium
COMPOUND W*
Acetic Acid, Glacial
Ether
Salicylic Acid
COMPOZ*
Methapyrilene
Pyrilamine
COMTREX*
Acetaminophen
Alcohol
Chlorpheniramine
Dextromethorphan
Phenylpropanolamine
COMYCIN*
Nystatin
Tetracycline
CONACETOL

Acetaminophen
CONAR*
Noscapine
Phenylephrine
CONAR EXPECTORANT*
Guaifenesin
Noscapine
Phenylephrine
CONAR SUSPENSION*
Noscapine
Phenylephrine
CONCENTRATED MILK OF MAGNESIA*
Glycerin
Magnesium Hydroxide
CONCEPTROL
Nonoxynol 9
CONCORDIN
Protriptyline
CONEX*
Chlorpheniramine
Guaifenesin
Phenylpropanolamine
CONEX DA*
Phenylpropanolamine
Phenyltoloxamine
CONEX LOZENGE*
Benzocaine
Cetylpyridinium
CONEX PLUS*
Acetaminophen
Phenylpropanolamine
Phenyltoloxamine
CONEX WITH CODEINE*
Chlorpheniramine
Codeine
Guaifenesin
Phenylpropanolamine
CONGESPIRIN
Dextromethorphan
CONGESPIRIN CHEWABLE COLD TABLETS FOR CHILDREN*
Acetaminophen
Phenylephrine
CONGESTAC*
Guaifenesin
Pseudoephedrine
CONGRESS JR.*
Guaifenesin
Pseudoephedrine
CONGRESS SR.*
Guaifenesin
Pseudoephedrine
CONRAY
Meglumine
CONRAY-325
Iothalamate Sodium
CONRAY-400
Iothalamate Sodium
CONSOTUSS*
Dextromethorphan
Doxylamine
CONSTANT-T
Theophylline
CONSTIBAN*
Casanthranol
Docusate Sodium
CONSULID
Sulfachlorpyridazine
CONTAC*
Chlorpheniramine
Phenylpropanolamine
CONTAC COUGH*
Dextromethorphan
Pseudoephedrine
CONTAC JR. CHILDRENS' COLD MEDICINE*
Acetaminophen
Dextromethorphan
Phenylpropanolamine
CONTAC NASAL MIST
Phenylephrine
CONTAC SEVERE COLD FORMULA*
Acetaminophen
Chlorpheniramine
Dextromethorphan
Pseudoephedrine
CONTAC SEVERE COLD FORMULA NIGHT STRENGTH*
Acetaminophen
Dextromethorphan
Doxylamine
Pseudoephedrine
CONTACTISOL
Methylcellulose
CONTIQUE ARTIFICIAL TEARS
Polyvinyl Alcohol
CONTIQUE DUAL WET*

Benzalkonium
Chloride
Edetic Acid
Polyvinyl Alcohol
CONTRABLEM*
Resorcinol
Sulfur
CONTROL
Phenylpropanolamine
CONVERZYME*
Amylase
Cellulase
Lipase
Protease
COPAVIN*
Codeine
Papaverine
COPE*
Aluminum Hydroxide
Aspirin
Magnesium Hydroxide
Methapyrilene
COPHENE*
Chlorpheniramine
Phenylephrine
Phenylpropanolamine
COPROLA
Docusate Sodium
COPSAMINE
Pyrilamine
COPTIN*
Sulfadiazine
Trimethoprim
CO-PYRONIL*
Chlorpheniramine
Pseudoephedrine
CORAMINE
Nikethamide
CORATHIEM
Cinnarizine
CORAX
Chlordiazepoxide
CORDAMINE*
Brompheniramine
Phenylephrine
CORDARONE
Amiodarone
CORDILATE
Erythrityl
Tetranitrate
CORDILOX
Verapamil
CORDRAN
Flurandrenolide
CORGARD
Nadolol
CORICIDIN*
Aspirin
Chlorpheniramine
CORICIDIN "D"*
Aspirin
Chlorpheniramine
Phenylpropanolamine
CORICIDIN ANTITUSSIVE*
Ammonium Chloride
Chlorpheniramine
Guaifenesin
Phenylpropanolamine
CORICIDIN DEMILETS*
Aspirin
Chlorpheniramine
Phenylephrine
CORICIDIN MEDILETS*
Aspirin
Chlorpheniramine
CORICIDIN NASAL SPRAY
Phenylephrine
CORLIN INFANT DROPS*
Alcohol
Chlorpheniramine
Sodium Salicylate
CORONEX
Isosorbide Dinitrate
COROPHYLLIN
Aminophylline
CORPHYLLIN
Aminophylline
CORQUE*
Hydrocortisone
Iodochlorhydroxyquin
CORRECTIVE MIXTURE*
Bismuth
Subsalicylate
Pepsin
Phenyl Salicylate
Zinc Phenolsulfonate
CORRECTIVE MIXTURE
WITH PAREGORIC*
Bismuth
Subsalicylate
Paregoric
Pepsin

Phenyl Salicylate
Zinc Phenolsulfonate
CORRECTOL*
Docusate Sodium
Phenolphthalein
CORRECTOL LIQUID
Phenolphthalein
CORSYM*
Chlorpheniramine
Phenylpropanolamine
CORTAID
Hydrocortisone
CORTAMED
Hydrocortisone
CORTAN
Prednisone
CORTATE
Desoxycorticosterone
CORT-DOME
Hydrocortisone
CORTEF
Hydrocortisone
CORTEF-F
Fludrocortisone
CORTELAN
Cortisone
CORTENEMA
Hydrocortisone
CORTHROSYN
Cosyntropin
CORTICAINE CREAM*
Dibucaine
Hydrocortisone
CORTICREME
Hydrocortisone
CORTIFOAM
Hydrocortisone
CORTIFORTE*
Ascorbic Acid
Caffeine
Chlorpheniramine
Phenacetin
Salicylamide
CORTIMENT
Hydrocortisone
CORTISPORIN CREAM*
Gramicidin
Hydrocortisone
Neomycin
Polymyxin B
CORTISPORIN OINTMENT*
Bacitracin
Hydrocortisone
Neomycin
Polymyxin B
CORTISPORIN OINTMENT OPHTHALMIC*
Bacitracin
Hydrocortisone
Neomycin
Polymyxin B
CORTISPORIN OPHTHALMIC SUSPENSION*
Hydrocortisone
Neomycin
Polymyxin B
CORTISPORIN OTIC SOLUTION*
Hydrocortisone
Neomycin
Polymyxin B
CORTISPORIN OTIC SUSPENSION*
Hydrocortisone
Neomycin
Polymyxin B
CORTISPRAY
Hydrocortisone
CORTISTAB
Cortisone
CORTIZONE-5
Hydrocortisone
CORTOGEN
Cortisone
CORTONE
Cortisone
CORT-QUIN*
Hydrocortisone
Iodoquinol
CORTRIL
Hydrocortisone
CORTROPHIN
Corticotropin
CORTROPHIN-ZINC
Corticotropin
CORTROSYN
Cosyntropin
CORTUSSIN
Griseofulvin
CORUTOL DH

Hydrocodone
CORUTOL EXPECTORANT
Guaifenesin
CORVOTONE
Nikethamide
CORYBAN-D*
Chlorpheniramine
Phenylpropanolamine
CORYBAN-D ANTITUSSIVE*
Dextromethorphan
Guaifenesin
Phenylephrine
CORYPHEN
Aspirin
CORYPHEN-CODEINE*
Aspirin
Codeine
CORYZA BRENGLE*
Acetaminophen
Pseudoephedrine
CORZIDE*
Bendroflumethiazide
Nadolol
CO-SALT*
Ammonium Chloride
Choline Bitartrate
Potassium Chloride
COSANYL COUGH*
Codeine
Pseudoephedrine
COSANYL DM IMPROVED FORMULA*
Dextromethorphan
Pseudoephedrine
COSCOPIN
Noscapine
COSCOTABS
Noscapine
COSLAN
Mefenamic Acid
COSMEGEN
Dactinomycin
COSPRIN
Aspirin
COSULFA
Sulfachlorpyridazine
COTAZYM
Pancrelipase
COTAZYME
Pancrelipase
COTINAZIN
Isoniazid
COTROL-D*
Chlorpheniramine
Pseudoephedrine
COTUSSIS*
Codeine
Terpin Hydrate
CO TYLENOL*
Acetaminophen
Chlorpheniramine
Pseudoephedrine
CO TYLENOL COLD FORMULA FOR CHILDREN*
Acetaminophen
Chlorpheniramine
Pseudoephedrine
COTYLENOL LIQUID COLD FORMULA*
Acetaminophen
Chlorpheniramine
Dextromethorphan
Pseudoephedrine
COUFARIN
Warfarin
COUMADIN
Warfarin
COUNTER PAIN RUB*
Eugenol
Menthol
Methyl Salicylate
COVANAMINE*
Chlorpheniramine
Phenylephrine
Phenylpropanolamine
Pyrilamine
COVANGESIC*
Acetaminophen
Chlorpheniramine
Phenylephrine
Phenylpropanolamine
Pyrilamine
COVAP*
Butabarbital
Pentaerythritol Tetranitrate
COVATIN
Captodiame
COVICONE*

Castor Oil
Dimethicone
Nitrocellulose
CO-XAN*
Codeine
Ephedrine
Guaifenesin
Theophylline
COZYME
Panthenol
CP2 TABLETS*
Aspirin
Caffeine
Phenacetin
CRASNITIN
Asparaginase
CREAMALIN*
Aluminum Hydroxide
Magnesium Oxide
CREMACOAT 1
Dextromethorphan
CREMACOAT 2
Guaifenesin
CREMACOAT 3*
Dextromethorphan
Guaifenesin
Phenylpropanolamine
CREMACOAT 4*
Dextromethorphan
Doxylamine
Phenylpropanolamine
CREMODIAZINE
Sulfadiazine
CREMOMETHAZINE
Sulfamethazine
CREMOSUXIDINE
Succinylsulfa-
thiazole
CREO-TERPIN*
Creosote
Terpin Hydrate
CROMEDAZINE
Chlorpromazine
C-RON*
Ascorbic Acid
Ferrous Fumarate
C-RON FORTE*
Ascorbic Acid
Ferrous Fumarate
C-RON FRECKLES*
Ascorbic Acid
Ferrous Fumarate
CRUEX
Calcium Undecylenate
CRUEX MEDICATED CREAM
Zinc Undecylenate
CRUEX MEDICATED POWDER
Calcium Undecylenate
CRYSTAPEN
Penicillin G
CRYSTICILLIN 300 A.S.
Penicillin G
Procaine
CRYSTICILLIN 600 A.S.
Penicillin G
Procaine
CRYSTODIGIN
Digitoxin
CRYSTOIDS
Hexylresorcinol
CRYSTWEL
Cyanocobalamin
C-TRAN
Chlordiazepoxide
CUEMID
Cholestyramine Resin
CUMERTILIN
Mercumatilin
CUMOPYRAN
Cyclocumarol
CUPREX*
Copper Oleate
Tetrahydronaphthalene
CUPRIMINE
Penicillamine
CURATIN
Doxepin
CURRETAB
Medroxyprogesterone
CUTEMOL*
Allantoin
Lanolin
Petrolatum
CUTICURA
Sulfur
CUTICURA MEDICATED
ACNE
Benzoyl Peroxide
CYANABIN
Cyanocobalamin

CYANTIN
  Nitrofurantoin
CYBIS
  Nalidixic Acid
CYCLAINE
  Hexylcaine
CYCLAMYCIN
  Troleandomycin
CYCLANFOUR
  Cyclandelate
CYCLAPEN
  Cyclacillin
CYCLAPEN-W
  Cyclacillin
CYCLINE-250
  Tetracycline
CYCLOBEC
  Dicyclomine
CYCLOCORT
  Amcinonide
CYCLOGYL
  Cyclopentolate
CYCLOMEN
  Danazol
CYCLOMYDRIL*
  Cyclopentolate
  Phenylephrine
CYCLOPAR
  Tetracycline
CYCLOSPASMOL
  Cyclandelate
CYDEL
  Cyclandelate
CYDRIL
  Levamfetamine
CYKLOKAPRON
  Tranexamic Acid
CYLERT
  Pemoline
CYLPHENICOL
  Chloramphenicol
CYNOMEL
  Liothyronine
CYREDIN
  Cyanocobalamin
CYSTEX*
  Benzoic Acid
  Methenamine
  Salicylamide
  Sodium Salicylate
CYSTO-CONRAY
  Meglumine
CYSTOGRAFIN
  Diatrizoate
    Meglumine
CYSTOSPAZ
  Hyoscyamine
CYTADREN
  Aminoglutethimide
CYTELLIN
  Sitosterols
CYTOFERIN*
  Ascorbic Acid
  Ferrous Sulfate
CYTOMEL
  Liothyronine
CYTOMINE
  Liothyronine
CYTOSAR
  Cytarabine
CYTOXAN
  Cyclophosphamide
CYVASO
  Cyclandelate
C3*
  Aspirin
  Caffeine
  Codeine
C4*
  Aspirin
  Caffeine
  Codeine

D

DACTIL
  Piperidolate
DAGENAN
  Sulfapyridine
DAKTARIN
  Miconazole
DALACIN C
  Clindamycin
DALCA*
  Magnesium Salicylate
  Phenylpropanolamine
DALFATOL
  Vitamin E
DALIDERM*

Salicylic Acid
Zinc Undecylenate
DALIDYNE*
Benzocaine
Benzyl Alcohol
Camphor
Chlorothymol
Menthol
Methylbenzethonium
Tannic Acid
DALLERGY*
Chlorpheniramine
Methscopolamine
Phenylephrine
DALMANE
Flurazepam
DALONE
Dexamethasone
DALTOSE
Vitamin E
D-AMP
Ampicillin
DANABOL
Methandrostenolone
DANDRID
Idoxuridine
DANEX
Pyrithione Zinc
DAN-GARD
Pyrithione Zinc
DANILONE
Phenindione
DANIVAC
Danthron
DANOCRINE
Danazol
DANTAFUR
Nitrofurantoin
DANTHROSS*
Danthron
Docusate Sodium
DANTOIN
Phenytoin
DANTRIUM
Dantrolene
DAONIL
Glyburide
DAPA
Acetaminophen
DAPASE
Acetaminophen
Salicylamide
DAPOTOM
Fluphenazine
DAPTAZOLE
Amiphenazole
DAQUIN
Chlorazanil
DARANIDE
Dichlorphenamide
DARAPRIM
Pyrimethamine
DARBID
Isopropamide
DARCIL
Phenethicillin
DARENTHIN
Bretylium
DARICON
Oxyphencyclimine
DARIFUR
Furaltadone
DARTAL
Thiopropazate
DARVOCET-N*
Acetaminophen
Propoxyphene
DARVOCET-N 100*
Acetaminophen
Propoxyphene
DARVON
Propoxyphene
DARVON COMPOUND-65*
Aspirin
Caffeine
Propoxyphene
DARVON-N
Propoxyphene
DARVON-N COMPOUND*
Aspirin
Caffeine
Propoxyphene
DARVON-N WITH ASA*
Aspirin
Propoxyphene
DARVON WITH A.S.A.*
Aspirin
Propoxyphene
D.A.S.
Aminosalicylate

DASIKON*
  Aspirin
  Atropine
  Caffeine
  Chlorpheniramine
DASIN*
  Aspirin
  Atropine
  Caffeine
  Camphor
DATHROID
  Thyroid
DATRIL
  Acetaminophen
DATRIL 500
  Acetaminophen
DAUNOBLASTIN
  Daunorubicin
DAWSON RUBBING COMPOUND
  Isopropyl Alcohol
DAXOLIN
  Loxapine
DAXOLIN C
  Loxapine
DAYALETS
  Vitamins, Multiple
DAYALETS PLUS IRON*
  Iron
  Vitamins, Multiple
DAY-BARB
  Butabarbital
DAYCARE*
  Acetaminophen
  Phenylpropanolamine
DBI
  Phenformin
D-CAINE
  Dibucaine
D.C.P.
  Dicalcium Phosphate
D.C.P. 340
  Dicalcium Phosphate
DDAVP
  Desmopressin
DEANER
  Deanol Acetamidobenzoate
DEANER-100
  Deanol Acetamidobenzoate
DEAPRIL-ST
  Ergoloid Mesylates
DEBRISAN
  Dextranomer
DEBROX
  Carbamide Peroxide
DECADERM
  Dexamethasone
DECADROL
  Dexamethasone
DECADRON
  Dexamethasone
DECADRON EYE-EAR SOLUTION
  Dexamethasone
DECADRON PHOSPHATE RESPIHALER
  Dexamethasone
DECA-DURABOLIN
  Nandrolone
DECAJET-L.A.
  Dexamethasone
DE-CAL
  Vitamins, Multiple
DECAMETH L.A.
  Dexamethasone
DECAPYRYN
  Doxylamine
DECASERPYL
  Methoserpidine
DECASERPYL PLUS*
  Hydrochlorothiazide
  Methoserpidine
DECASPRAY
  Dexamethasone
DECLINAX
  Debrisoquine
DECLOMYCIN
  Demeclocycline
DECLOSTATIN*
  Demeclocycline
  Nystatin
DECOHIST*
  Chlorpheniramine
  Phenylephrine
DECONADE*
  Chlorpheniramine
  Phenylpropanolamine
DECONAMINE*
  Chlorpheniramine
  Pseudoephedrine

DECONEX*
  Acetaminophen
  Phenylpropanolamine
DECONGESTABS*
  Chlorpheniramine
  Phenylephrine
  Phenylpropanolamine
  Phenyltoloxamine
DECONSMINE*
  Chlorpheniramine
  Pseudoephedrine
DECORTANCYL
  Prednisone
DECOSTRATE
  Desoxycorticosterone
DECUBITEX*
  Castor Oil
  Peruvian Balsam
  Propylene Glycol
  Scarlet Red
  Zinc Oxide
DECYCLINE
  Tetracycline
DEFICOL
  Bisacodyl
DEFINATE
  Docusate Sodium
DEGEST
  Phenylephrine
DEGEST-2
  Naphazoline
DEHAVAC*
  Allantoin
  Aminacrine
  Sulfanilamide
DEHIST*
  Atropine
  Chlorpheniramine
DEHYDROCHOLIN
  Dehydrocholic Acid
DEKABOLIN
  Nandrolone
DELACORT
  Hydrocortisone
DELALUTIN
  Hydroxyprogesterone
DELAPAV
  Papaverine
DELATESTRYL
  Testosterone
DELAVAN
  Methylbenzethonium
DELAXIN
  Methocarbamol
DELCID*
  Aluminum Hydroxide
  Magnesium Oxide
DELCOBESE
  Amphetamine
DELCOID
  Thyroid
DELESTROGEN
  Estradiol
DELFEN
  Nonoxynol 9
DELLADEC
  Dexamethasone
DELSYM
  Dextromethorphan
DELTA-CORTEF
  Prednisolone
DELTA-DOME
  Prednisone
DELTALIN
  Cholecalciferol
DELTAMINE
  Pemoline
DELTAMYCIN
  Tetracycline
DELTAPEN-VK
  Penicillin V
    Potassium
DELTASONE
  Prednisone
DELVEX
  Dithiazanine
DELVINAL
  Vinbarbital
DELYSID
  Lysergide
DEMASONE L.A.
  Dexamethasone
DEMASORB
  Dimethyl Sulfoxide
DEMAZIN*
  Chlorpheniramine
  Phenylephrine
DEMECLOR
  Demeclocycline
DEMER-IDINE

Meperidine
DEMEROL
Meperidine
DEMESO
Dimethyl Sulfoxide
DEMI-REGROTON*
Chlorthalidone
Reserpine
DEMO-CINEOL
Guaifenesin
DEMO-CINEOL ANTITUSSIVE
Dextromethorphan
DEMO-CINEOL EXPECTORANT
Guaifenesin
DEMSER
Metyrosine
DEMULEN*
Ethinyl Estradiol
Ethynodiol
DEMULEN 1/35*
Ethinyl Estradiol
Ethynodiol
DEMULEN-28*
Ethinyl Estradiol
Ethynodiol
DENDRID
Idoxuridine
DENOREX*
Coal Tar
Menthol
DENTAVITE*
Sodium Fluoride
Vitamins, Multiple
DENTITION
Benzocaine
DENTOCAINE
Benzocaine
DENTOJEL
Quinine
DEPAKENE
Valproic Acid
DEPAKOTE*
Valproate Sodium
Valproic Acid
DEPANATE
Estradiol
DEPEN TITRATABS
Penicillamine
DEPESTRO
Estradiol
DEP-GYNOGEN
Estradiol
DEPINAR
Cyanocobalamin
DEPLETITE
Diethylpropion
DEP MEDALONE
Methylprednisolone
DEPO-ACTH
Corticotropin
DEPOGEN
Estradiol
DEPO-HEPARIN SODIUM
Heparin
DEPO-MEDROL
Methylprednisolone
DEPO-PREDATE 80
Methylprednisolone
DEPO-PROVERA
Medroxyprogesterone
DEPO-TESTADIOL*
Estradiol
Testosterone
DEPO-TESTOSTERONE
Testosterone
DEPREX
Amitriptyline
DEPROIST*
Chlorpheniramine
Phenylpropanolamine
DEPROL*
Benactyzine
Meprobamate
DEPROLUTIN-250
Hydroxyprogesterone
DEPRONAL
Propoxyphene
DEQUADIN
Dequalinium
DEQUASINE*
Ascorbic Acid
Copper
Cysteine
Iodine
Iron
Lysine
Magnesium
Manganese
Racemethionine

Zinc
DERFON
Diethylpropion
DERIFIL
Chlorophyllin
DERMA+SOFT CREME
Salicylic Acid
DERMACOAT
Benzocaine
DERMACORT
Hydrocortisone
DERM-AID
Cetyl Alcohol
DERMALAR
Fluocinolone
DERMA MEDICONE-HC OINTMENT*
Benzocaine
Ephedrine
Hydrocortisone
Ichthammol
Menthol
Oxyquinoline
Zinc Oxide
DERMA MEDICONE OINTMENT*
Benzocaine
Ichthammol
Menthol
Oxyquinoline
Zinc Oxide
DERMAPHILL*
Aluminum Acetate
Camphor
Menthol
Phenol
DERMAREX*
Hydrocortisone
Iodochlorhydroxyquin
Pramoxine
DERMICORT
Hydrocortisone
DERMODEX 5 & 10 GEL
Benzoyl Peroxide
DERMOHEX
Hexachlorophene
DERMOLATE
Hydrocortisone
DERMOPLAST AEROSOL SPRAY*
Benzocaine
Menthol
DERMOVATE
Clobetasol
DERMOXYL
Benzoyl Peroxide
DERMTEX
Hydrocortisone
DERONIL
Dexamethasone
DESCOTONE
Desoxycorticosterone
DESENEX*
Undecylenic Acid
Zinc Undecylenate
DESENEX LIQUID
Undecylenic Acid
DESERIL
Methysergide
DESERNIL
Methysergide
DESEROL
Bromodiphenhydramine
DESFERAL
Deferoxamine
DESITIN OINTMENT*
Cholecalciferol
Vitamin A
Zinc Oxide
DESO-CREME*
Caprylic Acid
Zinc Undecylenate
DESOMEDINE
Hexamidine
DESOXEDRINE
Methamphetamine
DESOXYN
Methamphetamine
DESQUAM-X
Benzoyl Peroxide
DESYPHED
Methamphetamine
DESYREL
Trazodone
DETIGON
Chlophedianol
DE-TONE-2
Digitoxin
DEVELIN RETARD
Propoxyphene

DEVINES KOOL FOOT
Zinc Undecylenate
DEVROM
Bismuth Subgallate
DEWITT'S ANTACID POWDER*
Aluminum Hydroxide
Magnesium Carbonate
Magnesium Trisilicate
Sodium Bicarbonate
DEWITT'S BABY COUGH*
Ammonium Chloride
Glycerin
DEWITT'S OIL FOR EAR USE*
Cajeput Oil
Camphor
Menthol
Mineral Oil
Thyme Oil
DEWITT'S PILLS FOR BACKACHE & JOINT PAIN*
Caffeine
Potassium Nitrate
Salicylamide
DEX-A-DIET II
Phenylpropanolamine
DEXAMETH
Dexamethasone
DEXAMPEX
Dextroamphetamine
DEXAMYL*
Amobarbital
Dextroamphetamine
DEXASONE
Dexamethasone
DEXATRIM
Phenylpropanolamine
DEXEDRINE
Dextroamphetamine
DEXO-LA
Dexamethasone
DEXON
Dexamethasone
DEXONE
Dexamethasone
DEXTRAVEN
Dextran 150
DEXTRO-TUSS GG*
Dextromethorphan
Guaifenesin
DEXTROTUSSIN*
Ammonium Chloride
Ascorbic Acid
Dextromethorphan
Pheniramine
Phenylpropanolamine
DEY-DOSE
Isoetharine
D-FEDA
Pseudoephedrine
D.F.P.
Isoflurophate
D.H.E. 45
Dihydroergotamine
DHS ZINC
Pyrithione Zinc
DHT
Dihydrotachysterol
DIABETA
Glyburide
DIA BETA
Glyburide
DIABETORAL
Chlorpropamide
DIABEWAS
Tolazamide
DIABEXYL
Metformin
DIABINESE
Chlorpropamide
DIABISMUL*
Kaolin
Opium
Pectin
DIACTION*
Atropine
Diphenoxylate
DIADAX
Phenylpropanolamine
DI-ADEMIL
Hydroflumethiazide
DIA-EZE*
Bismuth Subgallate
Kaolin
DIAFEN
Diphenylpyraline
DIAGNEX BLUE

Azuresin
DIAHIST
Diphenhydramine
DIAL
Allobarbital
DIALOG*
Acetaminophen
Allobarbital
DIALOSE*
Carboxymethyl-cellulose
Docusate Potassium
DIALOSE
Docusate Potassium
DIALOSE PLUS*
Carboxymethyl-cellulose
Casanthranol
Docusate Potassium
DIALUME
Aluminum Hydroxide
DIAMOX
Acetazolamide
DIAMOX SEQUELS
Acetazolamide
DIANABOL
Methandrostenolone
DIAPARENE
Methylbenzethonium
DIAPID NASAL SPRAY
Lypressin
DIAQUA
Hydrochlorothiazide
DIA-QUEL*
Homatropine
Paregoric
Pectin
DIA-QUEL LIQUID*
Homatropine
Pectin
Tincture of Opium
DIAR-AID*
Attapulgite
Pectin
DIARKOTE*
Attapulgite
Belladonna Alkaloids
Pectin
DIARSED
Diphenoxylate
DIASONE
Sulfoxone
DIASONE SODIUM ENTERAB
Sulfoxone
DIASTIX
Glucose Oxidase Reagent
DIATRIN
Methaphenilene
DI-ATRO*
Atropine
Diphenoxylate
DIATROL*
Pectin
Sodium Bicarbonate
DIAZIL
Sulfamethazine
DI-AZO
Phenazopyridine
DIBENT
Dicyclomine
DIBENT-PB*
Dicyclomine
Phenobarbital
DIBENZYLINE
Phenoxybenzamine
DIBOTIN
Phenformin
DIBUCAINE OINTMENT
Dibucaine
DICAL-D WITH IRON*
Ergocalciferol
Ferric Pyrophosphate
DICAL-D WITH VITAMIN C
Vitamins, Multiple
DICALGIN
Calcium
DICARBOSIL
Calcium Carbonate
DICEN
Dicyclomine
DICETEL
Pinaverium
DICHLOREN
Mechlorethamine
DICHLOR-MAPHARSEN
Dichlorophenarsine
DICLOCIL
Dicloxacillin
DICODID
Hydrocodone
DICUMAN

Dicumarol
DICURIN PROCAINE*
Merethoxylline
Procaine
Theophylline
DI-DELAMINE*
Benzalkonium
Chloride
Diphenhydramine
Menthol
Tripelennamine
DIDREX
Benzphetamine
DIDRONEL
Etidronate Disodium
DIETAC*
Caffeine
Phenylpropanolamine
DIETAC DROPS
Phenylpropanolamine
DIETAC MAXIMUM STRENGTH
Phenylpropanolamine
DIETEC
Diethylpropion
DIET GARD
Phenylpropanolamine
DIETROL
Phendimetrazine
DIET-TRIM*
Carboxymethyl-
cellulose
Phenylpropanolamine
DIFFUSIN
Hyaluronidase
DI-GEL*
Aluminum Hydroxide
Magnesium Carbonate
Magnesium Oxide
Simethicone
DI-GENIK*
Estrone
Testosterone
DIGESTALIN*
Bismuth Subgallate
Charcoal, Activated
Pancreatin
Papain
Pepsin
DIGESTAMIC*
Atropine
Hyoscyamine
Papain
DIGESTIVE ENZYMES-PXP*
Pancrelipase
Pepsin
DIGIFORTIS
Digitalis
DIGIGLUSIN
Digitalis
DIGISIDIN
Digitoxin
DIGITALINE NATIVELLE
Digitoxin
DIGOLASE*
Amylase
Pancreatin
Proteinase
DIHYDREX
Diphenhydramine
DI-ISOPACIN*
Aminosalicylic Acid
Isoniazid
DILABIL
Dehydrocholic Acid
DILANCA
Pentaerythritol
Tetranitrate
DILANTIN
Phenytoin
DILAR
Paramethasone
DILART
Papaverine
DILATRATE-SR
Isosorbide Dinitrate
DILATYL
Nylidrin
DILAUDID
Hydromorphone
DILAUDID-HP
Hydromorphone
DILAVASE
Isoxsuprine
DILAX
Docusate Sodium
DILAX-250
Docusate Sodium
DILIN
Dyphylline
DILOCAINE
Lidocaine
DILOMINE

Dicyclomine
DILONE*
Acetaminophen
Caffeine
Phenyltoloxamine
DILOR
Dyphylline
DILOR G TABS*
Dyphylline
Guaifenesin
DILOSYN
Methdilazine
DILYN
Griseofulvin
DIMACID*
Calcium Carbonate
Magnesium Carbonate
DIMACOL*
Dextromethorphan
Guaifenesin
Pseudoephedrine
DIMALIX*
Brompheniramine
Phenylpropanolamine
DIMELIN
Acetohexamide
DIMELOR
Acetohexamide
DIMENEST
Dimenhydrinate
DIMENFORMON
Estradiol
DIMENTABS
Dimenhydrinate
DIMETANE
Brompheniramine
DIMETANE DECONGESTANT*
Brompheniramine
Phenylephrine
DIMETANE EXPECTORANT*
Brompheniramine
Guaifenesin
Phenylephrine
Phenylpropanolamine
DIMETANE EXPECTORANT-DC*
Brompheniramine
Guaifenesin
Phenylephrine
Phenylpropanolamine
DIMETANE EXTENTABS*
Brompheniramine
DIMETAPP ELIXIR*
Brompheniramine
Phenylephrine
Phenylpropanolamine
DIMETAPP EXTENTABS*
Brompheniramine
Phenylephrine
Phenylpropanolamine
DIMETAPP WITH CODEINE*
Brompheniramine
Codeine
Phenylephrine
Phenylpropanolamine
DIMOCILLIN-RT
Methicillin
DIMOTANE
Brompheniramine
DIMOTHYN
Dihydroxyaluminum Aminoacetate
DINACRIN
Isoniazid
DINATE
Dimenhydrinate
DIOCTALOSE*
Carboxymethylcellulose
Casanthranol
Docusate Sodium
DIOCTO*
Carboxymethylcellulose
Casanthranol
Docusate Sodium
DIOCTYL
Docusate Sodium
DIODINE
Iodine
DIODOQUIN
Iodoquinol
DIODRAST
Iodopyracet
DIOEZE
Docusate Sodium
DIOGYN
Estradiol
DIOGYN E
Ethinyl Estradiol

DIOGYNETS
  Estradiol
DIOLAX*
  Casanthranol
  Docusate Sodium
DIOLOXOL
  Mephenesin
DIOMEDICONE
  Docusate Sodium
DIONOSIL
  Propyliodone
DIOSUCCIN
  Docusate Sodium
DIO-SUL
  Docusate Sodium
DIOTHANE
  Diperodon
DIOTHRON*
  Casanthranol
  Docusate Sodium
DIOVAL
  Estradiol
DI-OVOCYLIN
  Estradiol
DIOVOL*
  Aluminum Hydroxide
  Magnesium Hydroxide
  Simethicone
DIOVOL EX*
  Aluminum Hydroxide
  Magnesium Hydroxide
D.I.P.
  Diethylpropion
DI-PARALENE
  Chlorcyclizine
DIPARCOL
  Diethazine
DIPAV
  Papaverine
DIPAXIN
  Diphenadione
DIPHEN
  Diphenhydramine
DIPHENADRIL
  Diphenhydramine
DIPHENATOL*
  Atropine
  Diphenoxylate
DIPHENYLAN
  Phenytoin
DIPROSONE
  Betamethasone
DIPSAN
  Calcium Carbimide
DIREMA
  Hydrochlorothiazide
DISALCID
  Salsalate
DISANTHROL*
  Casanthranol
  Docusate Sodium
DISIPAL
  Orphenadrine
DISOLAN*
  Docusate Sodium
  Phenolphthalein
DISOLAN FORTE*
  Carboxymethyl-
    cellulose
  Casanthranol
  Docusate Sodium
DISOMER
  Dexbrompheniramine
DISONATE
  Docusate Sodium
DISOPHROL*
  Dexbrompheniramine
  Pseudoephedrine
DISOPLEX*
  Carboxymethyl-
    cellulose
  Docusate Sodium
DI-SOSUL
  Docusate Sodium
DISPATABS
  Vitamin A
DI-SPAZ
  Dicyclomine
DISPOS-A-MED
  Isoetharine
DISTAMINE
  Penicillamine
DISULONE
  Dapsone
DISYNCRAN
  Methdilazine
DITAN
  Phenytoin
DITROPAN
  Oxybutynin

DITUBIN
  Isoniazid
DIUCARDIN
  Hydroflumethiazide
DIUCHLOR H
  Hydrochlorothiazide
DIULO
  Metolazone
DIUPRES*
  Chlorothiazide
  Reserpine
DIUPRES-250*
  Chlorothiazide
  Reserpine
DIURESE
  Trichlormethiazide
DIURETIN
  Theobromine
DIUREXAN
  Xipamide
DIURIL
  Chlorothiazide
DIU-SCRIP
  Hydrochlorothiazide
DIUTENSEN*
  Cryptenamine
  Methyclothiazide
DIUTENSEN-R*
  Methyclothiazide
  Reserpine
DIZMISS
  Meclizine
DIZYME*
  Betaine
  Glutamic Acid
  Pancreatin
  Pepsin
DM
  Dextromethorphan
D-MED-80
  Methylprednisolone
DM-4 CHILDREN'S COUGH CONTROL*
  Ammonium Chloride
  Dextromethorphan
  Potassium Guaiacolsulfonate
DM-8*
  Ammonium Chloride
  Dextromethorphan
  Potassium Guaiacolsulfonate
DOAK OIL
  Coal Tar
DOAK OIL FORTE
  Coal Tar
DOAN'S PILLS*
  Caffeine
  Magnesium Salicylate
DOANS RUB*
  Menthol
  Methyl Salicylate
DOBUTREX
  Dobutamine
DOCA ACETATE
  Desoxycorticosterone
DOCIBIN
  Cyanocobalamin
DOCTASE*
  Casanthranol
  Docusate Sodium
DOCTATE
  Docusate Sodium
DOCTATE-P*
  Danthron
  Docusate Sodium
DODDS HEMORAIDS
  Diperodon
DODDS PILLS
  Sodium Salicylate
DODECAMIN
  Cyanocobalamin
DODECAVITE
  Cyanocobalamin
DODEX
  Cyanocobalamin
DOFUS
  Acidophillus
DOLACET*
  Acetaminophen
  Propoxyphene
DOLANEX
  Acetaminophen
DOLANTAL
  Meperidine
DOLANTIN
  Meperidine
DOLCIN*
  Aspirin
  Calcium Succinate

DOLENE
\ Propoxyphene
DOLENE-AP-65*
Acetaminophen
Propoxyphene
DOLENE COMPOUND-65*
Aspirin
Caffeine
Propoxyphene
DOLICAINE
Lidocaine
DOLIPOL
Tolbutamide
DOLOBID
Diflunisal
DOLOMIDE
Salicylamide
DOLONIL*
Butabarbital
Hyoscyamine
Phenazopyridine
DOLOPHINE
Methadone
DOLOR*
Acetaminophen
Aspirin
Caffeine
DOLOXENE
Propoxyphene
DOLSED*
Atropine
Benzoic Acid
Hyoscyamine
Methenamine
Methylene Blue
Phenylsalicylate
DOMEBORO
Aluminum Acetate
DOMEFORM
Iodochlorhydroxyquin
DOMEFORM-HC*
Clioquinol
Hydrocortisone
DOME-PASTE BANDAGE*
Calamine
Zinc Oxide
DOMERINE*
Allantoin
Salicylic Acid
DOMMANATE
Dimenhydrinate
DONATUSSIN DROPS*
Chlorpheniramine
Guaifenesin
Phenylephrine
DONATUSSIN SYRUP*
Chlorpheniramine
Dextromethorphan
Guaifenesin
Phenylephrine
DONEX
Pyrithione Zinc
DONNAGEL*
Atropine
Hyoscyamine
Kaolin
Pectin
Scopolamine
DONNAGEL-MB*
Kaolin
Pectin
DONNAGEL-PG*
Atropine
Hyoscyamine
Kaolin
Opium
Pectin
Scopolamine
DONNAMOR ELIXIR*
Atropine
Hyoscyamine
Phenobarbital
Scopolamine
DONNATAL*
Atropine
Hyoscine
Hyoscyamine
Phenobarbital
DONNATAL EXTENTABS*
Atropine
Hyoscine
Hyoscyamine
Phenobarbital
DONNAZYME*
Atropine
Bile Salts
Hyoscyamine
Pancreatin
Pepsin
Phenobarbital

Scopolamine
DONPHEN*
Atropine
Hyoscyamine
Phenobarbital
Scopolamine
DOPAIDAN
Levodopa
DOPAMET
Methyldopa
DOPAR
Levodopa
DOPASTAT
Dopamine
DOPRAM
Doxapram
DORANTAMIN
Pyrilamine
DORAXIMIN
Dihydroxyaluminum Aminoacetate
DORBANE
Danthron
DORBANTYL*
Danthron
Docusate Sodium
DORBANTYL FORTE*
Danthron
Docusate Sodium
DORCOL PEDIATRIC*
Dextromethorphan
Guaifenesin
Phenylpropanolamine
DORCOSTRIN
Desoxycorticosterone
DORIDEN
Glutethimide
DORMAREX
Pyrilamine
DORMETHAN
Dextromethorphan
DORMIN
Methapyrilene
DORMISON
Meparfynol
DORMYTAL
Amobarbital
DORNOKINASE
Streptokinase
DORSACAINE
Benoxinate
DORSAPHYLLIN
Theophylline
DORSITAL
Pentobarbital
DORYL
Carbachol
DOSALUPENT
Metaproterenol
DOSS* (CANADA)
Danthron
Docusate Sodium
DOSS (USA)
Docusate Sodium
DOUBLE-E ALERTNESS
Caffeine
DOUBLE ISOPACIN*
Aminosalicylic Acid
Isoniazid
DOUBLE-T
Tetracycline
DOWMYCIN E
Erythromycin
DOXAN*
Danthron
Docusate Sodium
DOXAPRIL
Doxapram
DOXATONE
Desoxycorticosterone
DOXICAL
Docusate Calcium
DOXIDAN*
Danthron
Docusate Calcium
DOXINATE
Docusate Sodium
DOXINE*
Doxylamine
Pyridoxine
DOXYCHEL
Doxycycline
DOXY-II
Doxycycline
DOXY-LEMMON
Doxycycline
DOXY-TABS
Doxycycline
DOXY 100
Doxycycline

DOXY 200
  Doxycycline
DOZAR
  Methapyrilene
DRALSERP*
  Hydralazine
  Reserpine
DRALZINE
  Hydralazine
DRAMABAN
  Dimenhydrinate
DRAMAMINE
  Dimenhydrinate
DRAMILIN
  Dimenhydrinate
DRAMOCEN
  Dimenhydrinate
DRAMOJECT
  Dimenhydrinate
DRAPOLEX
  Cetrimide
DRAPOLEX CREAM
  Benzalkonium
    Chloride
DR. CALDWELL'S SENNA
    LAXATIVE
  Senna
DR. DRAKE'S
  Ipecac Fluidextract
DRENIFORM*
  Clioquinol
  Flurandrenolide
DRENISON
  Flurandrenolide
DRENUSIL
  Polythiazide
DRINOPHEN*
  Acetaminophen
  Aspirin
  Caffeine
  Phenylpropanolamine
DRISDOL
  Ergocalciferol
DRISTAMEAD LONG
  Xylometazoline
DRISTAN*
  Aspirin
  Chlorpheniramine
  Phenylephrine
DRISTAN ADVANCED
    FORMULA*
  Acetaminophen
  Chlorpheniramine
  Phenylpropanolamine
DRISTAN ANTITUSSIVE*
  Chlorpheniramine
  Dextromethorphan
  Phenylephrine
DRISTAN INHALER
  Propylhexedrine
DRISTAN LONG LASTING
    NASAL MIST
  Oxymetazoline
DRISTAN LONG LASTING
    VAPOR SPRAY
  Oxymetazoline
DRISTAN NASAL SPRAY*
  Pheniramine
  Phenylephrine
DRISTAN ULTRA*
  Acetaminophen
  Chlorpheniramine
  Dextromethorphan
  Pseudoephedrine
DRISTAN ULTRA COUGHS
    FORMULA*
  Acetaminophen
  Chlorpheniramine
  Dextromethorphan
  Pseudoephedrine
DRISTOL DELTALIN
  Ergocalciferol
DRITHOCREME
  Anthralin
DRIXINE
  Oxymetazoline
DRIXORAL*
  Dexbrompheniramine
  Pseudoephedrine
DRIZE*
  Chlorpheniramine
  Phenylpropanolamine
DROCORT
  Flurandrenolide
DROLBAN
  Dromostanolone
DROLEPTAN
  Droperidol
DROMISOL
  Dimethyl Sulfoxide
DROPSAL

Salicylamide
DROXARYL
Bufexamac
DROXINE L.A.
Dyphylline
DROXINE S.F.
Dyphylline
DROXOMIN
Hydroxocobalamin
DRY AND CLEAR
Benzoyl Peroxide
DRY AND CLEAR ACNE CREAM*
Salicylic Acid
Sulfur
DRY AND CLEAR ACNE MEDICATION
Salicylic Acid
DRY AND CLEAR CLEANSER
Salicylic Acid
DRYSOL*
Alcohol
Aluminum Chloride
DRYTEX
Salicylic Acid
DRYVAX
Smallpox Vaccine
D-SINUS*
Acetaminophen
Phenylpropanolamine
D-S-S
Docusate Sodium
D-S-S PLUS*
Casanthranol
Docusate Sodium
DTIC-DOME
Dacarbazine
D-TRAN
Diazepam
DUADACIN*
Acetaminophen
Chlorpheniramine
Phenylephrine
Pyrilamine
Salicylamide
DUAL FORMULA FEEN-A-MINT*
Docusate Sodium
Phenolphthalein
DUAPEN
Penicillin G Benzathine
DUCOBEE
Cyanocobalamin
DUCOBEE-HY
Hydroxocobalamin
DUFALONE
Dicumarol
DULARIN
Acetaminophen
DULCODOS*
Bisacodyl
Docusate Sodium
DULCOLAX
Bisacodyl
DUO-BARB*
Amobarbital
Secobarbital
DUO-CVP
Vitamins, Multiple
DUOFILM*
Lactic Acid
Salicylic Acid
DUOGASTRONE
Carbenoxolone
DUOGEN*
Estrone
Testosterone
DUOHALER*
Isoproterenol
Phenylephrine
DUO-HIST*
Dexbrompheniramine
Pseudoephedrine
DUO-MEDIHALER*
Isoproterenol
Phenylephrine
DUOPRIN*
Acetaminophen
Salicylamide
DUOSOL
Docusate Sodium
DUO-TRACH KIT
Lidocaine
DUOTRATE PLATEAU CAPS
Pentaerythritol Tetranitrate
DUPHALAC
Lactulose
DUPHASTON

Dydrogesterone
DUPHRENE*
Chlorpheniramine
Phenylephrine
Pyrilamine
DURABOLIN
Nandrolone
DURACILLIN
Penicillin G
DURACILLIN A.S.
Penicillin G
Procaine
DURACTON
Corticotropin
DURA-C 500 GRADUALS
Vitamins, Multiple
DURADYNE*
Acetaminophen
Aspirin
Caffeine
DURADYNE-FORTE*
Acetaminophen
Chlorpheniramine
Phenylephrine
Salicylamide
DURA-ESTRIN
Estradiol
DURAGEN
Estradiol
DURAGESIC*
Aspirin
Salsalate
DURALEX*
Chlorpheniramine
Pseudoephedrine
DURALONE-40
Methylprednisolone
DURALONE-80
Methylprednisolone
DURALUTIN
Hydroxyprogesterone
DURA-METH
Methylprednisolone
DURAMIST PM
Xylometazoline
DURAMORPH PF
Morphine
DURANEST
Etidocaine
DURAPAR
Papaverine
DURAPHYL
Theophylline
DURAQUIN
Quinidine
DURASAL
Magnesium Salicylate
DURATHESIA
Procaine
DURATION
Oxymetazoline
DURATION MENTHOLATED VAPOR SPRAY
Oxymetazoline
DURETIC
Methyclothiazide
DUREZE OTIC DROPS*
Acetic Acid
Benzalkonium Chloride
Hydrocortisone
Parachlorometa-xylenol
Pramoxine
Propylene Glycol
DURICEF
Cefadroxil
DUROMIN
Phentermine
DURRAX
Hydroxyzine
DUVADILIN
Isoxsuprine
DUVOID
Bethanechol
DV
Diethylstilbestrol
DV CREAM/SUPPOSITORIES
Dienestrol
DYAZIDE*
Hydrochlorothiazide
Triamterene
DYCHOLIUM
Dehydrocholic Acid
DYCILL
Dicloxacillin
DYCLONE
Dyclonine
DYFLEX
Dyphylline

DYFLEX G TABS*
  Dyphylline
  Guaifenesin
DYMELOR
  Acetohexamide
DYMENATE
  Dimenhydrinate
DYMENOL
  Dimenhydrinate
DYNAPEN
  Dicloxacillin
DYNAPHYLLINE
  Acefylline
DYNAPRIN
  Imipramine
DYNERIC
  Clomiphene
DYNOCTOL
  Docusate Sodium
DYNOSAL*
  Acetaminophen
  Aspirin
  Caffeine
DYRENIUM
  Triamterene
DYSNE-INHAL
  Epinephrine
DYSPAS
  Dicyclomine
DYTAC
  Triamterene

E

EARDRO*
  Antipyrine
  Benzocaine
EAR DROP BY MURINE*
  Carbamide Peroxide
  Glycerin
EASPRIN
  Aspirin
EAZOL
  Phosphorated
    Carbohydrate
EBSERPINE
  Reserpine
E-CARPINE*
  Epinephrine
  Pilocarpine
ECHODIDE
  Echothiophate Iodide
ECOBUTAZONE
  Phenylbutazone
ECODIDE
  Echothiophate Iodide
ECOLID
  Chlorisondamine
ECONOCHLOR OPHTHALMIC
  Chloramphenicol
ECONOPRED
  Prednisolone
ECOSTATIN
  Econazole
ECOTRIN
  Aspirin
E-CYPIONATE
  Estradiol
EDECRIN
  Ethacrynic Acid
E.D.T.A.
  Edetate Calcium
    Disodium
E.E.S.
  Erythromycin
    Ethylsuccinate
EFA STERI-OPT
  Sodium Chloride
EFED II*
  Caffeine
  Ephedrine
  Phenylpropanolamine
EFEDRA P.A.*
  Dexbrompheniramine
  Pseudoephedrine
EFEDRON NASAL JELLY
  Ephedrine
E-FEROL
  Vitamin E
EFFERSYLLIUM
  Plantago Seed
EFFICIN
  Magnesium Salicylate
EFFISAX
  Tybamate
EFODINE
  Povidone-Iodine
EFRICEL
  Phenylephrine
EFRICON*
  Ammonium Chloride

Chlorpheniramine
Codeine
Phenylephrine
Potassium
Guaiacolsulfonate
EFUDEX
Fluorouracil
E. IONATE P.A.
Estradiol
ELAQUA XX
Urea
ELASE*
Desoxyribonuclease
Fibrinolysin
ELASE-CHLOROMYCETIN OINTMENT*
Chloramphenicol
Desoxyribonuclease
Fibrinolysin
ELATROL
Amitriptyline
ELAVIL
Amitriptyline
ELDADRYL
Diphenhydramine
ELDEC KAPSEALS*
Minerals, Multiple
Vitamins, Multiple
ELDECORT
Hydrocortisone
ELDERCAPS*
Minerals, Multiple
Vitamins, Multiple
ELDERTONIC*
Minerals, Multiple
Vitamins, Multiple
ELDEZOL
Nitrofurazone
ELDISINE
Vindesine
ELDODRAM
Dimenhydrinate
ELDOPAQUE
Hydroquinone
ELDOQUIN
Hydroquinone
ELECTROCORTIN
Aldosterone
ELIXICON SUSPENSION
Theophylline
ELIXOPHYLLIN
Theophylline
ELIXOPHYLLIN-GG ORAL LIQUID
Guaifenesin
Theophylline
ELIXOPHYLLIN SR
Theophylline
ELKOSIN
Sulfisomidine
ELMARINE
Chlorpromazine
ELMOTIL*
Atropine
Diphenoxylate
E-LONATE P.A.
Estradiol
ELOXYL
Benzoyl Peroxide
EL PETN
Pentaerythritol Tetranitrate
ELRODORM
Glutethimide
ELSPAR
Asparaginase
ELTOR
Pseudoephedrine
ELTROXIN
Levothyroxine
ELZYME 303
Pancreatin
EMAGRIN*
Aspirin
Caffeine
Salicylamide
EMAGRIN FORTE*
Acetaminophen
Phenylephrine
Salicylamide
EMBINAL
Barbital
EMCYT
Estramustine
EMER-CIDE
Cresol
EMERDENT
Eugenol
EMEROID*
Bismuth Subcarbonate
Diperodon
Phenylephrine

Pyrilamine
Zinc Oxide
EMETE-CON
Benzquinamide
EMETROL
Invert Sugar
EMIVAN
Ethamivan
EMKO CONTRACEPTIVE FOAM
Nonoxynol 9
EMO-CORT
Hydrocortisone
EMOTIVAL
Lorazepam
EMPIRIN COMPOUND*
Aspirin
Caffeine
EMPIRIN WITH CODEINE*
Aspirin
Codeine
EMPLETS
Potassium Chloride
EMPRACET
Acetaminophen
EMPRACET WITH CODEINE PHOSPHATE NO. 3*
Acetaminophen
Codeine
EMPRACET WITH CODEINE PHOSPHATE NO. 4*
Acetaminophen
Codeine
EMPRACET-30*
Acetaminophen
Codeine
EMPRAZIL*
Aspirin
Caffeine
Pseudoephedrine
EMPRAZIL-C*
Aspirin
Caffeine
Codeine
Pseudoephedrine
EMUL-O-BALM*
Camphor
Menthol
Methyl Salicylate
E-MYCIN
Erythromycin
E-MYCIN E LIQUID
Erythromycin Ethylsuccinate
ENARAX*
Hydroxyzine
Oxyphencyclimine
ENCAPRIN
Aspirin
ENCARE
Nonoxynol 9
EN-CEBRIN*
Minerals, Multiple
Vitamins, Multiple
EN-CEBRIN F*
Folic Acid
Minerals, Multiple
Vitamins, Multiple
ENDECON*
Acetaminophen
Phenylpropanolamine
ENDEP
Amitriptyline
ENDOGRAFIN
Meglumine
ENDOTUSSIN-NN*
Ammonium Chloride
Dextromethorphan
Pyrilamine
ENDOTUSSIN-NN PEDIATRIC*
Ammonium Chloride
Dextromethorphan
ENDOXAN
Cyclophosphamide
ENDRATE DISODIUM
Edetate Calcium Disodium
ENDURON
Methyclothiazide
ENDURONYL*
Deserpidine
Methyclothiazide
ENDURONYL FORTE*
Deserpidine
Methyclothiazide
ENGLISH STYLE HEALTH SALTS
Magnesium Sulfate
ENGRAN-HP
Vitamins, Multiple
ENICOL

Chloramphenicol
ENISYL
Lysine
ENO*
Sodium Bicarbonate
Sodium Citrate
Sodium Tartrate
ENOVID*
Mestranol
Norethynodrel
ENOVID-E*
Mestranol
Norethynodrel
ENOXA*
Atropine
Diphenoxylate
ENRUMAY
Pyrilamine
ENSIDON
Opipramol
ENTACYL
Piperazine
ENTAIR*
Guaifenesin
Theophylline
ENTERIC COATED ASA
Aspirin
ENTEX*
Guaifenesin
Phenylephrine
Phenylpropanolamine
ENTEX LA*
Guaifenesin
Phenylpropanolamine
ENTOZYME*
Bile Salts
Pancreatin
Pepsin
ENTROMONE
Gonadotropin, Chorionic
ENTROPHEN
Aspirin
ENTROPHEN WITH CODEINE*
Aspirin
Codeine
ENTROSALYL
Sodium Salicylate
ENTUREN
Sulfinpyrazone
ENTUSS EXPECTORANT & LIQUID*
Guaifenesin
Hydrocodone
ENTUSUL
Sulfisoxazole
ENZACTIN
Triacetin
ENZEON
Chymotrypsin
ENZODASE
Hyaluronidase
ENZYMACOL*
Amylase
Bile Salts
Iron
Lipase
Protease
ENZYPAN*
Bile Salts
Pancreatin
Pepsin
E-PAM
Diazepam
EPANUTIN
Phenytoin
EPHEDSOL
Ephedrine
EPHYNAL
Vitamin E
EPICEL
Phenylephrine
EPICLASE
Phenacemide
EPI-CLEAR*
Benzoyl Peroxide
Sulfur
EPI-CLEAR SCRUB CLEANSER
Aluminum Oxide
EPICORT
Hydrocortisone
EPIDOSIN
Valethamate
EPIFOAM
Hydrocortisone
EPIFORM-HC*
Hydrocortisone
Iodochlorhydroxyquin
EPIFRIN
Epinephrine

EPILIM
  Valproate Sodium
E-PILO*
  Epinephrine
  Pilocarpine
E-PILO-1
  Epinephrine
  Pilocarpine
E-PILO-2
  Epinephrine
  Pilocarpine
EPIMORPH
  Morphine
EPIMYCIN "A"*
  Bacitracin
  Diperodon
  Neomycin
  Polymyxin B
EPINAL
  Epinephrine
EPIPEN JR.
  Epinephrine
EPITRATE
  Epinephrine
E.P. MYCIN
  Oxytetracycline
EPONTOL
  Propanidid
EPPY
  Epinephryl Borate
EPPY/N
  Epinephryl Borate
EPROLIN
  Vitamin E
EPSAMON
  Aminocaproic Acid
EPSIKAPRON
  Aminocaproic Acid
EPSILAN-M
  Vitamin E
EPSOM SALT
  Magnesium Sulfate
EPTOIN
  Phenytoin
EQUAGESIC*
  Aspirin
  Ethoheptazine
  Meprobamate
EQUANIL
  Meprobamate
EQUANITRATE*
  Meprobamate
  Pentaerythritol
    Tetranitrate
EQUILET
  Calcium Carbonate
EQUIPOISE
  Hydroxyzine
EQUIVERT
  Buclizine
ERADACIL
  Rosoxacin
ERAMYCIN
  Erythromycin
    Stearate
ERANTIN
  Propoxyphene
ERCAF*
  Caffeine
  Ergotamine
ERCATAB*
  Caffeine
  Ergotamine
ERGENYL
  Valproic Acid
ERGOBASINE
  Ergonovine
ERGOBEL*
  Ergotamine
  Hyoscyamine
  Phenobarbital
ERGOCAF*
  Caffeine
  Ergotamine
ERGOKLININE
  Ergotamine
ERGOMAR
  Ergotamine
ERGOSTAT
  Ergotamine
ERGOTRATE
  Ergonovine
ERILAX
  Bisacodyl
ERIMAG
  Magnesium Gluconate
ERIVIT C
  Ascorbic Acid
ERYC
  Erythromycin

ERYC
Erythromycin
ERYDERM
Erythromycin
ERYMYCIN
Erythromycin
ERYPAR
Erythromycin Stearate
ERYPED
Erythromycin
ERY-TAB
Erythromycin
ERYTHROCIN
Erythromycin
ERYTHROCIN STEARATE FILMTAB
Erythromycin Stearate
ERYTHROGRAN
Erythromycin
ERYTHROGUENT
Erythromycin
ERYTHROMID
Erythromycin
ESBALOID
Bethanidine
ESBATAL
Bethanidine
ESCHATIN
Adrenal Cortex Extract
ESCOT*
Aluminum Hydroxide
Bismuth Aluminate
Magnesium Carbonate
Magnesium Trisilicate
ESERINE SULFATE
Physostigmine
ESGIC*
Acetaminophen
Butalbital
Caffeine
ESIDRIX
Hydrochlorothiazide
ESIMIL*
Guanethidine
Hydrochlorothiazide
ESKABARB
Phenobarbital
ESKADIAZINE
Sulfadiazine
ESKALITH
Lithium Carbonate
ESKALITH CR
Lithium Carbonate
ESKASERP
Reserpine
ESKATROL*
Dextroamphetamine
Prochlorperazine
ESOMEDINA
Hexamidine
ESOPHOTRAST
Barium
ESORB
Vitamin E
ESOTERICA
Hydroquinone
ESPECOL
Phosphorated Carbohydrate
ESPERSON
Desoximetasone
ESPOTABS
Phenolphthalein
ESTABS
Estrogens, Esterified
ESTAR
Coal Tar
ESTATE
Estradiol
ESTENCILLINE
Penicillin G
ESTEQUA
Estrone
ESTERTEST H.S.*
Estrogens, Esterified
Methyltestosterone
ESTINYL
Ethinyl Estradiol
ESTOMUL-M*
Aluminum Hydroxide
Magnesium Carbonate
Magnesium Oxide
ESTRACE
Estradiol

ESTRA-CYP
  Estradiol
ESTRA-D
  Estradiol
ESTRADURIN
  Polyestradiol
ESTRAGUARD
  Dienestrol
ESTRALDINE
  Estradiol
ESTRATAB
  Estrogens,
    Esterified
ESTRATEST*
  Estrogens,
    Esterified
  Methyltestosterone
ESTRAVAL P.A.
  Estradiol
ESTRAVAL 2X
  Estradiol
ESTRIVIN
  Rose Petal Aqueous
ESTROCON
  Conjugated Estrogens
ESTROJECT-L.A.
  Estradiol
ESTROJECT-2
  Estrone
ESTROMED
  Estrogens,
    Esterified
ESTRONOL
  Estrone
ESTROSYN
  Diethylstilbestrol
ESTROVIS
  Quinestrol
ESTRUSOL
  Estrone
ETA-LENT
  Ethaverine
ETAPHYLLINE
  Acefylline
ETHAMIDE
  Ethoxzolamide
ETHAQUIN
  Ethaverine
ETHATAB
  Ethaverine
ETHINORAL
  Ethinyl Estradiol
ETHIODAN
  Iophendylate
ETHIODOL
  Ethiodized Oil
ETHNINE
  Pholcodine
ETHNINE SIMPLEX
  Pholcodine
ETHOPHYLLINE
  Aminophylline
ETHRANE
  Enflurane
ETHRIL
  Erythromycin
    Stearate
ETHRIL 250
  Erythromycin
    Stearate
ETIBI
  Ethambutol
ETICYLOL
  Ethinyl Estradiol
ETOPHYLATE
  Acefylline
E-TOPLEX
  Vitamin E
ETRAFON*
  Amitriptyline
  Perphenazine
ETRAFON-A*
  Amitriptyline
  Perphenazine
ETRAFON FORTE*
  Amitriptyline
  Perphenazine
ETRENOL
  Hycanthone
EUDATINE
  Pargyline
EUDOL
  Oxycodone
EUFLAVINE
  Acriflavine
EUGLUCON
  Glyburide
EUHYPNOS FORTE
  Temazepam
EULISSIN

Decamethonium
EUMOVATE
Clobetasone
EUNOCTAL
Amobarbital
EUNURETROL
Ephedrine
EUPHENEX*
Acetaminophen
Phenyltoloxamine
EUPHTHALMINE
Eucatropine
EURAX
Crotamiton
EURESOL
Resorcinol
EUSAPRIM
Co-Trimoxazole
EUTHROID
Liotrix
EUTONYL
Pargyline
EUTRON*
Methyclothiazide
Pargyline
EVAC-Q-KIT*
Carbon Dioxide
Magnesium Citrate
Phenolphthalein
EVAC-Q-KWIK*
Bisacodyl
Magnesium Citrate
Phenolphthalein
EVAC-U-GEN
Phenolphthalein
EVENTIN
Propylhexedrine
EVERONE
Testosterone
EVESTRONE
Conjugated Estrogens
EVEX
Estrogens, Esterfied
EVIPAL
Hexobarbital
E-VISTA
Hydroxyzine
EX-APAP*
Acetaminophen
Aspirin
Caffeine
EXCEDRIN*
Acetaminophen
Aspirin
Caffeine
EXCEDRIN P.M.*
Acetaminophen
Pyrilamine
EXDOL
Acetaminophen
EX-LAX
Phenolphthalein
EX-LAX EXTRA GENTLE*
Docusate Sodium
Phenolphthalein
EX-LAX PILLS
Phenolphthalein
EXNA
Benzthiazide
EXNA-R*
Benzthiazide
Reserpine
EX-OBESE
Phendimetrazine
EXOCAINE CREAM
Trolamine Salicylate
EXSEL
Selenium Sulfide
EXTENDAC*
Chlorpheniramine
Pheniramine
Phenylpropanolamine
EXTENDRYL*
Chlorpheniramine
Methscopolamine
Phenylephrine
EXTRA GENTLE EX-LAX*
Docusate Sodium
Phenolphthalein
EXZIT*
Resorcinol
Sulfur
EXZIT MEDICATED CLEANSER*
Salicylic Acid
Sulfur
EYE COOL
Phenylephrine
EYEPHRINE*
Phenylephrine

Zinc Sulfate
E1
Epinephrine
E1/2
Epinephrine
E2
Epinephrine

F

FACTORATE
Antihemophilic Factor
FACTREL
Gonadorelin
FALAPEN
Penicillin G
FANSIDAR*
Pyrimethamine
Sulfadoxine
FASIGYN
Tinidazole
FASTIN
Phentermine
FASTON
Dimenhydrinate
FEBRINOL
Acetaminophen
FEBROGESIC
Acetaminophen
FEDAHIST*
Chlorpheniramine
Pseudoephedrine
FEDAHIST EXPECTORANT*
Chlorpheniramine
Guaifenesin
Pseudoephedrine
FEDAHIST SYRUP*
Chlorpheniramine
Pseudoephedrine
FEDRAZIL*
Chlorcyclizine
Pseudoephedrine
FEEN-A-LAX
Phenolphthalein
FEEN-A-MINT
Phenolphthalein
FEEN-A-MINT GUM
Phenolphthalein
FEEN-A-MINT PILLS*
Docusate Sodium
Phenolphthalein
FEIBA IMMUNO
Anti-inhibitor coagulant complex
FELDENE
Piroxicam
FELLOZINE
Promethazine
FELSOL POWDER
Antipyrine
FELSULES
Chloral Hydrate
FEMADOL
Propoxyphene
FEMCAPS*
Acetaminophen
Atropine
Caffeine
Ephedrine
FEMERGIN
Ergotamine
FEMGUARD*
Allantoin
Aminacrine
Sulfanilamide
FEMIDINE
Povidone-Iodine
FEMINAID
Vitamins, Multiple
FEMININS
Vitamins, Multiple
FEMINONE
Ethinyl Estradiol
FEMIRON
Ferrous Fumarate
FEMIRON WITH VITAMINS*
Ferrous Fumarate
Vitamins, Multiple
FEMOGEN
Estrone
FEMOGEN CYP
Estradiol
FEMOGEX
Estradiol
FEMOTRONE
Progesterone
FENAMIZOL
Amiphenazole
FENDOL*
Acetaminophen

Phenylephrine
Salicylamide
FENDON
Acetaminophen
FENICOL
Chloramphenicol
FENISTIL
Dimethindene
FENOPRON
Fenoprofen
FENTAZIN
Perphenazine
FENYLHIST
Diphenhydramine
FE-O.D.*
Ascorbic Acid
Ferrous Fumarate
FEOSOL
Ferrous Sulfate
FEOSOL SPANSULES
Ferrous Sulfate
FEOSTAT
Ferrous Fumarate
F-E-P CREME*
Hydrocortisone
Iodochlorhydroxyquin
Pramoxine
FE-PLUS
Iron
FERANCEE*
Ascorbic Acid
Ferrous Fumarate
Sodium Ascorbate
FERANCEE-HP*
Ascorbic Acid
Ferrous Fumarate
Sodium Ascorbate
FERAPLEX LIQUID*
Iron
Vitamin B Complex
FERGON
Ferrous Gluconate
FERGON WITH C CAPLETS*
Ascorbic Acid
Ferrous Gluconate
FER-IN-SOL
Ferrous Sulfate
FER-IN-SOL DROPS,
Ferrous Sulfate
FERMALOX
Ferrous Sulfate
FERMENTOL
Pepsin
FERMINATE-10
Estradiol
FERNDEX
Dextroamphetamine
FERNHIST*
Chlorpheniramine
Phenylpropanolamine
Pyrilamine
FERNISOLONE-P
Prednisolone
FERNISONE
Prednisone
FERO-FOLIC-500*
Ascorbic Acid
Folic Acid
Iron
FERO-GRAD
Ferrous Sulfate
FERO-GRADUMET
Ferrous Sulfate
FERO-GRAD-500*
Ferrous Sulfate
Sodium Ascorbate
FEROSORB-C*
Ascorbic Acid
Ferrous Fumarate
FEROTON
Ferrous Fumarate
FERRALET
Ferrous Gluconate
FERRITRINSIC
Vitamins, Multiple
FERROBID*
Ascorbic Acid
Ferrous Fumarate
FERROID
Ferrous Gluconate
FERROLIP
Ferrocholinate
FERROLIP PLUS
Vitamins, Multiple
FERRONORD
Ferroglycine Sulfate
FERRO-SEQUELS*
Docusate Sodium
Ferrous Fumarate
FERROSPAN
Iron Dextran
FERROSULPH

Ferrous Sulfate
FERSAMAL
Ferrous Fumarate
FERTINIC
Ferrous Gluconate
FESOFOR
Ferrous Sulfate
FESTAL*
Amylase
Bile Salts
Hemicellulase
Lipase
Protease
FESTALAN*
Amylase
Atropine
Lipase
Protease
FEXIMAC
Bufexamac
FIBOCIL
Aprindine
FIBORAN
Apridine
FIBRINDEX
Thrombin
FIBROGEN
Fibrinogen
FILAIR
Terbutaline
FILIBON*
Minerals, Multiple
Vitamins, Multiple
FINAC
Sulfur
FINAL STEP
Povidone-Iodine
FIOGESIC*
Carbaspirin Calcium
Pheniramine
Phenylpropanolamine
Pyrilamine
FIORINAL*
Aspirin
Butalbital
Caffeine
FIORINAL-C1/2*
Aspirin
Butalbital
Caffeine
Codeine
FIORINAL-C1/4*
Aspirin
Butalbital
Caffeine
Codeine
FIORINAL WITH CODEINE*
Aspirin
Butalbital
Caffeine
FIRST SIGN NASAL DECONGESTANT
Pseudoephedrine
FIVENT
Cromolyn Sodium
FIZRIN POWDER
Aspirin
FLACID*
Aluminum Hydroxide
Magnesium Carbonate
Magnesium Hydroxide
Simethicone
FLAGYL
Metronidazole
FLAGYLSTATIN*
Metronidazole
Nystatin
FLAMAZINE
Silver Sulfadiazine
FLAVEDRIN MILD*
Aminacrine
Ephedrine
FLAVOQUIN
Amodiaquine
FLAVORCEE
Ascorbic Acid
FLEET BABYLAX
Glycerin
FLEET BAGENEMA
Castile Soap
FLEET BAROBAG
Barium
FLEET BISACODYL ENEMA
Bisacodyl
FLEET ENEMA*
Sodium Biphosphate
Sodium Phosphate
FLEET ENEMA MINERAL OIL
Mineral Oil

FLEET ENEMA OIL RETENTION
Mineral Oil
FLEET ORAL
Barium
FLEET PEDIATRIC ENEMA*
Sodium Biphosphate
Sodium Phosphate
FLEET PREP KIT*
Bisacodyl
Phospho-soda
FLEET PREP KIT 2*
Bisacodyl
Phospho-soda
FLEET PREP KIT 3*
Bisacodyl
Phospho-soda
FLEET PREP KIT 4*
Bisacodyl
Castor Oil
FLEET PREP KIT 5*
Bisacodyl
Castor Oil
FLEET PREP KIT 6*
Bisacodyl
Castor Oil
FLENAC
Fenclofenac
FLETCHER'S CASTORIA
Senna
FLEXAPHEN*
Acetaminophen
Chlorzoxazone
FLEXERIL
Cyclobenzaprine
FLEXOJECT
Orphenadrine
FLEXON
Orphenadrine
FLINTSTONES
Vitamins, Multiple
FLINTSTONES PLUS IRON*
Iron
Vitamins, Multiple
FLONATRIL
Clorexolone
FLORAQUIN
Iodoquinol
FLORIDA FOAM IMPROVED*
Aluminum Acetate
Benzalkonium Chloride
Boric Acid
FLORINEF ACETATE
Fludrocortisone
FLORONE
Diflorasone Diacetate
FLOROPRYL
Isoflurophate
FLORVITE*
Sodium Fluoride
Vitamins, Multiple
FLO-TABS
Sodium Fluoride
FLOZENGES
Sodium Fluoride
FLUAGEL
Aluminum Hydroxide
FLUANXOL
Flupentixol
FLUCLOX
Floxacillin
FLUCORT
Flumethasone
FLUDESTRIN
Testolactone
FLUDROCORTONE
Fludrocortisone
FLUIDEX PLUS
Phenylpropanolamine
FLUIDIL
Cyclothiazide
FLUOCIN CREAM
Fluocinolone
FLUOCINOLONE ACETONIDE
Fluocinolone
FLUODERM
Fluocinolone
FLUOGEN
Influenza Virus Vaccine
FLUONID
Fluocinolone
FLUOR-A-DAY
Sodium Fluoride
FLUORESCITE
Fluorescein
FLUORETYL
Sodium Fluoride

FLUORIDENT
  Sodium Fluoride
FLUORINSE
  Sodium Fluoride
FLUORITAB
  Sodium Fluoride
FLUOR-L-STRIP A.T.
  Fluorescein
FLUOROMAR
  Fluroxene
FLUOROPLEX
  Fluorouracil
FLUOTHANE
  Halothane
FLURA-DROPS
  Sodium Fluoride
FLURESS*
  Benoxinate
  Chlorobutanol
  Fluorescein
  Povidone
FLUROBATE GEL
  Betamethasone
FLUROSYN
  Fluocinolone
FLUTEX
  Triamcinolone
FLUTONE
  Triamcinolone
FLUVIN
  Hydrochlorothiazide
FLUZONE
  Influenza Virus
    Vaccine
FML LIQUIFILM
  Fluorometholone
FOILLE
  Benzocaine
FOLBAL
  Folic Acid
FOLBESYN
  Vitamins, Multiple
FOLDINE
  Folic Acid
FOLIGAN
  Allopurinol
FOLLUTEIN
  Gonadotropin,
    Chorionic
FOLVITE
  Folic Acid
FOLVRON*
  Ferrous Sulfate
  Folic Acid
FOMAC
  Hexachlorophene
FOMAC FOAM
  Salicylic Acid
FOMNIPEN
  Ampicillin
FORANE
  Isoflurane
FORBAXIN
  Methocarbamol
FORDUSTIN
  Methylbenzethonium
FORHISTAL
  Dimethindene
FORMAC
  Salicylic Acid
FORMATRIX*
  Ascorbic Acid
  Estrogens, Esterfied
  Methyltestosterone
FORMIN
  Methenamine
FORMTONE-HC*
  Clioquinol
  Hydrocortisone
FORMULA MAGSIC*
  Magnesium Carbonate
  Mineral Oil
FORMULA 405
  Pregnenolone
FORMULA 44*
  Dextromethorphan
  Doxylamine
FORMULA 44 COUGH DISCS
  Dextromethorphan
FORMULA 44-D*
  Dextromethorphan
  Guaifenesin
  Phenylpropanolamine
FORMULE A
  Vitamin A
FORMULEX
  Dicyclomine
FORPEN
  Penicillin G
FORTALGESIC

Pentazocine
FORTAZ
Ceftazidime
FORTESPAN
Vitamins, Multiple
FORTICILLIN
Penicillin G
FORTIOR-2B*
Pyridoxine
Thiamine
FORTOMBRINE 'M'
Meglumine
FORTRAL
Pentazocine
FOSFREE*
Calcium
Iron
Vitamins, Multiple
FOSTEX BPO 5%
Benzoyl Peroxide
FOSTEX CAKE*
Salicylic Acid
Sulfur
FOSTEX CM
Sulfur
FOSTEX CREAM*
Salicylic Acid
Sulfur
FOSTEX MEDICATED CLEANSER*
Salicylic Acid
Sulfur
FOSTRIL
Sulfur
FOYGEN
Estrone
FRANOCIDE
Diethylcarbamazine
FREEZONE*
Ether
Salicylic Acid
Zinc Chloride
FRENANTOL
Paroxypropione
FRENQUEL
Azacyclonol
FREPP ANTISEPTIC
Povidone-Iodine
FRUCTINES-VICHY
Phenolphthalein
FUADIN
Stibophen
FUA-MED
Nitrofurantoin
FUCIDIN
Fusidic Acid
FUDR
Floxuridine
FUDR
Floxuridine
FUL-GLO
Fluorescein
FULLUTEIN
Gonadotropin, Chorionic
FULVICIN P/G
Griseofulvin
FULVICIN-U/F
Griseofulvin
FUMA DROPS
Ferrous Fumarate
FUMARAL ELIXIR AND SPANCAPS*
Ascorbic Acid
Ferrous Fumarate
Ferrous Sulfate
FUMASORB
Ferrous Fumarate
FUMERIN
Ferrous Fumarate
FUNDUSCEIN-10
Fluorescein
FUNGACETIN
Triacetin
FUNGIDERM
Undecylenic Acid
FUNGIZONE
Amphotericin B
FUNGOID
Triacetin
FUNGOID TINCTURE
Triacetin
FUNG-O-SPRAY*
Benzocaine
Hexachlorophene
Zinc Undecylenate
FUNGOTIC*
Acetic Acid
Benzalkonium Chloride

Hydrocortisone
Parachlorometaxylenol
Pramoxine
FURACIN
Nitrofurazone
FURACIN SOLUBLE DRESSING
Nitrofurazone
FURADANTIN
Nitrofurantoin
FURALAN
Nitrofurantoin
FURAMIDE
Diloxanide Furoate
FURAN
Nitrofurantoin
FURANEX
Nitrofurantoin
FURATINE
Nitrofurantoin
FURATOIN
Nitrofurantoin
FUROSIDE
Furosemide
FUROXONE
Furazolidone
FURSEMIDE
Furosemide
FYDALIN
Carbromal

G

GAIAPECT
Guaifenesin
GAMASTAN
Gobulin, Immune
GAMENE
Lindane
GAMIMUNE
Globulin, Immune
GAMMACORTEN
Dexamethasone
GAMMAR
Gobulin, Immune
GAMOPHEN
Hexachlorophene
GAMULIN RH
Rh D Immune Globulin, Human
GANAL
Fenfluramine
GANATREX
Vitamins, Multiple
GANPHEN
Promethazine
GANTANOL
Sulfamethoxazole
GANTRISIN
Sulfisoxazole
GANTRISIN CREAM
Sulfisoxazole
GARAMYCIN
Gentamicin
GARAMYCIN OPHTHALMIC
Gentamicin
GARAMYCIN OTIC
Gentamicin
GARDENAL
Phenobarbital
GASTICANS*
Pancreatin
Papain
Sodium Bicarbonate
GASTRIX
Oxyphencyclimine
GASTRODIAGNOST
Pentagastrin
GASTROGRAFIN*
Diatrizoate Meglumine
Diatrizoate Sodium
Iodine
GASTROVIST
Diatrizoate Meglumine
GASTROZEPIN
Pirenzepine
GASTROZEPINE
Pirenzepine
GAS-X
Simethicone
GAVISCON ANTACID*
Aluminum Hydroxide
Magnesium Trisilicate
GAVISCON-2 ANTACID*
Aluminum Hydroxide
Magnesium Trisilicate
GAYSAL*

Acetaminophen
Aluminum Hydroxide
Butabarbital
Phenobarbital
Salicylate
GAYSAL-S*
Acetaminophen
Aluminum Hydroxide
Salicylate
GBH
Lindane
GEE GEE
Guaîfenesin
GELTABS
Ergocalciferol
GELUMINA*
Aluminum Hydroxide
Magnesium Trisilicate
GEL-UNIX
Barium
GELUSIL*
Aluminum Hydroxide
Magnesium Oxide
Simethicone
GELUSIL EXTRA STRENGTH LIQUID*
Aluminum Hydroxide
Magnesium Hydroxide
GELUSIL II*
Aluminum Hydroxide
Magnesium Oxide
Simethicone
GELUSIL M*
Aluminum Hydroxide
Magnesium Oxide
Simethicone
GEMNISYN*
Acetaminophen
Aspirin
GEMONIL
Metharbital
GENAPEX
Gentian Violet
GENECILLIN-VK-500
Penicillin V Potassium
GENECILLIN-400
Penicillin G
GENESERP
Reserpine
GENOPTIC*
Benzalkonium Chloride
Gentamicin
GENTALLINE
Gentamicin
GENTALYN
Gentamicin
GENTICIN
Gentamicin
GENTLAX
Senna
GENTLAX B
Senna
GENTLAX S*
Docusate Sodium
Senna
GENTRAN 40
Dextran 40
GENTRAN 75
Dextran 75
GEOCILLIN
Carbenicillin
GEOPEN
Carbenicillin
GEOPEN ORAL
Carbenicillin
GERALIX LIQUID
Vitamins, Multiple
GERAVITE ELIXIR*
Alcohol
Cyanocobalamin
Lysine
Niacinamide
Pentylenetetrazol
Riboflavin
Thiamine
GERIAMIC
Vitamins, Multiple
GERILETS
Vitamins, Multiple
GERILIQUID
Niacin
GERIMAL
Ergoloid Mesylates
GERIPLEX
Vitamins, Multiple
GERIPLEX-FS KAPSEALS
Vitamins, Multiple
GERIPLEX-FS LIQUID
Vitamins, Multiple

GERITINIC
  Vitamins, Multiple
GERITOL
  Vitamins, Multiple
GERITOL JUNIOR
  Vitamins, Multiple
GERITOL JUNIOR LIQUID
  Vitamins, Multiple
GERITOL LIQUID
  Vitamins, Multiple
GERIX ELIXIR*
  Alcohol
  Vitamins, Multiple
GERIZYME
  Vitamins, Multiple
GERMA-MEDICA
  Hexachlorophene
GERMANIN
  Suramin
GERMICIN
  Benzalkonium
    Chloride
GERM-I-TOL
  Benzalkonium
    Chloride
GER-O-FOAM*
  Benzocaine
  Methyl Salicylate
GESINAL
  Medroxyprogesterone
GESTANIN
  Allylestrenol
GESTANON
  Allylestrenol
GESTASOL DRY
  Gonadotropin
GESTEROL
  Progesterone
GEVILON
  Hexacyclonate
GEVRABON
  Vitamins, Multiple
GEVRAL
  Vitamins, Multiple
GEVRAL PROTEIN
  Vitamins, Multiple
GEVRAL T
  Vitamins, Multiple
GEVRITE
  Vitamins, Multiple
GEXANE
  Lindane
GG-CEN
  Guaifenesin
G G TUSSIN
  Guaifenesin
GINSOPAN*
  Chlorpheniramine
  Phenylephrine
  Phenylpropanolamine
  Pyrilamine
GIQUEL
  Propantheline
GITALIGIN
  Gitalin
GLANIL
  Cinnarizine
GLAUCON
  Epinephrine
GLAUCOSTAT
  Aceclidine
GLOBUCID
  Sulfaethidole
GLUCAMIDE
  Chlorpropamide
GLUCODEX
  Dextrose
GLUCOPHAGE
  Metformin
GLUCOSOL
  Glucose
GLUCOTROL
  Glipizide
GLUCURONE
  Glucurolactone
GLUKOR INJECTION*
  Chlorobutanol
  Glutamic Acid
  Gonadotropin,
    Chorionic
  Procaine
  Thiamine
GLUTAN HYDROCHLORIDE
  Glutamic Acid
GLUTOFAC*
  Minerals, Multiple
  Vitamins, Multiple
GLYATE
  Guaifenesin
GLYCATE*

Aminoacetic Acid
Calcium Carbonate
GLYCEROL-T*
Guaifenesin
Theophylline
GLYCOGEL*
Aluminum Hydroxide
Calcium Carbonate
Magnesium Carbonate
GLYCOLIXIR
Aminoacetic Acid
GLYCOPYRROLATE*
Glycopyrrolate
Phenobarbital
GLYCOTUSS
Guaifenesin
GLYDM*
Dextromethorphan
Guaifenesin
GLY-OXIDE
Carbamide Peroxide
GLYROL
Glycerin
GLYSENNID
Sennosides A and B
GLYSENNID NORSENNA
Senna
GLYTINIC*
Glycine
Iron
Vitamins, Multiple
GLYTUSS
Guaifenesin
G-MYCIN
Tetracycline
GOLDEN BOUNTY B COMPLEX WITH VITAMIN C
Iron
Vitamins, Multiple
GOLDEN BOUNTY MULTIVITAMIN SUPPLEMENT WITH IRON
Vitamins, Multiple
GONADIN
Gonadotropin, Serum
GONADOGEN
Gonadotropin, Serum
GOODY'S HEADACHE POWDER*
Aspirin
Caffeine
GORDOFILM*
Lactic Acid
Salicylic Acid
GORDOGESIC CREAM
Methyl Salicylate
GRAMACAL
Calcium
GRAMODERM
Gramicidin
GRANULEX*
Castor Oil
Peruvian Balsam
Trypsin
GRAPEFRUIT DIET PLAN WITH DIADAX
Phenylpropanolamine
GRAPEFRUIT DIET PLAN WITH DIADAX CHEWABLE EXTRA STRENGTH
Phenylpropanolamine
GRAPEFRUIT DIET PLAN WITH DIADAX EXTRA STRENGTH VITAMIN FORTIFIED
CONTINUOUS ACTION
Phenylpropanolamine
GRAPEFRUIT DIET PLAN WITH DIADAX VITAMIN FORTIFIED CONTINUOUS ACTION
Phenylpropanolamine
GRAVIDOX
Pyridoxine
GRAVIGEN
Estrone
GRAVOL
Dimenhydrinate
G-RECILLIN
Penicillin G
G-RECILLIN-T
Penicillin G
GRIFULVIN-V
Griseofulvin
GRIPELIN
Carbenicillin
GRISACTIN
Griseofulvin

GRISACTIN ULTRA
  Griseofulvin
GRISOVIN-FP
  Griseofulvin
GRISOWEN
  Griseofulvin
GRIS-PEG
  Griseofulvin
G-TUSSIN DM*
  Dextromethorphan
  Guaifenesin
GT-250
  Tetracycline
GT-500
  Tetracycline
GUAIAHIST TT
    TEMPOTROL*
  Guaifenesin
  Phenylephrine
GUAIANESIN
  Guaifenesin
GUAIFED*
  Guaifenesin
  Pseudoephedrine
GUAIMID*
  Dextromethorphan
  Guaifenesin
GUIAPHED ELIXIR*
  Ephedrine
  Guaifenesin
  Phenobarbital
  Theophylline
GVS VAGINAL
  Gentian Violet
G-W EMULSOIL
  Castor Oil
GYNECORT
  Hydrocortisone
GYNE-LOTRIMIN
  Clotrimazole
GYNERGEN
  Ergotamine
GYNETONE*
  Ethinyl Estradiol
  Methyltestosterone
GYNOGEN
  Estrone
GYNOL
  Nonoxynol
GYNO-PEVARYL 150
  Econazole
GYNOPLIX
  Acetarsone
GYNOREST
  Dydrogesterone
GYNOTERAX
  Chlorquinaldol
GYNOVULES
  Iodoquinol
G-11
  Hexachlorophene
G-2*
  Acetaminophen
  Butabarbital
G-200
  Guaifenesin
G-3*
  Acetaminophen
  Butabarbital
  Codeine

H

HAIR POWER
  Pyrithione Zinc
HAL-CHLOR
  Chlorpheniramine
HALCIDERM
  Halcinonide
HALCION
  Triazolam
HALDOL
  Haloperidol
HALDRATE
  Paramethasone
HALDRONA
  Paramethasone
HALDRONE
  Paramethasone
HALDRONE-F
  Flurandrenolide
HALENOL EXTRA STRENGTH
  Acetaminophen
HALEY'S M-O*
  Magnesium Hydroxide
  Mineral Oil
HALINONE
  Bromindione
HALLS*

Dextromethorphan
Phenylpropanolamine
HALODRIN*
Ethinyl Estradiol
Fluoxymesterone
HALOG
Halcinonide
HALOTESTIN
Fluoxymesterone
HALOTEX
Haloprogin
HARMONYL
Deserpidine
HASACODE*
Acetaminophen
Codeine
HASP*
Atropine
Hyoscyamine
Phenobarbital
Scopolamine
HAZOL
Oxymetazoline
H-BIG
Hepatitis B Immune Globulin
HC-FORM*
Hydrocortisone
Iodochlorhydroxyquin
HC-JEL
Hydrocortisone
HCV CREME*
Hydrocortisone
Iodochlorhydroxyquin
H.E.A.
Ergoloid Mesylates
HEAD & CHEST COLD MEDICINE*
Guaifenesin
Phenylpropanolamine
HEAD & SHOULDERS
Pyrithione Zinc
HEADWAY*
Acetaminophen
Chlorpheniramine
Phenylpropanolamine
HEALON
Sodium Hyaluronate
HEB-CORT
Hydrocortisone
HEDULIN
Phenindione
HEET ANALGESIC LINIMENT*
Alcohol
Camphor
Methyl Salicylate
Oleoresin Capsicum
HEET SPRAY ANALGESIC*
Camphor
Menthol
Methyl Nicotinate
Methyl Salicylate
HEMATON
Ferrous Fumarate
HEMOCYTE
Ferrous Fumarate
HEMOCYTE-F*
Ferrous Fumarate
Folic Acid
HEMOCYTE INJECTION*
Benzyl Alcohol
Cyanocobalamin
Ferrous Fumarate
Folic Acid
Phenol
HEMOCYTE PLUS TABULES*
Ferrous Fumarate
Minerals, Multiple
Vitamins, Multiple
HEMOFIL
Antihemophilic Factor
HEMO-VITE*
Ferrous Fumarate
Intrinsic Factor
Vitamins, Multiple
HENOTAL
Phenobarbital
HEPAHYDRIN
Dehydrocholic Acid
HEPALEAN
Heparin
HEPARINAR
Heparin
HEPATHROM
Heparin
HEP-B-GAMMAGEE
Hepatitis B Immune Globulin, Human

HEPCOVITE
  Cyanocobalamin
HEP-LOCK
  Heparin
HEPP-IRON DROPS*
  Biotin
  Cyanocobalamin
  Iron
  Pyridoxine
  Thiamine
HEPTAVAX-B
  Hepatitis B Vaccine
HEPTEDRINE
  Tuaminoheptane
HEPTIN
  Tuaminoheptane
HEPTUNA PLUS*
  Ferrous Sulfate
  Minerals, Multiple
  Vitamin B Complex
HERISAN
  Zinc Oxide
HERISAN ANTIBIOTIC
  Neomycin
HERPLEX
  Idoxuridine
HERPLEX-D LIQUIFILM
  Idoxuridine
HESPAN
  Hetastarch
HETRAZAN
  Diethylcarbamazine
HEXA-BETALIN
  Pyridoxine
HEXADERM CREAM MODIFIED
  Hydrocortisone
HEXADERM I.Q. MODIFIED CREAM*
  Clioquinol
  Hydrocortisone
HEXADROL
  Dexamethasone
HEXALET
  Methenamine Sulfosalicylate
HEXAMEAD-PH
  Hexachlorophene
HEXATHIDE
  Hexamethonium
HEXAVIBEX
  Pyridoxine
HEXODORM
  Calcium Cyclobarbital
HEXOMEDINE
  Hexamidine
HEXORAL
  Hexetidine
HEXYPHEN
  Trihexyphenidyl
HIBANIL
  Chlorpromazine
HI-BEE WITH C
  Vitamins, Multiple
HIBICARE
  Chlorhexidine
HIBICLENS
  Chlorhexidine
HIBISTAT
  Chlorhexidine
HIBITANE
  Chlorhexidine
HIBITANE TINCTURE*
  Chlorhexidine
  Isopropyl Alcohol
HI-FIBRAN
  Plantago Seed
HILL CORTAC LOTION*
  Hydrocortisone
  Isopropyl Alcohol
  Resorcinol
  Sulfur
  Zinc Oxide
HILL-SHADE LOTION*
  Alcohol
  Aminobenzoic Acid
HI-PEN
  Penicillin V Potassium
HIPIRIN
  Aspirin
HIPREX
  Methenamine Hippurate
HISERPIA
  Reserpine
HISPRIL
  Diphenylpyraline
HISTABID DURACAP*

Chlorpheniramine
Phenylpropanolamine
HISTA-CLOPANE*
Cyclopentamine
Methapyrilene
HISTA-COMPOUND NO.5*
Chlorpheniramine
Phenylephrine
Salicylamide
HISTADYL
Methapyrilene
HISTADYL EC*
Ammonium Chloride
Codeine
Ephedrine
Methapyrilene
HISTAJECT*
Atropine
Chlorpheniramine
HISTALET*
Chlorpheniramine
Pseudoephedrine
HISTALET DM*
Chlorpheniramine
Dextromethorphan
Pseudoephedrine
HISTALET FORTE*
Chlorpheniramine
Phenylephrine
Phenylpropanolamine
Pyrilamine
HISTALOG
Betazole
HISTALON
Chlorpheniramine
HISTAN
Pyrilamine
HISTA-NIL
Diphenylpyraline
HISTANTIL
Promethazine
HISTA-PHEN-S.A.*
Chlorpheniramine
Methscopolamine
Phenylephrine
HISTARALL*
Dexbrompheniramine
Pseudoephedrine
HISTASPAN
Chlorpheniramine
HISTASPAN-D*
Chlorpheniramine
Methscopolamine
Phenylephrine
HISTASPAN-P*
Chlorpheniramine
Phenylephrine
HISTASPAN-PLUS*
Chlorpheniramine
Phenylephrine
HISTATAB*
Chlorpheniramine
Phenylephrine
HISTATAPP ELIXIR*
Brompheniramine
Phenylephrine
Phenylpropanolamine
HISTATAPP T.D.*
Brompheniramine
Phenylephrine
Phenylpropanolamine
HISTA-VADRIN*
Chlorpheniramine
Phenylephrine
Phenylpropanolamine
HISTERONE 100
Testosterone
HISTERONE 50
Testosterone
HISTEX
Chlorpheniramine
HISTIONEX
Phenyltoloxamine
HISTIVITE-D*
Ammonium Chloride
Dextromethorphan
Ephedrine
Methapyrilene
HISTORAL*
Chlorpheniramine
Methscopolamine
Pseudoephedrine
HISTOR-D SYRUP*
Chlorpheniramine
Phenylephrine
HISTOR-D TIMECELLES*
Chlorpheniramine
Methscopolamine
Phenylephrine
HISTOSAL*

Acetaminophen
Caffeine
Phenylpropanolamine
Pyrilamine
HISTOSTAB
Antazoline
HI-TEMP
Acetaminophen
HMS LIQUIFILM
Medrysone
HOLD*
Benzocaine
Dextromethorphan
HOLD LIQUID COUGH SUPPRESSANT*
Dextromethorphan
Phenylpropanolamine
HOLD 4 HOUR COUGH SUPPRESSANT
Dextromethorphan
HOLOCAINE
Phenacaine
HOMAGENETS AORAL
Vitamin A
HOMAPIN
Homatropine
HOMATRISOL
Homatropine
HOMATROCEL
Homatropine
HOMO-TET
Tetanus Immune Globulin, Human
HONVOL
Diethylstilbestrol
HORMESTRIN
Estrone
HORMOGEN-A
Estrone
HORMOGEN DEPOT
Estradiol
HORMONIN*
Estradiol
Estriol
Estrone
HOSTA 'P'
Tetracycline
HOSTAGINAN
Prenylamine
HOSTA 500
Tetracycline
HOT LEMON*
Acetaminophen
Chlorpheniramine
Phenylephrine
HOURNAZE*
Chlorpheniramine
Pseudoephedrine
H.P. ACTHAR GEL
Corticotropin
HQC
Hydroquinone
H-STADUR
Chlorpheniramine
HTO STAINLESS MANZAN HEMORRHOIDAL TISSUE OINTMENT*
Allantoin
Benzocaine
Ephedrine
Phenol
Zinc Oxide
HUMAFAC
Antihemophilic Factor
HUMAGEL
Paromomycin
HUMAN N
Insulin Human
HUMAN R
Insulin Human
HUMATIN
Paromomycin
HUMORSOL
Demecarium
HUMULIN
Insulin Human
HUMULIN N
Insulin Human
HUNGREX PLUS*
Caffeine
Phenylpropanolamine
HURRICAINE
Benzocaine
HU-TET
Tetanus Immune Globulin, Human
HYAMINE 1622
Benzethonium Chloride

HYAMINE 3500
Benzalkonium Chloride
HYAZYME
Hyaluronidase
HYBEPHEN*
Atropine
Hyoscyamine
Phenobarbital
Scopolamine
HYCODAN*
Homatropine
Hydrocodone
HYCOMINE*
Hydrocodone
Phenylpropanolamine
HYCOTUSS*
Guaifenesin
Hydrocodone
HYDELTRA
Prednisolone
HYDELTRASOL
Prednisolone
HYDELTRA-T.B.A.
Prednisolone
HYDERGINE
Ergoloid Mesylates
HYDERM
Hydrocortisone
HYDOXIN
Pyridoxine
HYDRA
Phenylephrine
HYDRAP-ES*
Hydralazine
Hydrochlorothiazide
Reserpine
HYDRA-SPRAY
Xylometazoline
HYDRATE
Dimenhydrinate
HYDRAZOL
Acetazolamide
HYDREA
Hydroxyurea
HYDRENOX
Hydroflumethiazide
HYDREX
Benzthiazide
HYDRIL COUGH
Diphenhydramine
HYDRIODIC ACID COUGH
Hydrogen Iodide
HYDRIONIC
Glutamic Acid
HYDRISALIC
Salicylic Acid
HYDRO-AQUIL
Hydrochlorothiazide
HYDROCARE
Papain
HYDROCHLOR 50
Hydrochlorothiazide
HYDROCIL
Plantago Seed
HYDROCIL FORTIFIED*
Casanthranol
Plantago Seed
HYDROCIL INSTANT
Plantago Seed
HYDROCIL PLAIN
Plantago Seed
HYDRO-CORTILEAN
Hydrocortisone
HYDROCORTONE
Hydrocortisone
HYDROCORTONE ACETATE
Hydrocortisone
HYDRO-CORTONE ACETATE OPHTHALMIC
Hydrocortisone
HYDRODIURIL
Hydrochlorothiazide
HYDROL
Mineral Oil
HYDROLOSE
Methylcellulose
HYDROMAL
Hydrochlorothiazide
HYDROMAX SYRUP*
Alcohol
Ephedrine
Hydroxyzine
Theophylline
HYDROMEDIN
Ethacrynic Acid
HYDROMOX
Quinethazone
HYDROPHED TABS*
Ephedrine

Hydroxyzine
Theophylline
HYDROPRES*
Hydrochlorothiazide
Reserpine
HYDROQUIN*
Clioquinol
Hydrocortisone
HYDROQUINE
Dihydroquinidine
HYDRO-SALURIC
Hydrochlorothiazide
HYDROSERP*
Hydrochlorothiazide
Reserpine
HYDROSERPINE*
Hydrochlorothiazide
Reserpine
HYDROSTERONE
Hydroxyprogesterone
HYDROTENSIN*
Hydrochlorothiazide
Reserpine
HYDROTRICINE
Tyrothricin
HYDROXO B12
Hydroxocobalamin
HYDRO-Z
Hydrochlorothiazide
HYDROZIDE
Hydrochlorothiazide
HY-FLOW*
Benzalkonium Chloride
Hydroxyethyl-cellulose
Polyvinyl Alcohol
HYGEOL
Sodium Hypochlorite
HYGROTON
Chlorthalidone
HYGROTON-RESERPINE*
Chlorthalidone
Reserpine
HYKINONE
Menadione
HYKOLEX
Dehydrocholic Acid
HYLATE-TABS*
Guaifenesin
Theophylline
HYLOREL
Guanadrel
HYLUTIN
Hydroxyprogesterone
HYMORPHAN
Hydromorphone
HYOSOPHEN*
Atropine
Hyoscyamine
Phenobarbital
Scopolamine
HY-PAM
Hydroxyzine
HYPAQUE
Dextrothyroxine
HYPAQUE M*
Diatrizoate Sodium
Meglumine
HYPAQUE ORAL
Diatrizoate Sodium
HYPAQUE SODIUM
Diatrizoate Sodium
HYPERAB
Rabies Immune Globulin, Human
HYPERETIC
Hydrochlorothiazide
HYPER HEP
Hepatitis B Immune Globulin, Human
HYPEROPTO
Sodium Chloride
HYPERSAL OPHTHALMIC
Sodium Chloride
HYPERSTAT
Diazoxide
HYPERTENSIN
Angiotensin Amide
HYPER-TET
Tetanus Immune Globulin, Human
HYPERTUSSIS
Pertussis Immune Globulin, Human
HYPLEX
Vitamins, Multiple
HYPNODOL
Barbital
HYPNOLONE

Phenobarbital
HYPNOMIDATE
Etomidate
HYPNOREX
Lithium Carbonate
HYPNOTAL
Pentobarbital
HYPOVASE
Prazosin
HYP RHO-D
RH D Immune Globulin, Human
HYPROVAL P.A.
Hydroxyprogesterone
HYPTOR
Methaqualone
HYPTRAN*
Phenyltoloxamine
Secobarbital
HYPTROL
Secobarbital
HYREX
Vitamins, Multiple
HYREXIN
Diphenhydramine
HYSEPTINE
Methylbenzethonium
HYSER PLUS*
Hydralazine
Hydrochlorothiazide
Reserpine
HYSONE OINTMENT*
Clioquinol
Hydrocortisone
HYTAKEROL
Dihydrotachysterol
HYTINIC
Polysaccharide-Iron Complex
HYTONE
Hydrocortisone
HYTUSS
Guaifenesin
HYTUSS 2X
Guaifenesin
HYVA
Gentian Violet
HYVA VAGINAL
Gentian Violet
HYWOLFIA
Rauwolfia Serpentina
HYZINE-50
Hydroxyzine
HYZYD
Isoniazid
HY-12
Hydroxocobalamin
H2 CORT
Hydrocortisone

I

IBARIL
Desoximetasone
IBATAL
Pentobarbital
IBERET
Vitamins, Multiple
IBERET ORAL SOLUTION
Vitamins, Multiple
IBERET-500
Vitamins, Multiple
IBERET-500 ORAL SOLUTION
Vitamins, Multiple
IBEROL
Vitamins, Multiple
IBIOTON
Chlorpheniramine
ICE MINT
Lanolin
ICE-O-DERM
Chloroxylenol
ICE-O-DERM GEL
Benzalkonium Chloride
ICE-O-DERM LOTION
Chloroxylenol
ICE-O-DERM SKIN CLEANSER
Chloroxylenol
ICHTHYOL
Ichthammol
ICY HOT*
Menthol
Methyl Salicylate
IDROCRINE
Dehydrocholic Acid
IDULIAN

Azatadine
IGROTON
Chlorthalidone
IKTORIVIL
Clonazepam
ILETIN LENTE
Insulin Zinc
Suspension
ILETIN REGULAR
Insulin Regular
ILETIN SEMILENTE
Insulin Zinc
[Suspension] Prompt
ILETIN ULTRALENTE
Insulin Zinc
[Suspension]
Extended
ILIDAR
Azapetine
ILOPAN
Dexpanthenol
Panthenol
ILOSOFT
Docusate Sodium
ILOSONE
Erythromycin
ILOTYCIN
Erythromycin
ILOZYME
Pancrelipase
ILVIN
Brompheniramine
I.L.X. B12*
Ascorbic Acid
Ferrous Gluconate
Vitamin B Complex
I.L.X. B12 ELIXIR*
Alcohol
Iron
Vitamin B Complex
IMAP
Fluspirilene
IMAVATE
Imipramine
IMFERON
Iron Dextran
IMIDAN
Thalidomide
IMMU-G
Gobulin, Immune
IMMUGLOBIN
Gobulin, Immune
IMMUNE GLOBULIN
Gobulin, Immune
IMMUNE SERUM GLOBULIN
GAMMAR
Gobulin, Immune
IMODIUM
Loperamide
IMOGAM RABIES
Rabies Immune
Globulin, Human
IMOTEP*
Chlorpheniramine
Phenylephrine
IMOVAC
Human Diploid Cell
Rabies Vaccine
IMOVAC RABIES
Rabies Vaccine, Human
IMPERACIN
Oxytetracycline
IMPRIL
Imipramine
IMURAN
Azathioprine
IMURIL
Azathioprine
INABRIN
Ibuprofen
INAMYCIN
Novobiocin
INAPASADE-SQ*
Aminosalicylic Acid
Isoniazid
INAPSINE
Droperidol
INCREMIN WITH IRON*
Iron
Vitamins, Multiple
INDERAL
Propranolol
INDERAL-LA
Propranolol
INDERIDE*
Hydrochlorothiazide
Propranolol
INDOCID
Indomethacin
INDOCIN

Indomethacin
INDOCIN SR
Indomethacin
INDOCORT*
Hydrocortisone
Iodochlorhydroxyquin
INDOKLON
Flurothyl
INDO-LEMMON
Indomethacin
INDOMED
Indomethacin
INDOMEE
Indomethacin
INDON
Phenindione
INESTRA
Ethinyl Estradiol
INFANTOL PINK*
Bismuth Subsalicylate
Opium
Pectin
Zinc Phenolsulfonate
INFILTRASE
Hyaluronidase
INFLAMASE
Prednisolone
INFROCIN
Indomethacin
INH
Isoniazid
INHISTON
Pheniramine
INNOVAR*
Droperidol
Fentanyl
INOCOR
Amrinone
INOCOR IV
Amrinone
INODOR
Bismuth Subgallate
INPAS
Pasiniazid
INSIDON
Opipramol
INSIPIDIN
Vasopressin
INSOMNAL
Diphenhydramine
INSORAL
Phenformin
INSTANT MIX METAMUCIL*
Citric Acid
Plantago Seed
Sodium Bicarbonate
INSULASE
Chlorpropamide
INSULATARD
Insulin [Suspension] Isophane
INSULIN LENTE
Insulin Zinc Suspension
INSULIN SEMILENTE
Insulin Zinc [Suspension] Prompt
INSULIN ULTRALENTE
Insulin Zinc [Suspension] Extended
INTAL
Cromolyn Sodium
INTASEDOL
Butabarbital
INTENSIN*
Acetaminophen
Chlorpheniramine
Pseudoephedrine
INTERCEPT
Nonoxynol
INTRABUTAZONE
Phenylbutazone
INTRASED
Amobarbital
INTRAZINE
Promazine
INTROPIN
Dopamine
INVERSINE
Mecamylamine
IODEX
Iodine
IODINE RATION
Vitamins, Multiple
IODOCHLOROL
Chloriodized Oil
IODOCORT CREAM*
Clioquinol

Hydrocortisone
IODO-NIACIN*
Niacinamide
Hydroiodide
Potassium Iodide
IODOSONE*
Hydrocortisone
Iodochlorhydroxyquin
IODOTOPE
Sodium Iodide
IODOTOPE THERAPEUTIC
Sodium Iodide
IONAMIN
Phentermine
IONAX
Benzalkonium
Chloride
IONIL
Pyrithione Zinc
IONIL-T
Zinc pyrithione
IOP
Epinephrine
IOQUIN SUSPENSION
Iodoquinol
IPERDIUREN
Trichlormethiazide
IPHYLLIN
Dyphylline
IPRENOL
Isoproterenol
IPROVERATRIL
Verapamil
IPSATOL
Iodinated Glycerol
IRCON
Ferrous Fumarate
IRGASAN DP 300
Triclosan
IRIDIL
Oxyphenbutazone
IROLONG*
Ascorbic Acid
Ferrous Fumarate
IROMIN-G*
Calcium
Ferrous Gluconate
Vitamins, Multiple
IRONATE
Ferrous Gluconate
IRONIZED YEAST*
Ferrous Sulfate
Thiamine
IRON WITH C*
Ascorbic Acid
Ferrous Fumarate
I-SEDRIN PLAIN
Ephedrine
ISET
Oxprenolol
ISMELIN
Guanethidine
ISMELIN-ESIDRIX*
Guanethidine
Hydrochlorothiazide
ISMOTIC
Isosorbide
ISOBEC
Amobarbital
ISO-BID
Isosorbide Dinitrate
ISOBUTAL*
Acetaminophen
Butalbital
ISOCAINE
Mepivacaine
ISOCLOR*
Chlorpheniramine
Pseudoephedrine
ISODETTES SUPER*
Benzocaine
Cetalkonium
ISODINE
Povidone-Iodine
ISOGARD
Isosorbide Dinitrate
ISOGEN COMPOUND*
Ephedrine
Phenobarbital
Potassium Iodide
Theophylline
ISOGEN COMPOUND ELIXIR*
Alcohol
Ephedrine
Phenobarbital
Potassium Iodide
Theophylline
ISOJECT-STREPTOMYCIN
Streptomycin
ISOKET
Isosorbide Dinitrate
ISOLYN

Isoniazid
ISOMETH
Isometheptene
ISONORIN
Isoproterenol
ISO-PERAZINE TR*
Isopropamide
Prochlorperazine
ISOPHRIN
Phenylephrine
ISOPRINOSINE
Inosiplex
ISOPRO T.D.*
Isopropamide
Prochlorperazine
ISOPTIN
Verapamil
ISOPTO ALKALINE
Methylcellulose
ISOPTO ATROPINE
Atropine
ISOPTO CARBACHOL
Carbachol
ISOPTO CARBACHOL OPHTHALMIC
Carbachol
ISOPTO CARPINE
Pilocarpine
ISOPTO CETAMIDE
Sulfacetamide
ISOPTO CETAPRED*
Prednisolone
Sulfacetamide
ISOPTO ESERINE
Physostigmine
ISOPTO FENICOL
Chloramphenicol
ISOPTO-FRIN
Phenylephrine
ISOPTO HOMATROPINE
Homatropine
ISOPTO HYOSCINE
Scopolamine
ISOPTO PLAIN
Methylcellulose
ISOPTO TEARS
Methylcellulose
ISORDIL
Isosorbide Dinitrate
ISORDIL TEMBIDS
Isosorbide Dinitrate
ISORDIL TITRADOSE
Isosorbide Dinitrate
ISOTAMINE
Isoniazid
ISOTIL TABS*
Noscapine
Theophylline
ISOTOL
Mannitol
ISOTRATE
Isosorbide Dinitrate
ISOTRATE TIMECELLES
Isosorbide Dinitrate
ISOVAL
Bromisovalum
ISOVEX-100
Ethaverine
ISOXYL
Tiocarlide
ISTIZIN
Danthron
ISUPREL
Isoproterenol
ISUPREL COMPOUND ELIXIR*
Alcohol
Ephedrine
Phenobarbital
Potassium Iodide
Theophylline
ISUPREL-NEO MISTOMETER*
Isoproterenol
Phenylephrine
ITURAN
Nitrofurantoin
IVADANTIN
Nitrofurantoin
IVAREST*
Benzocaine
Calamine
Pyrilamine
IVY-CHEX*
Benzalkonium Chloride
Salicylate

J

JANIMINE
Imipramine

JATRONEURAL
  Trifluoperazine
JATROPUR
  Triamterene
JAY C
  Ascorbic Acid
JAY LEITH
  Cholecalciferol
JAYLETH
  Cholecalciferol
J-DANTIN
  Nitrofurantoin
JECTOFER
  Iron Sorbitex
JECTO SAL
  Sodium
    Thiosalicylate
JEFRON
  Polyferose
JELLIN
  Fluocinolone
JENAMICIN
  Gentamicin
JEN-BALM*
  Eucalyptus Oil
  Menthol
  Methyl Salicylate
JERI-BATH OIL*
  Keratin
  Mineral Oil
JERI-LOTION*
  Keratin
  Lanolin
  Mineral Oil
JOCKEX
  Calcium
    Undecylenate

K

KABIKINASE
  Streptokinase
KAFOCIN
  Cephaloglycin
KALMADOL
  Alverine
KALYMIN
  Pyridostigmine
KAMU JAY
  Ascorbic Acid
KAMYCINE
  Kanamycin
KANABRISTOL
  Kanamycin
KANECIDIN
  Kanamycin
KANK-A*
  Benzocaine
  Benzoin Compound
  Cetylpyridinium
KANONE
  Menadione
KANTREX
  Kanamycin
KANULASE*
  Bile Salts
  Glutamic Acid
  Pancreatin
  Pepsin
KAOCHLOR
  Potassium Chloride
KAOCHLOR CONCENTRATE
  Potassium Chloride
KAOCHLOR EFF*
  Potassium
    Bicarbonate
  Potassium Chloride
KAOCHLOR S-F
  Potassium Chloride
KAOCHLOR 10%
  Potassium Chloride
KAOCHLOR 20%
  Potassium Chloride
KAO-CON*
  Kaolin
  Pectin
KAODENE*
  Bismuth
    Subsalicylate
  Carboxymethyl-
    cellulose
  Kaolin
  Pectin
KAODONNA*
  Belladonna Alkaloids
  Kaolin
  Pectin
KAODONNA-PG*
  Belladonna Alkaloids

Kaolin
Paregoric
Pectin
KAOLIN PECTIN SUSPENSION*
Carboxymethylcellulose
Kaolin
Pectin
KAOMEAD*
Kaolin
Pectin
KAOMEAD WITH BELLADONNA*
Belladonna Alkaloids
Kaolin
Pectin
KAON
Potassium Gluconate
KAON-CL
Potassium Chloride
KAON CL-10
Potassium Chloride
KAO-NOR
Potassium Gluconate
KAOPECTATE*
Kaolin
Pectin
KAOPECTATE CONCENTRATE*
Kaolin
Pectin
KA-PEN
Penicillin G
KAPILON
Menadiol
KAPPADIONE
Menadiol
KAPPAXIN
Menadione
KARIDIUM
Sodium Fluoride
KASOF
Docusate Potassium
KATO POWDER
Potassium Chloride
KAVRIN
Papaverine
KAY CIEL
Potassium Chloride
KAYEXALATE
Sodium Polystyrene Sulfonate
KAYLIXIR
Potassium Gluconate
KAYQUINONE
Menadione
KAYTRATE
Pentaerythritol Tetranitrate
K-CILLIN 250
Penicillin G
K-CILLIN 500
Penicillin G
KEFF*
Betaine
Potassium Bicarbonate
Potassium Carbonate
Potassium Chloride
KEFGLYCIN
Cephaloglycin
KEFLEX
Cephalexin
KEFLIN
Cephalothin
KEFLIN NEUTRAL
Cephalothin
KEFLODIN
Cephaloridine
KEFLORIDIN
Cephaloridine
KEFORAL
Cephalexin
KEFSPOR
Cephaloridine
KEFZOL
Cefazolin
KELL-E
Vitamin E
KEMADRIN
Procyclidine
KEMICETINE
Chloramphenicol
KEMITHAL
Thialbarbital
KEMSOL
Dimethyl Sulfoxide
KENAC
Triamcinolone

KENACOMB*
  Gramicidin
  Neomycin
  Nystatin
  Triamcinolone
KENACORT
  Triamcinolone
KENALOG
  Triamcinolone
KENALOG-E
  Triamcinolone
KENALOG IN ORABASE
  Triamcinolone
KERALYT
  Salicylic Acid
KERASOL BATH OIL*
  Lanolin
  Mineral Oil
KERECID
  Idoxuridine
KERID EAR DROP*
  Glycerin
  Propylene Glycol
  Urea
KESSADROX*
  Aluminum Hydroxide
  Magnesium Hydroxide
KESTRIN
  Conjugated Estrogens
KESTRONE
  Estrone
KETAJECT
  Ketamine
KETALAR
  Ketamine
KETASET
  Ketamine
KETHAMED
  Pemoline
KETOCHOL
  Dehydrocholic Acid
KETOSTIX
  Sodium Nitroprusside Reagent
KEVADON
  Thalidomide
K-FLEX
  Orphenadrine
K-FORTE POTASSIUM SUPPLEMENT WITH VITAMIN C CHEWABLE*
  Ascorbic Acid
  Potassium Chloride
KHAROPHENE
  Acetarsone
KHELISEM
  Khellin
KHELLOYD
  Khellin
KIDDIES PEDIATRIC*
  Ammonium Chloride
  Potassium Guaiacolsulfonate
KIDDISAN*
  Chlorpheniramine
  Phenylephrine
  Salicylamide
KIDROLASE
  Asparaginase
KIE*
  Ephedrine
  Potassium Iodide
KINESED*
  Atropine
  Hyoscyamine
  Phenobarbital
  Scopolamine
KINEVAC
  Sincalide
KINIDINE
  Quinidine
KININE
  Quinine
KIRKRINAL
  Trichlormethiazide
KIT 1*
  Bisacodyl
  Phospho-soda
KLARON*
  Salicylic Acid
  Sulfur
KLAVI CORDAL
  Nitroglycerin
KLEER CHEWABLE*
  Chlorpheniramine
  Dextromethorphan
  Phenylephrine
KLEER COMP*
  Guaifenesin
  Phenylpropanolamine
  Salicylamide
KLEV

Sodium Salicylate
KLOR
Potassium Chloride
K-LOR
Potassium Chloride
KLOR-CON
Potassium Chloride
KLOR-CON/25
Potassium Chloride
KLORVESS EFFERVESCENT GRANULES*
Potassium Bicarbonate
Potassium Chloride
KLORVESS 10%*
Potassium Bicarbonate
Potassium Chloride
KLOTRIX
Potassium Chloride
K-LYTE
Potassium Bicarbonate
K-LYTE CL*
Potassium Bicarbonate
Potassium Chloride
K-LYTE CL 50*
Potassium Bicarbonate
Potassium Chloride
K-LYTE DS*
Potassium Bicarbonate
Potassium Chloride
K-MED
Potassium Tartrate
KOATE
Antihemophilic Factor
KOLANTYL*
Aluminum Hydroxide
Magnesium Hydroxide
Magnesium Oxide
KOLEPHRIN*
Acetaminophen
Caffeine
Chlorpheniramine
Phenylephrine
Salicylamide
KOLEPHRIN GG*
Dextromethorphan
Guaifenesin
KOLTON
Piprinhydrinate
KOLYUM LIQUID/POWDER*
Potassium Chloride
Potassium Gluconate
KOMED*
Isopropyl Alcohol
Salicylic Acid
Sodium Thiosulfate
KOMED HC*
Hydrocortisone
Isopropyl Alcohol
Salicylic Acid
Sodium Thiosulfate
KOMEX
Sodium Tetraborate Decahydrate
KONAKION
Phytonadione
KONDREMUL*
Chondrus
Mineral Oil
KONDREMUL PLAIN
Mineral Oil
KONDREMUL WITH CASCARA SAGRADA*
Cascara Sagrada
Chondrus
Mineral Oil
KONDREMUL WITH PHENOLPHTHALEIN*
Chondrus
Mineral Oil
Phenolphthalein
KONLAX
Docusate Sodium
KONSYL
Plantago Seed
KONYNE
Factor IV complex
KOPHANE COUGH & COLD FORMULA*
Ammonium Chloride
Chlorpheniramine
Dextromethorphan
Phenylpropanolamine
KORIGESIC*
Caffeine
Chlorpheniramine

Phenylephrine
Phenylpropanolamine
Salicylamide
KORONOEX
Nonoxynol
KOROSTATIN VAGINAL
Nystatin
KORO-SUFF VAGINAL CREAM
Sulfisoxazole
K-P*
Kaolin
Pectin
K-PEK*
Kaolin
Pectin
K-PEN
Penicillin G
K-PHOS M.F.*
Potassium Acid Phosphate
Sodium Acid Phosphate
K-PHOS NEUTRAL*
Potassium Acid Phosphate
Sodium Acid Phosphate
Sodium Phosphate
K-PHOS NO.2*
Potassium Acid Phosphate
Sodium Acid Phosphate
K-PHOS ORIGINAL
Potassium Acid Phosphate
KREM*
Calcium Carbonate
Magnesium Carbonate
KRIPTIN
Pyrilamine
KRONOFED-A KRONOCAPS*
Chlorpheniramine
Pseudoephedrine
KRONOHIST KRONOCAPS*
Chlorpheniramine
Phenylpropanolamine
Pyrilamine
K-TAB
Potassium Chloride
KUDROX*
Aluminum Hydroxide
Magnesium Carbonate
Magnesium Oxide
KUTRASE*
Amylase
Cellulase
Hyoscyamine
Lipase
Phenyltoloxamine
Protease
KU-ZYME*
Amylase
Cellulase
Lipase
Protease
KU-ZYME HP
Pancrelipase
KWELL
Lindane
KWELLADA
Lindane
KWELLS
Scopolamine
KYNEX
Sulfamethoxypyridazine
K-10
Potassium Chloride

L

LABID
Theophylline
LACO
Bisacodyl
LACRIL
Methylcellulose
LACTAID
Lactase
LACTINEX*
Lactobacillus acidophilus
Lactobacillus bulgaricus
LACT-IRON
Lactase
LACTRASE

Lactase
L.A.DEZONE
Dexamethasone
L.A.E. 20
Estradiol
L. A. FORMULA*
Dextrose
Plantago Seed
LAMPIT
Nifurtimox
LAMPRENE
Clofazimine
LANACANE MEDICATED CREME*
Benzocaine
Resorcinol
LANACORT
Hydrocortisone
LANATUSS*
Chlorpheniramine
Guaifenesin
Phenylpropanolamine
LANATUSS EXPECTORANT*
Chlorpheniramine
Guaifenesin
Phenylpropanolamine
LANAZETS*
Benzocaine
Cetylpyridinium
LAN-DOL
Meprobamate
LAN-E
Vitamin E
LANE'S PILLS
Casanthranol
LANIAZID
Isoniazid
LANOPHYLLIN
Theophylline
LANOPHYLLINE-GG CAPSULES*
Guaifenesin
Theophylline
LANOXICAPS
Digoxin
LANOXIN
Digoxin
LANVIS
Thioguanine
LANVISONE*
iodochlorhydroxyquin
Hydrocortisone
LAPAV GRADUALS
Papaverine
LARDET EXPECTORANT TABS*
Ephedrine
Guaifenesin
Phenobarbital
Theophylline
LARDET TABS*
Ephedrine
Phenobarbital
Theophylline
LARDOPA
Levodopa
LARGACTIL
Chlorpromazine
LARGON
Propiomazine
LAROBEC
Vitamins, Multiple
LARODOPA
Levodopa
LAROTID
Amoxicillin
LAROXYL
Amitriptyline
LARPOSE
Lorazepam
LARYLGAN THROAT SPRAY*
Antipyrine
Pyrilamine
Sodium Caprylate
LARYNGINE
Cetylpyridinium
LASAN POMADE
Anthralin
LASAN UNGUENT
Anthralin
LASERDIL
Isosorbide Dinitrate
LASILIX
Furosemide
LASIX
Furosemide
LAUD-IRON PLUS CHEWING*
Cyanocobalamin
Ferrous Fumarate

LAUDOLISSIN
  Laudexium
    Methylsulfate
LAUN-IRON
  Ferrous Fumarate
LAURO*
  Boric Acid
  Sodium Chloride
LAURON
  Aurothioglycanide
LAVATAR
  Coal Tar
LAVOPTIK EYE WASH*
  Benzalkonium
    Chloride
  Sodium Biphosphate
  Sodium Chloride
  Sodium Phosphate
LAXATYL*
  Danthron
  Docusate Sodium
LAXINATE
  Docusate Sodium
LAXINEX 100
  Docusate Sodium
LAXSIL*
  Magnesium Hydroxide
  Simethicone
LAXUR
  Furosemide
L-CAINE
  Lidocaine
L.C.D.
  Coal Tar
L-DOPA
  Levodopa
LEDERCILLIN VK
  Penicillin V
    Potassium
LEDERMYCIN
  Demeclocycline
LEDERPLEX
  Vitamins, Multiple
LEMBROL
  Diazepam
LEMISERP
  Reserpine
LENETRAN
  Mephenoxalone
LENSINE EXTRA
    STRENGTH*
  Benzalkonium
    Chloride
  Edetic Acid
LENS-MATE*
  Benzalkonium
    Chloride
  Edetic Acid
  Hydroxypropyl
    Methylcellulose
  Polyvinyl Alcohol
LENSRINS*
  Edetic Acid
  Sodium Chloride
  Thimerosal
LENS-WET*
  Edetic Acid
  Polyvinyl Alcohol
  Thimerosal
LENTARD
  Insulin Zinc
    Suspension
LENTE ILETIN
  Insulin Zinc
    Suspension
LENTE INSULIN
  Insulin Zinc
    Suspension
LENTIN
  Carbachol
LEPTAZOL
  Pentylenetetrazol
LERITINE
  Anileridine
LES-CAV
  Sodium Fluoride
LETHIDRONE
  Nalorphine
LETHOPHEROL*
  Selenium Sulfide
  Vitamin E
LETTER
  Levothyroxine
LEUKERAN
  Chlorambucil
LEUKOMYCIN
  Chloramphenicol
LEVADOL
  Propoxyphene
LEVAMINE
  Hyoscyamine
LEVATE

Amitriptyline
LEVISUL
Sulfadimethoxine
LEVO-DROMORAN
Levorphanol
LEVOID
Levothyroxine
LEVOL
Benactyzine
LEVOPA
Levodopa
LEVOPHED
Levarterenol
LEVOPROME
Methotrimeprazine
LEVOTHROID
Levothyroxine
LEVSIN
Hyoscyamine
LEVSINEX TIMECAPS
Hyoscyamine
LEVSINEX WITH PHENOBARBITAL TIMECAPS*
Hyoscyamine
Phenobarbital
LEVSIN-PB
Phenobarbital
LEVSIN WITH PHENOBARBITAL*
Hyoscyamine
Phenobarbital
LEVUCAL
Calcium Levulinate
LEXXOR
Hydrochlorothiazide
L-GLUTAVITE*
Iron
Vitamin B Complex
LIBIGEN
Gonadotropin
LIBRAX*
Chlordiazepoxide
Clidinium
LIBRELEASE
Chlordiazepoxide
LIBRITABS
Chlordiazepoxide
LIBRIUM
Chlordiazepoxide
LIDAFORM-HC*
Hydrocortisone
Iodochlorhydroxyquin
Lidocaine
LIDA-MANTLE
Lidocaine
LIDANAR
Mesoridazine
LIDEMOL
Fluocinonide
LIDEX
Fluocinonide
LIDINIUM*
Chlordiazepoxide
Clidinium
LIDOCICLINA
Rolitetracycline
LIDOJECT
Lidocaine
LIDONE
Molindone
LIDOPEN AUTO-INJECTOR
Lidocaine
LIDOSPORIN OTIC SOLUTION*
Lidocaine
Polymyxin B
LIFENE
Phensuximide
LIKUDEN
Griseofulvin
LIMBIAL
Oxazepam
LIMBITROL*
Amitriptyline
Chlordiazepoxide
LIMIT
Phendimetrazine
LIMONADE ASEPTA
Sodium Tartrate
LIMONADE RODECA
Sodium Tartrate
LINCOCIN
Lincomycin
LINGRAINE
Ergotamine
LINGUSORBS
Progesterone
LINODIL
Inositol Niacinate
LIORESAL
Baclofen

LIORESAL DS
  Baclofen
LIPIODOL
  Iodized Oil
LIPOFLAVONOID
  Vitamins, Multiple
LIPO GANTRISIN
  Sulfisoxazole Acetyl
LIPO GANTRISM
  Sulfisoxazole
LIPO-HEPIN
  Heparin
LIPO-LUTIN
  Progesterone
LIPO-NICIN*
  Niacin
  Vitamins, Multiple
LIPOSID
  Clofibrate
LIPOTRIAD
  Vitamins, Multiple
LIPRINAL
  Clofibrate
LIP THERAPY
  Petrolatum
LIQUAEMIN
  Heparin
LIQUAMAR
  Phenprocoumon
LIQUAPEN
  Penicillin G
LIQUAPRES*
  Hydrochlorothiazide
  Reserpine
LIQUI-CEE
  Sodium Ascorbate
LIQUID ANTACID*
  Aluminum Hydroxide
  Magnesium Hydroxide
LIQUID-ANTIDOSE
  Charcoal, Activated
LIQUID GERITONIC
  Vitamins, Multiple
LIQUI-DOSS*
  Docusate Sodium
  Mineral Oil
LIQUIFILM TEARS
  Polyvinyl Alcohol
LIQUIFILM WETTING*
  Benzalkonium
    Chloride
  Hydroxypropyl
    Methylcellulose
  Polyvinyl Alcohol
LIQUIMAT
  Sulfur
LIQUIPRIN
  Acetaminophen
LIQUIPRIN SUSPENSION
  Acetaminophen
LIQUITAL
  Phenobarbital
LIQUITUSSIN
  Guaifenesin
LIQUITUSSIN DM*
  Dextromethorphan
  Guaifenesin
LIQUIX-C*
  Acetaminophen
  Codeine
LIQUOPHYLLINE
  Theophylline
LISPAMOL
  Aminopromazine
LISTACORT
  Prednisone
LISTEREX GOLDEN LOTION
  Salicylic Acid
LISTEREX HERBAL LOTION
  Salicylic Acid
LISTERINE
  Hexylresorcinol
LISTERINE COUGH
    CONTROL
  Benzocaine
LISTICA
  Hydroxyphenamate
LITALIR
  Hydroxyurea
LITEC
  Pizotyline
LITHANE
  Lithium Carbonate
LITHIZINE
  Lithium Carbonate
LITHOBID
  Lithium Carbonate
LITHONATE
  Lithium Carbonate
LITHONATE-S
  Lithium Citrate
LITHOSTAT

Acetohydroxamic Acid
LITHOTABS
Lithium Carbonate
LIVITAMIN
Vitamins, Multiple
LIXAMINOL
Aminophylline
LIXOLIN
Theophylline
LMD 10%
Dextran 40
LOBAC*
Acetaminophen
Chlorzoxazone
LOBANA*
Corn Starch
Methylbenzethonium
Sodium Bicarbonate
LOCACORTEN
Flumethasone
LOCACORTEN-VIOFORM*
Flumethasone
Iodochlorhydroxyquin
LOCOID
Hydrocortisone
LOCON*
Benzalkonium Chloride
Coal Tar
LOCORTEN
Flumethasone
LODRANE
Theophylline
LOESTRIN*
Ethinyl Estradiol
Norethindrone
LOFENALAC
Vitamins, Multiple
LOFENE*
Atropine
Diphenoxylate
LOFLO*
Atropine
Diphenoxylate
LOMIDINE
Pentamidine
LOMOTIL*
Atropine
Diphenoxylate
LOMUDAL
Cromolyn Sodium
LONALAC*
Minerals, Multiple
Vitamins, Multiple
LONAVAR
Oxandrolone
LONITEN
Minoxidil
LONOX*
Atropine
Diphenoxylate
LO/OVRAL*
Ethinyl Estradiol
Norgestrel
LOPID
Gemfibrozil
LOPRESS
Hydralazine
LOPRESSOR
Metoprolol
LOPROX
Ciclopirox
LOPURIN
Allopurinol
LORAX
Lorazepam
LORELCO
Probucol
LORFAN
Levallorphan
LORIDINE
Cephaloridine
LORINAL
Chloral Hydrate
LORISAL
Magnesium Salicylate
LOROTHIDOL
Bithionol
LOROXIDE ACNE LOTION*
Benzoyl Peroxide
Chlorhydroxyquinoline
LOROXIDE-HC LOTION*
Benzoyl Peroxide
Chlorhydroxyquinoline
Hydrocortisone
LORUSIL
Aminopromazine
LO-SAL*
Calcium Carbonate
Magnesium Hydroxide

LOSEL 250
  Selenium Sulfide
LOTENSE
  Polythiazide
LOTIO ALSULFA
  Sulfur
LOTRIMIN
  Clotrimazole
LO-TROL*
  Atropine
  Diphenoxylate
LOTUSATE
  Talbutal
LO-TUSSIN*
  Codeine
  Guaifenesin
  Pseudoephedrine
LOWILA CAKE*
  Boric Acid
  Mineral Oil
  Urea
LOW QUEL*
  Atropine
  Diphenoxylate
LOXAPAC
  Loxapine
LOXITANE
  Loxapine
LOZOL
  Indapamide
LTS
  Levothyroxine
LUBRIDERM*
  Glycerin
  Lanolin
  Mineral Oil
LUCOFEN
  Chlorphentermine
LUCORTEUM
  Progesterone
LUDIOMIL
  Maprotiline
LUFA
  Vitamins, Multiple
LUF-ISO
  Isoproterenol
LUFYLINE-EPG TABS*
  Dyphylline
  Ephedrine
  Guaifenesin
  Phenobarbital
LUFYLLIN
  Dyphylline
LUFYLLINE G TABS*
  Dyphylline
  Guaifenesin
LUGOL'S SOLUTION*
  Iodine
  Potassium Iodide
LULLAMIN
  Methapyrilene
LUMINAL
  Phenobarbital
LURIDE
  Sodium Fluoride
LURIDE LOZI-TABS
  Sodium Fluoride
LUTEINOL
  Progesterone
LUTOCYLIN
  Progesterone
LUTOCYLOL
  Ethisterone
LUTREXIN
  Lututrin
LUTROMONE
  Progesterone
LV PENICILLIN
  Penicillin V
    Potassium
LYCORAL
  Chloral Hydrate
LYNORAL
  Ethinyl Estradiol
LYOPHRIN
  Epinephrine
LYSIVANE
  Ethopropazine
LYSODREN
  Mitotane
LYSPAFEN
  Pentapiperide
LYTEERS
  Methylcellulose

M

MAALOX*
  Aluminum Hydroxide

Magnesium Hydroxide
MAALOX #1*
Aluminum Hydroxide
Magnesium Hydroxide
MAALOX #2*
Aluminum Hydroxide
Magnesium Hydroxide
MAALOX PLUS*
Aluminum Hydroxide
Magnesium Hydroxide
Simethicone
MACRODANTIN
Nitrofurantoin
MACRODEX
Dextran 70
MADRIBON
Sulfadimethoxine
MAGACIN*
Ascorbic Acid
Glutamic Acid
Magnesium
Niacin
Niacinamide
MAGAN
Magnesium Salicylate
MAGCYL*
Danthron
Docusate Sodium
MAGCYL
Poloxamer 188
MAGENION
Magnesium Hydroxide
MAGMALIN*
Aluminum Hydroxide
Magnesium Hydroxide
MAGNACORT
Hydrocortamate
MAGNA GEL*
Aluminum Hydroxide
Magnesium Hydroxide
MAGNAMYCIN
Carbomycin
MAGNATRIL*
Aluminum Hydroxide
Magnesium Oxide
Magnesium Trisilicate
MAGNELIUM
Magnesium Chloride
MAGNESIA AND ALUMINA ORAL SUSPENSION*
Aluminum Oxide
Magnesium Oxide
MAGNESIUM ROUGIER
Magnesium Glucoheptonate
MAG-OX 400
Magnesium Oxide
MAG-5
Magnesium Sulfate
MAJEPTIL
Thioproperazine
MAKAROL
Diethylstilbestrol
MAKOZ
Caffeine
MALATAL*
Atropine
Hyoscyamine
Phenobarbital
Scopolamine
MALCOTRAN
Homatropine
MALDEX*
Belladonna
Methenamine Mandelate
Salicylamide
MALGESIC
Phenylbutazone
MALGESIC-ALK
Phenylbutazone
MALLAMINT
Calcium Carbonate
MALLISOL
Povidone-Iodine
MALLOPHENE
Phenazopyridine
MAL-O-FEM CYP
Estradiol
MALOGEN
Testosterone
MALOGEN AQUASPENSION
Testosterone
MALOGEX
Testosterone
MALOTUSS
Guaifenesin
MALTLEVOL*
Iron
Vitamins, Multiple

MALTLEVOL-M*
  Minerals, Multiple
  Vitamins, Multiple
MALTLEVOL 12*
  Iron
  Vitamins, Multiple
MALTSUPEX
  Malt Soup Extract
MANDALAY
  Methenamine
    Mandelate
MANDELAMINE
  Methenamine
    Mandelate
MANDELETS
  Methenamine
    Mandelate
MANDOL
  Cefamandole
MANEXIN
  Mannitol Hexanitrate
MANITE
  Mannitol Hexanitrate
MANNEX
  Mannitol Hexanitrate
MANTADIL*
  Chlorcyclizine
  Hydrocortisone
MANTICOR
  Hydrocortisone
MANURIL
  Hydrochlorothiazide
MAOLATE
  Chlorphenesin
MAOX
  Magnesium Oxide
MAPHARSEN
  Oxophenarsine
MAPHARSIDE
  Oxophenarsine
MARAX*
  Ephedrine
  Hydroxyzine
  Theophylline
MARAZIDE
  Benzthiazide
MARBAXIN-750
  Methocarbamol
MARBLEN*
  Calcium Carbonate
  Magnesium Carbonate
MARBORAN
  Methisazone
MARCAINE
  Bupivacaine
MARCUMAR
  Phenprocoumon
MARELINE
  Amitriptyline
MAREVAN
  Warfarin
MAREZINE
  Cyclizine
MARFANIL
  Mafenide
MARFLEX
  Orphenadrine
MARINOL
  Dronabinol
MARMINE
  Dimenhydrinate
MARPLAN
  Isocarboxazid
MARSILID
  Iproniazid
MARZINE
  Cyclizine
MASTERID
  Dromostanolone
MASTERIL
  Dromostanolone
MASTERONE
  Dromostanolone
MATERNA*
  Minerals, Multiple
  Vitamins, Multiple
MATROPINAL*
  Homatropine
  Phenobarbital
MATROPINAL FORTE
    INSERTS*
  Homatropine
  Phenobarbital
MATROPINAL INSERTS*
  Homatropine
  Phenobarbital
MATULANE
  Procarbazine
MAXAMAG SUSPENSION*
  Aluminum Hydroxide

Magnesium Oxide
MAXERAN
Metoclopramide
MAXIBOLIN
Ethylestrenol
MAXIDEX
Dexamethasone
MAXIDEX OPHTHALMIC
Dexamethasone
MAXI-E
Vitamin E
MAXIFLOR
Diflorasone Diacetate
MAXIGESIC*
Acetaminophen
Codeine
Promethazine
MAXIMED
Protriptyline
MAXIMUM CRAMP RELIEF*
Acetaminophen
Pamabrom
Pyrilamine
MAXIPEN
Phenethicillin
MAXITATE
Mannitol Hexanitrate
MAXOLON
Metoclopramide
MAXZIDE*
Hydrochlorothiazide
Triamterene
MAYEPTIL
Thioproperazine
MAYTREX
Tetracycline
MAZANOR
Mazindol
MAZON*
Benzoic Acid
Coal Tar
Resorcinol
Salicyclic Acid
M-B TABS
Methylene Blue
M-CILLIN D 400
Penicillin G
MD-76
Diatrizoate Meglumine
MEADACHE*
Acetaminophen
Caffeine
Phenyltoloxamine
Salicylamide
MEASURIN
Aspirin
MEBARAL
Mephobarbital
MEBROIN*
Mephobarbital
Phenytoin
MEBUTAL
Butabarbital
MECHOLYL
Methacholine
MECLAN
Meclocycline Sulfosalicylate
MECLOMEN
Meclofenamate
MECOSTRIN CHLORIDE
Tubocurarine Dimethyl Ether
MEDACHE*
Acetaminophen
Caffeine
Phenyltoloxamine
Salicylamide
MED-DEPO
Methylprednisolone
MEDICATED FACE CONDITIONER
Salicylic Acid
MEDICATED FOOT POWDER*
Benzoic Acid
Chlorothymol
Salicylic Acid
MEDICOAL
Charcoal
MEDICONE DRESSING CREAM*
Benzocaine
Hydroxyquinoline
MEDICONET*
Benzalkonium Chloride
Lanolin
MEDICYCLINE
Tetracycline

MEDIGESIC PLUS*
  Acetaminophen
  Butalbital
  Caffeine
MEDIHALER-EPI
  Epinephrine
MEDIHALER-ERGOTAMINE
  Ergotamine
MEDIHALER-ISO
  Isoproterenol
MEDIHALER-TETRACAINE
  Tetracaine
MEDILIUM
  Chlordiazepoxide
MEDIMET-250
  Methyldopa
MEDINAL
  Barbital
MEDIPHEN
  Phenobarbital
MEDIPLAST
  Salicylic Acid
MEDIQUELL
  Dextromethorphan
MEDI-QUIK*
  Alcohol
  Benzalkonium
    Chloride
  Lidocaine
MEDITRAN
  Meprobamate
MEDIZINC
  Zinc Sulfate
MEDOMIN
  Heptabarbital
MEDRALONE-40
  Methylprednisolone
MEDRALONE-80
  Methylprednisolone
MEDRATE
  Methylprednisolone
MEDROCORT
  Medrysone
MEDROL
  Methylprednisolone
MEDROL ACETATE
  Methylprednisolone
MEDROL ACNE LOTION*
  Aluminum
    Chlorohydrate
  Methylprednisolone
  Sulfur
MEDROL TOPICAL
  Methylprednisolone
MEDRONE
  Methylprednisolone
MEFEDINA
  Meperidine
MEFOXIN
  Cefoxitin
MEGA-B
  Vitamin B Complex
MEGACE
  Megestrol
MEGACILLIN
  Penicillin G
MEGACILLIN SUSPENSION
  Penicillin G
    Benzathine
MEGADON
  Nitrazepam
MEGADOSE*
  Minerals, Multiple
  Vitamins, Multiple
MEGAPEN
  Penicillin G
MEGAPHEN
  Chlorpromazine
MEGIMIDE
  Bemegride
MELANEX
  Hydroquinone
MEL-B
  Melarsoprol
MELFIAT
  Phendimetrazine
MELFIAT-105 UNICELLES
  Phendimetrazine
MELIPRAMIN
  Imipramine
MELLARIL
  Thioridazine
MELLARIL-S
  Thioridazine
MELLINESE
  Chlorpropamide
MELLITOL
  Tolbutamide
MELOXINE
  Methoxsalen

MELTEX*
Hydroquinolone
Titanium Dioxide
MELTROL
Phenformin
MELTROL-50
Phenformin
MEMBRETTES
Progesterone
MENAVAL-10
Estradiol
MENEST
Estrogens, Esterified
MENFORMON A
Estrone
MENIC*
Niacin
Pentylenetetrazol
MENOMUNE A
Meningococcal Polysaccharide Vaccine
MENOMUNE-A/C
Meningococcal Polysaccharide Vaccine
MENOSPASM
Dicyclomine
MENOTAB
Conjugated Estrogens
MENOTROL
Esterified Estrogens
MENRIUM
Chlordiazepoxide
MENTA-BAL
Mephobarbital
MENTHOLATUM TOOTHACHE REMEDY
Eugenol
MENTHOL CHLORASEPTIC*
Phenol
Phenolate Sodium
MEONINE
Racemethionine
MEPAVLON
Meprobamate
MEP-E
Meprobamate
MEPEDYL
Piprinhydrinate
MEPERGAN*
Meperidine
Promethazine
MEPHENAMINE
Orphenadrine
MEPHORAL
Mephobarbital
MEPHSON
Mephenesin
MEPHYTON
Phytonadione
MEPILIN*
Ethinyl Estradiol
Methyltestosterone
MEPRED
Methylprednisolone
MEPROGESIC*
Aspirin
Ethoheptazine
Meprobamate
MEPRO-HEX*
Meprobamate
Tridihexethyl
MEPROSPAN
Meprobamate
MEPROSPAN-400
Meprobamate
MEPROTABS
Meprobamate
MEQUELON
Methaqualone
MEQUIN
Methaqualone
MERACTINOMYCIN
Dactinomycin
MERATRAN
Pipradrol
MERAVIL
Amitriptyline
MERBENTYL
Dicyclomine
MERCARDON
Meralluride
MERCAZOLE
Methimazole
MERCLORAN
Chlormerodrin
MERCODINONE
Hydrocodone

MERCODOL WITH
DECAPRYN*
Codeine
Doxylamine
Phenylephrine
MERCUHYDRIN
Meralluride
MERCUROCHROME*
Benzalkonium
Chloride
Merbromin
MERCUROCHROME II*
Benzalkonium
Chloride
Isopropyl Alcohol
Lidocaine
Menthol
MERCUROXYL
Chlormerodrin
MERITAL
Nomifensine
MERLENATE*
Phenylmercuric
Nitrate
Undecylenic Acid
MEROCET
Cetylpyridinium
MERODICEIN
Meralein
MERSOL
Thimerosal
MERSYNDOL WITH
CODEINE*
Acetaminophen
Codeine
Doxylamine
MERTESTATE
Testosterone
MERTHIOLATE
Thimerosal
MERUVAX II
Rubella Virus
Vaccine
MER/29
Triparanol
MESANTOIN
Mephenytoin
MESOPIN
Homatropine
MESTINON
Pyridostigmine
MESTINON BROMIDE
Pyridostigmine
METACEN
Indomethacin
METAHYDRIN
Trichlormethiazide
METALEX-P
Pentylenetetrazol
METAMINE
Trolnitrate
METAMUCIL
Plantago Seed
METANDREN
Methyltestosterone
METAPHEN
Nitromersol
METAPREL
Metaproterenol
METASEP
Parachlorometa-
xylenol
METASEP MEDICATED
SHAMPOO
Parachlorometa-
xylenol
METASPAS
Dihexyverine
METASTAB
Methylprednisolone
METATENSIN*
Reserpine
Trichlormethiazide
METED SHAMPOO*
Salicylic Acid
Sulfur
METED 2 SHAMPOO*
Salicylic Acid
Sulfur
METHAMPEX
Methamphetamine
METHANDINE
Methenamine
METHEDRINE
Methamphetamine
METHIDATE
Methylphenidate
METHISCHOL
Vitamins, Multiple
METHIUM
Hexamethonium
METHOCARBAMOL W/ASA*

Aspirin
Methocarbamol
METHOCEL
Methylcellulose
METHOFANE
Methoxyflurane
METHOPTO*
Benzalkonium Chloride
Methylcellulose
METHORATE
Dextromethorphan
METHOSARB
Calusterone
METHOSTAN
Methandriol
METHOXA-DOME
Methoxsalen
METHO-500
Methocarbamol
METHULOSE
Methylcellulose
METHYLONE
Methylprednisolone
METHYLOSE
Methylcellulose
METICORTELONE
Prednisolone
METICORTEN
Prednisone
METI-DERM
Prednisolone
METIMYD*
Prednisolone
Sulfacetamide
METOPIRONE
Metyrapone
METOSYN
Fluocinonide
METRA
Phendimetrazine
METRASPRAY
Tetracaine
METRAZOL
Pentylenetetrazol
METRETON
Prednisolone
METROMYCIN
Oleandomycin
METRYL
Metronidazole
METUBINE IODIDE
Metocurine Iodide
METYCAINE
Piperocaine
MEVAL
Diazepam
MEVANIN-C*
Minerals, Multiple
Vitamins, Multiple
MEXATE
Methotrexate
MEXITIL
Mexiletine
MEZLIN
Mezlocillin
MG-BLUE
Methylene Blue
MG-PLUS
Magnesium
MICATIN
Miconazole
MI-CEBRIN*
Minerals, Multiple
Vitamins, Multiple
MI-CEBRIN T*
Minerals, Multiple
Vitamins, Multiple
MICLO-ZYME
Glutamic Acid
MICRAININ*
Aspirin
Meprobamate
MICREST
Diethylstilbestrol
MICRHOGAM
Gobulin, Immune
MICROCORT
Hydrocortisone
MICRO-K
Potassium Chloride
MICROLUT
Norgestrel
MICRONASE
Glyburide
MICRONEFRIN
Epinephrine
MICRONOR
Norethindrone
MICROSUL
Sulfamethizole
MICROSUL-A*

Phenazopyridine
Sulfamethizole
MICROSULFON
Sulfadiazine
MICROSYN*
Resorcinol
Salicylic Acid
MICROVAL
Levonorgestrel
MICTOBEN
Oxycodone
MICTROL
Bethanechol
MIDAMOR
Amiloride
MIDATANE EXPECTORANT*
Brompheniramine
Guaifenesin
Phenylpropanolamine
MIDATAP*
Brompheniramine
Phenylephrine
Phenylpropanolamine
MIDICEL
Sulfamethoxy-pyridazine
MIDOL*
Aspirin
Caffeine
Cinnamedrine
MIDRAN DECONGESTANT*
Acetaminophen
Chlorpheniramine
Phenylephrine
Salicylamide
MIDRIN*
Acetaminophen
Dichloralphenazone
Isometheptene Mucate
MIELUCIN
Busulfan
MIFLEX*
Acetaminophen
Chlorzoxazone
MIGRAL*
Caffeine
Cyclizine
MIGRALAM*
Acetaminophen
Caffeine
Isometheptene Mucate
MIGRASTAT*
Caffeine
Ergotamine
MIGRISTENE
Fonazine
MIKEDIMIDE
Bemegride
MILES NERVINE
Pyrilamine
MILIBIS
Glycobiarsol
MILKINOL*
Docusate Sodium
Mineral Oil
MILK OF MAGNESIA
Magnesium Hydroxide
MILK OF MAGNESIA-CASCARA SUSPENSION*
Cascara Sagrada
Magnesium Hydroxide
MILONTIN
Phensuximide
MILPATH*
Meprobamate
Tridihexethyl
MILPREM
Meprobamate
MILSPAN
Meprobamate
MILTOWN
Meprobamate
MILTRATE*
Meprobamate
Pentaerythritol Tetranitrate
MINIHIST
Pyrilamine
MINI-LIX
Aminophylline
MINIPRESS
Prazosin
MINIRIN
Desmopressin
MINIZIDE*
Polythiazide
Prazosin
MINOCIN
Minocycline

MINOTAL*
  Acetaminophen
  Butabarbital
MINTEZOL
  Thiabendazole
MINUTEMAN
  Vitamins, Multiple
MINUT-RUB*
  Camphor
  Menthol
  Methyl Salicylate
MIOCARPINE
  Pilocarpine
MIOCHOL
  Acetylcholine
MIOSTAT
  Carbachol
MI-PILO
  Pilocarpine
MIRADON
  Anisindione
MIRAPRONT
  Phentermine
MISSION PRENATAL*
  Calcium
  Folic Acid
  Iron
  Vitamins, Multiple
MISTURA C
  Carbachol
MISTURA D
  Phenylephrine
MISTURA E
  Epinephrine
MISTURA P
  Pilocarpine
MITHRACIN
  Mithramycin
MITOCIN-C
  Mitomycin
MITROLAN
  Polycarbophil
MITRONAL
  Cinnarizine
MITY-MYCIN*
  Bacitracin
  Diperodon
  Neomycin
  Polymyxin B
MITY-QUIN CREAM*
  Clioquinol
  Hydrocortisone
MIXTARD*
  Insulin [Suspension]
    Isophane
  Insulin Zinc
    [Suspension]
    Extended
M-M-RII
  Measles, Mumps and
    Rubella Virus
    Vaccine
MOBAN
  Molindone
MOBENOL
  Tolbutamide
MOBIDIN
  Salicylate
MOBIGESIC*
  Magnesium Salicylate
  Phenyltoloxamine
MOBISYL CREME
  Trolamine Salicylate
MODANE*
  Danthron
  Plantago Seed
MODANE BULK
  Plantago Seed
MODANE MILD
  Danthron
MODANE PLUS*
  Danthron
  Docusate Sodium
MODANE SOFT
  Docusate Sodium
MODECATE
  Fluphenazine
MODERIL
  Rescinnamine
MODICON*
  Ethinyl Estradiol
  Norethindrone
MODITEN
  Fluphenazine
MODRASTANE
  Trilostane
MODUMATE
  Arginine
MODURET*
  Amiloride

Hydrochlorothiazide
MODURETIC*
Amiloride
Hydrochlorothiazide
MOEBIQINE
Iodoquinol
MOGADON
Nitrazepam
MOLATOC-CST*
Casanthranol
Docusate Sodium
MOLCICLINA
Methacycline
MOLEVAC
Pyrvinium Pamoate
MOL-IRON
Ferrous Sulfate
MOL-IRON WITH VITAMIN C*
Ascorbic Acid
Ferrous Sulfate
MOLOFAC
Docusate Sodium
MOMENTUM*
Aspirin
Phenyltoloxamine
Salsalate
MONACET WITH CODEINE*
Aspirin
Caffeine
Codeine
MONACRIN
Aminacrine
MONILE
Racemethionine
MONISTAT
Miconazole
MONISTAT 3
Miconazole
MONISTAT 7 VAGINAL CREAM
Miconazole
MONOCAINE
Butethamine
MONOCID
Cefonicid
MONOCORTIN
Paramethasone
MONODRAL
Penthienate
MONO-KAY
Phytonadione
MONOLATE
Monoethanolamine
MONOTARD
Insulin Zinc Suspension
MONOTARD, HUMAN
Insulin Zinc, Human
MONOTARD MC
Insulin Zinc
MONOTEN
Phenelzine
MONSTER VITAMINS
Vitamins, Multiple
MONSTER VITAMINS & IRON*
Ferrous Fumarate
Vitamins, Multiple
MORONAL
Nystatin
MORO PILLS
Ferrous Fumarate
MOR-TUSSIN P.E.*
Guaifenesin
Pseudoephedrine
M.O.S.
Morphine
MOSATIL
Edetate Calcium Disodium
MOSEGOR
Pizotyline
MOTILIUM
Domperidone
MOTILYN
Panthenol
MOTION-AID
Dimenhydrinate
MOTION CURE
Meclizine
MOTRIN
Ibuprofen
MOTUSSIN
Guaifenesin
MOXACIN
Amoxicillin
MOXAM
Moxalactam
MOXILEAN
Amoxicillin
M-P

Methapyrilene
M-PREDNISOL
Methylprednisolone
M-R-VAXII
Measles and Rubella Virus Vaccine
MR VAX II
Rubella Virus Vaccine
MSC TRIAMINIC*
Methscopolamine
Pheniramine
Phenylpropanolamine
Pyrilamine
MSG-600
Magnesium Salicylate
MUCILLIUM
Plantago Seed
MUCILOSE
Plantago Seed
MUCINUM-F
Senna
MUCOMYST
Acetylcysteine
MUCOPLEX
Vitamins, Multiple
MUDRANE*
Aminophylline
Ephedrine
Phenobarbital
Potassium Iodide
MUDRANE GG*
Aminophylline
Ephedrine
Guaifenesin
Phenobarbital
MUDRANE GG ELIXIR*
Ephedrine
Guaifenesin
Phenobarbital
Theophylline
MUDRANE GG-2*
Aminophylline
Guaifenesin
MUDRANE-2*
Aminophylline
Potassium Iodide
MULTICEBRIN
Vitamins, Multiple
MULTIFUGE
Piperazine
MULTISCRUB*
Salicylic Acid
Sulfur
MULTI-SYMPTOM*
Brompheniramine
Dextromethorphan
Pseudoephedrine
MULVIDREN SOFTABS
Vitamins, Multiple
MUMPSVAX
Mumps Virus Vaccine
MURACIN
Methylthiouracil
MURACINE
Tetracycline
MUREL
Valethamate
MURIAMIC
Glutamic Acid
MURINE EAR DROPS*
Glycerin
Methylcellulose
MURINE EAR WAX REMOVAL SYSTEM/MURINE EAR DROPS*
Carbamide Peroxide
Glycerin
MURINE PLUS
Tetrahydrozoline
MURINE 2
Tetrahydrozoline
MURIPSIN*
Glutamic Acid
Pepsin
MUROCAL
Homatropine
MUROCOLL
Atropine
Epinephrine
MURO-128
Sodium Chloride
MUSTARGEN
Mechlorethamine
MUTAMYCIN
Mitomycin
M.V.I.
Vitamins, Multiple
M.V.I.-12
Vitamins, Multiple
M.V.M. LIQUID
Vitamins, Multiple

MYADEC
  Vitamins, Multiple
MYAMBUTOL
  Ethambutol
MY-B-DEN
  Adenosine
MYCELEX
  Clotrimazole
MYCELEX-G
  Clotrimazole
MYCELEX TROCHE
  Clotrimazole
MYCHEL
  Chloramphenicol
MYCIFRADIN
  Neomycin
MYCIFRADIN SULFATE
  Neomycin
MYCIGUENT*
  Chlorobutanol
  Neomycin
MYCIL
  Chlorphenesin
MYCIN
  Chloramphenicol
MYCINETTES*
  Benzocaine
  Cetylpyridinium
MYCINETTES SUGAR FREE*
  Benzocaine
  Cetylpyridinium
  Terpin Hydrate
MYCITRACIN*
  Bacitracin
  Neomycin
  Polymyxin B
MYCIVIN
  Lincomycin
MYCOLOG*
  Gramicidin
  Neomycin
  Nystatin
  Triamcinolone
MYCOQUIN
  Iodochlorhydroxyquin
MYCORT
  Hydrocortisone
MYCOSTATIN
  Nystatin
MYCO TRIACET CREAM & OINTMENT*
  Gramicidin
  Neomycin
  Nystatin
  Triamcinolone
MYDFRIN
  Phenylephrine
MYDPLEGIC
  Cyclopentolate
MYDRAPRED OPHTHALMIC*
  Atropine
  Benzalkonium Chloride
  Boric Acid
  Prednisolone
MYDRIACYL
  Tropicamide
MYDRILATE
  Cyclopentolate
MYELODIL
  Iophendylate
MYGEL*
  Aluminum Hydroxide
  Magnesium Hydroxide
  Simethicone
MYIDONE
  Primidone
MYLANTA*
  Aluminum Hydroxide
  Magnesium Hydroxide
  Simethicone
MYLANTA II*
  Aluminum Hydroxide
  Magnesium Hydroxide
  Simethicone
MYLANTA-2 EXTRA STRENGTH*
  Aluminum Hydroxide
  Magnesium Hydroxide
  Simethicone
MYLAXEN
  Hexafluorenium
MYLEPSINE
  Primidone
MYLERAN
  Busulfan
MYLICON
  Simethicone
MYLICON 80
  Simethicone
MYOBID
  Papaverine

MYOCALM*
Acetaminophen
Phenyltoloxamine
Salicylamide
MYOCALM REVISED II*
Acetaminophen
Phenyltoloxamine
MYOCARDOL
Pentaerythritol Tetranitrate
MYOCHRYSINE
Gold Sodium Thiomalate
MYOCON
Nitroglycerin
MYODIL
Iophendylate
MYOFLEX
Trolamine Salicylate
MYOFORTE*
Acetaminophen
Chlorzoxazone
MYOLIN
Orphenadrine
MYOTONACHOL
Bethanechol
MYOTROL
Orphenadrine
MYRINGACAINE
Mercufenol
MYSOLINE
Primidone
MYSONE
Hydrocortisone
MYSTECLIN-F*
Amphotericin B
Tetracycline
MYSURAN
Ambenonium
MYTELASE
Ambenonium
MYTOLON
Benzoquinonium
MYTRATE
Epinephrine
MYTREX*
Gramicidin
Nystatin
Triamcinolone

N

NAC
Acetylcysteine
NACK
Chlordiazepoxide
NACLEX
Benzthiazide
NACTATE
Poldine
NACTON
Poldine
NADOPEN-V
Penicillin V Potassium
NADOSTINE
Nystatin
NADOZONE
Phenylbutazone
NAFCIL
Nafcillin
NAFRINE
Oxymetazoline
NALATE
Sodium Thiosalicylate
NALDECON*
Chlorpheniramine
Phenylephrine
Phenylpropanolamine
Phenyltoloxamine
NALDECON-CX*
Codeine
Guaifenesin
Phenylpropanolamine
NALDECON-EX PEDIATRIC*
Guaifenesin
Phenylpropanolamine
NALDEGESIC*
Acetaminophen
Pseudoephedrine
NALDELATE*
Chlorpheniramine
Phenylephrine
Phenylpropanolamine
Phenyltoloxamine
NALDETUSS*
Dextromethorphan
Phenylpropanolamine
Phenyltoloxamine

NALFON
  Fenoprofen
NALGESIC
  Fenoprofen
NALLINE
  Nalorphine
NALLPEN
  Nafcillin
NALUTRON
  Progesterone
NAPAP
  Acetaminophen
NAPHCON
  Naphazoline
NAPHCON FORTE
  Naphazoline
NAPRIL PLATEAU CAPS*
  Chlorpheniramine
  Phenylephrine
  Phenylpropanolamine
  Pyrilamine
NAPROSYN
  Naproxen
NAP TABS
  Vitamins, Multiple
NAPTRATE
  Pentaerythritol
    Tetranitrate
NAQUA
  Trichlormethiazide
NAQUIVAL*
  Reserpine
  Trichlormethiazide
NARCAN
  Naloxone
NARCOZEP
  Flunitrazepam
NARDELZINE
  Phenelzine
NARDIL
  Phenelzine
NARIDAN
  Oxyphencyclimine
NARPHEN
  Phenazocine
NARSPAN*
  Chlorpheniramine
  Methscopolamine
  Phenylephrine
NASAHIST*
  Chlorpheniramine
  Phenylephrine
  Phenylpropanolamine
NASAHIST II*
  Atropine
  Chlorpheniramine
NASAL
  Sodium Chloride
NASALCROM
  Cromolyn Sodium
NASALIDE
  Flunisolide
NASALSPAN*
  Chlorpheniramine
  Pseudoephedrine
NASALSPAN EXPECTORANT*
  Dextromethorphan
  Guaifenesin
  Pseudoephedrine
NASDRO NO.3
  Ephedrine
NASE-X
  Phenylephrine
NASMIL
  Cromolyn Sodium
NASODILAN
  Isoxsuprine
NASO MIST
  Phenylephrine
NATABEC
  Vitamins, Multiple
NATACILLINE
  Hetacillin
NATACOMP-FA*
  Minerals, Multiple
  Vitamins, Multiple
NATACYN
  Natamycin
NATAFORT FILMSEAL*
  Minerals, Multiple
  Vitamins, Multiple
NATALINS
  Vitamins, Multiple
NATIGOXINE NATIVELLE
  Digoxin
NATI-K NATIVELLE
  Potassium Tartrate
NATIONAL LAXATIVE
  Magnesium Citrate
NATISEDINE NATIVELLE

Quinidine
Phenylethyl-
barbiturate
NATOPHEROL
Vitamin E
NATRASCORB
Ascorbic Acid
NATRIMAX
Hydrochlorothiazide
NATULAN
Procarbazine
NATURACIL
Plantago Seed
NATURAL THERATAB
Vitamins, Multiple
NATURE'S REMEDY CANDY
COATED
Cascara Sagrada
NATURE'S REMEDY
JUNIORS
Cascara Sagrada
NATURE'S REMEDY
REGULAR
Cascara Sagrada
NATURETIN
Bendroflumethiazide
NATURSLIM II*
Minerals, Multiple
Vitamins, Multiple
NAUSEAL
Dimenhydrinate
NAUSEATOL
Dimenhydrinate
NAUSETROL
Phosphorated
Carbohydrate
NAUTAMINE
Diphenhydramine
NAVANE
Thiothixene
NAXEN
Naproxen
NAZAC TIMED-
DISINTEGRATION
DECONGESTANT*
Chlorpheniramine
Pheniramine
Phenylpropanolamine
N.B.P.*
Bacitracin
Neomycin
Polymyxin B
N.D. CLEAR T.D.*
Chlorpheniramine
Pseudoephedrine
ND-GESIC*
Acetaminophen
Chlorpheniramine
Phenylephrine
Pyrilamine
N.D.-STAT*
Atropine
Chlorpheniramine
NEBCIN
Tobramycin
NEBRALIN
Pentobarbital
NEBS
Acetaminophen
NECTADON
Noscapine
NEFROLAN
Clorexolone
NEFROSUL
Sulfachlorpyridazine
NEGGRAM
Nalidixic Acid
NEKO
Mercuric Iodide
NELEX-100
Pentylenetetrazol
NEMA
Tetrachloroethylene
NEMASOL
Aminosalicylic Acid
NEMBUTAL
Pentobarbital
NEO-ANTERGEN
Pyrilamine
NEO-BARB
Butabarbital
NEO-BETALIN 12
Hydroxocobalamin
NEOBIOTIC
Neomycin
NEOCAINE
Procaine
NEO-CALGLUCON
Vitamins, Multiple
NEO-CALGLUCON SYRUP

Calcium
NEO-CALME
Diazepam
NEO-CASTADERM*
Alcohol
Boric Acid
Phenol
Resorcin
NEOCHOLAN
Dehydrocholic Acid
NEOCIN
Neomycin
NEO-COBEFRIN
Propoxycaine
NEO-CODEMA
Hydrochlorothiazide
NEO-COROVAS
Pentaerythritol Tetranitrate
NEO-CORT-DOME*
Hydrocortisone
Neomycin
NEO-CORTEF*
Hydrocortisone
Neomycin
NEO-CULTOL
Mineral Oil
NEOCYLATE*
Aminobenzoic Acid
Potassium Salicylate
NEODECADRON*
Dexamethasone
Neomycin
NEO-DELTA-CORTEF*
Chlorobutanol
Neomycin
Prednisolone
NEO-DIBETIC
Tolbutamide
NEODRINE
Methamphetamine
NEODROL
Stanolone
NEODYNE
Ethyl Dibunate
NEO-EPININE
Isoproterenol
NEO-ESTRONE
Esterified Estrogens
NEOFOL B-12
Vitamins, Multiple
NEOHETRAMINE
Thonzylamine
NEO-HOMBREOL
Methyltestosterone
NEO-HYDELTRASOL*
Neomycin
Prednisolone
NEOHYDRIN
Chlormerodrin
NEO-HYDRO*
Antipyrine
Dibucaine
Glycerin
Hydrocortisone
Neomycin
Polymyxin B
NEO-LARYNGOBIS
Bismuth Dipropylacetate
NEOLAX*
Dehydrocholic Acid
Docusate Sodium
NEOLIN
Penicillin G
NEOLINE
Aspirin
NEOLOID
Castor Oil
NEO-MAL
Propoxyphene
NEO-MEDROL*
Chlorobutanol
Methylprednisolone
Neomycin
NEOMEDROL ACNE LOTION*
Aluminum Chlorohydrate
Methylprednisolone
Neomycin
NEO-MERCAZOLE
Carbimazole
NEOMIXIN*
Bacitracin
Neomycin
Polymyxin B
NEO-NACLEX
Bendroflumethiazide
NEONAL
Butethal

NEO-OXYLONE*
  Fluorometholone
  Neomycin
NEOPAP SUPPRETTES
  Acetaminophen
NEOPHIBAN*
  Guaifenesin
  Phenylpropanolamine
  Phenyltoloxamine
NEOPHYL
  Dyphylline
NEOPIRINE CO. NO.35*
  Aspirin
  Caffeine
NEOPIRINE CO. WITH CODEINE*
  Aspirin
  Caffeine
  Codeine
NEOPIRINE NO.25
  Aspirin
NEOPLATIN
  Cisplatin
NEO-POLYCIN*
  Bacitracin
  Neomycin
  Polymyxin B
NEOQUESS INJECTABLE
  Dicyclomine
NEOQUESS TABLETS*
  Atropine
  Hyoscyamine
  Phenobarbital
  Scopolamine
NEO-RENAL
  Furosemide
NEORHIBAN*
  Acetaminophen
  Phenylpropanolamine
  Phenyltoloxamine
NEO-RUBEX
  Cyanocobalamin
NEOSAR
  Cyclophosphamide
NEO-SERP
  Reserpine
NEO-SILVOL
  Silver Iodide Colloidal
NEOSONE*
  Chlorobutanol
  Cortisone
  Neomycin
NEOSORB PLUS*
  Aluminum
  Magnesium
NEOSPORIN*
  Bacitracin
  Neomycin
  Polymyxin B
NEOSPORIN-G CREAM*
  Gramicidin
  Neomycin
  Polymyxin B
NEOSPORIN G.U. IRRIGANT*
  Neomycin
  Polymyxin B
NEOSTREPTAL
  Sulfadimethoxine
NEO-SYNALAR*
  Fluocinolone
  Neomycin
NEO-SYNEPHRINE
  Phenylephrine
NEO-SYNEPHRINE COMPOUND*
  Acetaminophen
  Phenylephrine
  Thenyldiamine
NEO-SYNEPHRINE EYE DROPS
  Phenylephrine
NEO-SYNEPHRINE II
  Xylometazoline
NEO-SYNEPHRINE 12-HOUR
  Oxymetazoline
NEOTAL*
  Neomycin
  Polymyxin B
NEOTEP*
  Chlorpheniramine
  Phenylephrine
NEO-TETRINE
  Tetracycline
NEO-THRYCEX*
  Bacitracin
  Neomycin
  Polymyxin B
NEOTHYLLINE

Dyphylline
NEOTHYLLINE-GG*
Dyphylline
Guaifenesin
NEO-TRAN
Meprobamate
NEO-TRIC
Metronidazole
NEOZIN*
Phenylephrine
Zinc Sulfate
NEO-ZOLINE
Phenylbutazone
NEPHRIL
Polythiazide
NEPHROFLOW
Iodohippurate
NEPHRONEX
Nitrofurantoin
NEPHROX SUSPENSION*
Aluminum Hydroxide
Mineral Oil
NEPTAZANE
Methazolamine
NERVINE
Methapyrilene
NERVINE EFFERVESCENT
Methapyrilene
NERVOCAINE
Lidocaine
NESACAINE
Chloroprocaine
NESACAINE-CE
Chlorprocaine
NETHAMINE
Etafedrine
NETROMYCIN
Netilmicin
NEULACTIL
Periciazine
NEULEPTIL
Periciazine
NEURO B-12 FORTE INJECTABLE*
Cyanocobalamin
Pyridoxine
Thiamine
NEURO B-12 INJECTABLE*
Cyanocobalamin
Thiamine
NEUROSEDINE
Butabarbital
NEUT
Sodium Bicarbonate
NEUTRACOMP*
Aluminum Hydroxide
Magnesium Trisilicate
NEUTRALCA-S*
Aluminum
Magnesium
NEUTRALOX*
Aluminum
Magnesium
NEUTRAPEN
Penicillinase
NEUTRA-PHOS*
Phosphorus
Potassium
NEUTRA-PHOS-K*
Phosphorus
Potassium
NEUTRAPHYLLINE
Dyphylline
NEUTRASIL
Magnesium Trisilicate
NEUTRATAR
Coal Tar
NEUTROGENA ACNE-DRYING GEL*
Isopropyl Alcohol
Witch Hazel
NEW FRESHNESS
Acetic Acid
NEWPHRINE
Phenylephrine
NIACOL
Nicotinyl Alcohol
NIAMID
Nialamide
NIARB SUPER*
Ascorbic Acid
Magnesium
Niacinamide
NICAMIN
Niacin
NICEL
Methylcellulose
NICLOCIDE

Niclosamide
NICOBID
Niacin
NICOCAP
Niacin
NICOLAR
Niacin
NICO-METRAZOL*
Niacin
Pentylenetetrazol
NICONACID
Niacin
NICONYL
Isoniazid
NICORETTE
Nicotine
NICO-SPAN
Niacin
NICOTINEX ELIXIR
Niacin
NICO-VERT*
Dimenhydrinate
Niacin
NICOZOL*
Niacin
Pentylenetetrazol
NICO-400
Niacin
NIDATON
Isoniazid
NIFEREX
Polysaccharide-Iron Complex
NIFEREX-PN*
Minerals, Multiple
Vitamins, Multiple
NIFEREX WITH VITAMIN C*
Ascorbic Acid
Polysaccharide-Iron Complex
Sodium Ascorbate
NIFEREX-150
Iron
NIFEREX-150 FORTE*
Cyanocobalamin
Folic Acid
Iron
NIFURAN
Nitrofurantoin
NIGRACAP
Chloral Hydrate
NIKETHYL
Nikethamide
NIKOBAN
Lobeline
NIKORIN
Nikethamide
NIL*
Allantoin
Aminacrine
Sulfanilamide
NILAIN*
Acetaminophen
Aspirin
Caffeine
NILATIL
Itramin Tosylate
NILCOL*
Chlorpheniramine
Dextromethorphan
Guaifenesin
Phenylpropanolamine
NILEVAR
Norethandrolone
NILPRIN
Acetaminophen
NILSTAT
Nystatin
NINOL
Racemethionine
NIONG
Nitroglycerin
NIORIC
Pentylenetetrazol
NIOSPAZ
Dicyclomine
NIPRIDE
Sodium Nitroprusside
NISENTIL
Alphaprodine
NISOLONE
Methylprednisolone
NITE REST*
Aminoxide Hydrobromide
Methapyrilene
NITRANITOL
Mannitol Hexanitrate
NITRETAMINE

Trolnitrate
NITREX
Nitrofurantoin
NITRO-BID OINTMENT
Nitroglycerin
NITRO-BID PLATEAU CAPS
Nitroglycerin
NITROBON
Nitroglycerin
NITROCAP T.D.
Nitroglycerin
NITRODAN
Nitrofurantoin
NITRODISC
Nitroglycerin
NITRO-DUR
Nitroglycerin
NITROGLYN
Nitroglycerin
NITROLIN
Nitroglycerin
NITROL OINTMENT
Nitroglycerin
NITRONET
Nitroglycerin
NITRONG
Nitroglycerin
NITROPRESS
Sodium Nitroprusside
NITROSPAN
Nitroglycerin
NITROSTABILIN
Nitroglycerin
NITROSTAT
Nitroglycerin
NITROSTAT IV
Nitroglycerin
NITRO-T.D.
Nitroglycerin
NITROTEST
Nitroglycerin
NIVEA SKIN OIL*
Lanolin
Mineral Oil
Petrolatum
NIZORAL
Ketoconazole
N-N COUGH*
Ammonium Chloride
Chlorpheniramine
Dextromethorphan
Potassium Guaiacolsulfonate
NOAN
Diazepam
NOBESE
Phenylpropanolamine
NOBESINE
Diethylpropion
NOBRIUM
Medazepam
NOCTAMID
Lormetazepam
NOCTEC
Chloral Hydrate
NODAPTON
Glycopyrrolate
NODOZ
Caffeine
NOGEST*
Atropine
Chlorpheniramine
NOGRAM
Nalidixic Acid
NOLAMINE*
Chlorpheniramine
Phenindamine
Phenylpropanolamine
NOLUDAR
Methyprylon
NOLVADEX
Tamoxifen
NONSUL JELLY
Benzalkonium Chloride
NOOTROPIL
Piracetam
NORADRYL
Diphenhydramine
NORAFED*
Pseudoephedrine
Triprolidine
NORAIAC*
Aluminum Hydroxide
Bismuth Aluminate
Magnesium Carbonate
Magnesium Trisilicate
NORALAC*
Aluminum Hydroxide

Bismuth Aluminate
Magnesium Carbonate
Magnesium Trisilicate
NORAMINIC SYRUP*
Chlorpheniramine
Phenylpropanolamine
NORATUSS*
Ammonium Chloride
Codeine
Potassium Guaiacolsulfonate
Terpin Hydrate
NORAZINE
Promazine
NORCET*
Acetaminophen
Hydrocodone
NORDETTE*
Ethinyl Estradiol
Levonorgestrel
NORDRYL
Diphenhydramine
NOREL PLUS*
Acetaminophen
Chlorpheniramine
Phenylpropanolamine
Phenyltoloxamine
NOREL PLUS INJECTION*
Atropine
Chlorpheniramine
Phenylpropanolamine
NORFEMAC
Bufexamac
NORFIN
Nalorphine
NORFLEX
Orphenadrine
NORGEIS FORTE*
Aspirin
Caffeine
Orphenadrine
NORGESIC*
Aspirin
Caffeine
Orphenadrine
NORGESIC FORTE*
Aspirin
Caffeine
Orphenadrine
NORGLYCIN
Tolazamide
NORIDAY
Norethindrone
NORIMEX
Vitamins, Multiple
NORIMEX-PLUS
Vitamins, Multiple
NORINYL 1+35*
Ethinyl Estradiol
Norethindrone
NORINYL 1+50*
Mestranol
Norethindrone
NORINYL 1+80*
Mestranol
Norethindrone
NORINYL 2*
Mestranol
Norethindrone
NORISODRINE
Isoproterenol
NORITREN
Nortriptyline
NORLAC
Vitamins, Multiple
NORLESTRIN*
Ethinyl Estradiol
Norethindrone
NOR-LIEF*
Ascorbic Acid
Chlorpheniramine
Phenylephrine
NORLUTATE
Norethindrone
NORLUTIN
Norethindrone
NORMACID*
Betaine
Pepsin
NORMATANE*
Brompheniramine
Phenylephrine
Phenylpropanolamine
NORMATANE EXPECTORANT*
Brompheniramine
Guaifenesin
Phenylpropanolamine
NOR-MIL*
Atropine

Diphenoxylate
NORMOCYTIN
Cyanocobalamin
NORMODYNE
Labetalol
NORODIN
Methamphetamine
NOROXINE
Levothyroxine
NORPACE
Disopyramide
NORPACE CR
Disopyramide
NORPANTH
Propantheline
NORPRAMIN
Desipramine
NOR-PRES
Hydralazine
NOR-Q.D.
Norethindrone
NORSENA
Senna
NOR-TET
Tetracycline
NORTUSSIN
Guaifenesin
NORZINE
Promazine
NOSCATUSS
Noscapine
NOSCOSED
Chlorpheniramine
NOSTRIL
Phenylephrine
NOSTRILLA
Phenylephrine
NOVACEBRIN WITH FLUORIDE*
Sodium Fluoride
Vitamins, Multiple
NOVADEX
Dexamethasone
NOVAFED
Pseudoephedrine
NOVAFED A*
Chlorpheniramine
Pseudoephedrine
NOVAHISTEX*
Diphenylpyraline
Phenylephrine
NOVAHISTINE*
Chlorpheniramine
Phenylpropanolamine
NOVAHISTINE DH*
Chlorpheniramine
Codeine
Phenylpropanolamine
NOVAHISTINE DMX*
Dextromethorphan
Guaifenesin
Pseudoephedrine
NOVAHISTINE ELIXIR*
Chlorpheniramine
Phenylpropanolamine
NOVAHISTINE EXPECTORANT*
Chlorpheniramine
Codeine
Guaifenesin
Phenylpropanolamine
NOVAHISTINE FORTIS*
Chlorpheniramine
Phenylephrine
NOVAHISTINE LP*
Chlorpheniramine
Phenylephrine
NOVAHISTINE SINUS*
Chlorpheniramine
Pseudoephedrine
NOVA-KELP
Iodine
NOVAMOR*
Chlorpheniramine
Phenylpropanolamine
NOVAMO-SECOBARB*
Amobarbital
Secobarbital
NOVAMOXIN
Amoxicillin
NOVANTRONE*
Bacitracin
Mitoxantrone
Polymyxin B
NOVA-PHASE
Aspirin
NOVA-PHASE WITH PHENO*
Aspirin
Phenobarbital
NOVA-PHENICOL OPHTHALMIC

Chloramphenicol
NOVA-PHENO
Phenobarbital
NOVA-PRED
Prednisolone
NOVA-RECTAL
Pentobarbital
NOVA-RUBI
Cyanocobalamin
NOVASEN
Aspirin
NOVATRIN
Homatropine
NOVATROPINE
Homatropine
NOVESINE
Benoxinate
NOVOAMPICILLIN
Ampicillin
NOVOBUTAMIDE
Tolbutamide
NOVOBUTAZONE
Phenylbutazone
NOVOCAIN
Propoxycaine
NOVOCAMID
Procainamide
NOVOCHLORHYDRATE
Chloral Hydrate
NOVOCHLOROCAP
Chloramphenicol
NOVOCICLINA
Demeclocycline
NOVO-CIMETINE
Cimetidine
NOVOCLOXIN
Cloxacillin
NOVOCOLCHINE
Colchicine
NOVO-CYCLO
Cyclopentolate
NOVODIAZEPAM
Diazepam
NOVODIGOXIN
Digoxin
NOVODIMENATE
Dimenhydrinate
NOVODIPAM
Diazepam
NOVO-DOPARIL*
Hydrochlorothiazide
Methyldopa
NOVO E
Vitamin E
NOVOFERROGLUC
Ferrous Gluconate
NOVOFERROSULFA
Ferrous Sulfate
NOVOFIBRATE
Clofibrate
NOVO-FLUPAM
Flurazepam
NOVOFLURAZINE
Trifluoperazine
NOVOFOLACID
Folic Acid
NOVOFUMAR
Ferrous Fumarate
NOVOFURAN
Nitrofurantoin
NOVOHEXIDYL
Trihexyphenidyl
NOVOHYDRAZIDE
Hydrochlorothiazide
NOVOHYDROCORT
Hydrocortisone
NOVOMEDOPA
Methyldopa
NOVOMEPRO
Meprobamate
NOVO-METHACIN
Indomethacin
NOVO-MUCILAX
Plantago Seed
NOVONAPROX
Naproxen
NOVONIACIN
Niacin
NOVONIDAZOL
Metronidazole
NOVOPEN
Penicillin G
NOVOPEN-G
Penicillin G
NOVOPEN-V
Penicillin V Potassium
NOVOPEN-V-500
Penicillin V Potassium

NOVOPHENIRAM
  Chlorpheniramine
NOVOPOXIDE
  Chlordiazepoxide
NOVOPRAMINE
  Imipramine
NOVO-PRANOL
  Propranolol
NOVOPROPAMIDE
  Chlorpropamide
NOVOPROPANTHIL
  Propantheline
NOVOPROPOXYN
  Propoxyphene
NOVOPROPOXYN COMPOUND*
  Aspirin
  Caffeine
  Propoxyphene
NOVORIDAZINE
  Thioridazine
NOVORYTHRO
  Erythromycin
NOVOSEMIDE
  Furosemide
NOVOSOXAZOLE
  Sulfisoxazole
NOVO-SPIROTON
  Spironolactone
NOVOTETRA
  Tetracycline
NOVOTHALIDONE
  Chlorthalidone
NOVOTRIAMZIDE*
  Hydrochlorothiazide
  Triamterene
NOVO-TRIAMZIDE*
  Hydrochlorothiazide
  Triamterene
NOVO-TRIMEL
  Co-Trimoxazole
NOVOTRIPTYN
  Amitriptyline
NOVRAD
  Levopropoxyphene
NOZINAN
  Methotrimeprazine
NPH ILETIN
  Insulin [Suspension]
    Isophane
NPH INSULIN
  Insulin [Suspension]
    Isophane
NP-27 CREAM*
  Benzoic Acid
  Hydroxyquinoline
  Salicylic Acid
NP-27 LIQUID*
  Benzoic Acid
  Chlorothymol
  Salicylic Acid
NP-27 POWDER*
  Benzoic Acid
  Salicylic Acid
NP-27 SPRAY POWDER
  Zinc Undecylenate
N-TOIN
  Nitrofurantoin
NTZ
  Phenylephrine
NUBAIN
  Nalbuphine
NUCOFED*
  Codeine
  Pseudoephedrine
NUCOFED PEDIATRIC
    EXPECTORANT*
  Codeine
  Guaifenesin
  Pseudoephedrine
NU-FLOW
  Parachlorometa-
    xylenol
NU-IRON
  Iron
NU-IRON-V*
  Iron
  Vitamins, Multiple
NUITAL
  Etymemazine
NUJOL
  Mineral Oil
NUKLORENE
  Chloramine-T
NULICAINE
  Lidocaine
NUMORPHAN
  Oxymorphone
NUMZIDENT*
  Benzocaine
  Oil of Cloves

Peppermint
NUM-ZIT JEL*
Benzocaine
Menthol
NUPERCAINAL
Dibucaine
NUPERCAINAL SUPPOSITORIES
Dibucaine
NUPERCAINE
Dibucaine
NUPERLONE
Dibucaine
NUPRIN
Ibuprofen
NURAN
Cyproheptadine
NUTRACORT
Hydrocortisone
NUTRAJEL
Aluminum Hydroxide
NUTRAMAG*
Aluminum Oxide
Magnesium Hydroxide
NUTRAPLUS
Urea
NUVAC
Bisacodyl
NUVOLA MEDICATED SHAMPOO
Undecylenic Acid
NYADERM
Nystatin
NYAMIK 15*
Pangamate Calcium
Pangamic Acid
NYCTAL
Carbromal
NYDRAZID
Isoniazid
NYLESTIN
Ethinyl Estradiol
NYQUIL*
Acetaminophen
Doxylamine
Ephedrine
NYQUIL NIGHTTIME COLDS MEDICINE*
Acetaminophen
Dextromethorphan
Doxylamine
Ephedrine
NYSOLONE*
Gramicidin
Neomycin
Nystatin
Triamcinolone
NYSTAFORM-HC*
Hydrocortisone
Iodochlorhydroxyquin
Nystatin
NYSTAFORM OINTMENT*
Iodochlorhydroxyquin
Nystatin
NYTILAX
Senna
NYTOL(CANADA)
Diphenhydramine
NYTOL(U.S.A.)
Methapyrilene

O

O'FLEX
Orphenadrine
OBALAN
Phendimetrazine
OBEDRIN-LA
Methamphetamine
OBEPAR
Phendimetrazine
OBEPHEN
Phentermine
OBERMINE
Phentermine
OBESAMEAD
Phentermine
OBESTAT
Phenylpropanolamine
OBESTIN
Phentermine
OBESTROL
Phendimetrazine
OBETROL*
Amphetamine
Dextroamphetamine
OBEVAL
Phendimetrazine
OBEZINE

Phendimetrazine
O.B. LIQUID
Chloroxylenol
OBOTAN
Dextroamphetamine
OBRON-6
Vitamins, Multiple
OCEAN MIST
Sodium Bicarbonate
OCTIN
Isometheptene
OCTOCAINE
Lidocaine
OCUSERT
Pilocarpine
OCUSERT PILO
Pilocarpine
OCUSOL DROPS
Tetrahydrozoline
ODOR-SCRIP
Methionine
ODRINEX*
Methylcellulose
Phenylpropanolamine
OEDEMIN
Acetazolamide
OESTRILIN
Conjugated Estrogens
OESTRILIN WITH METHYLTESTOSTERONE*
Conjugated Estrogens
Methyltestosterone
OFF-EZY
Salicylic Acid
OGEN
Estropipate
OLICIN
Troleandomycin
OMEX*
Acetaminophen
Phenylpropanolamine
OMNIBEL*
Atropine
Butabarbital
Hyoscyamine
Scopolamine
OMNIBESEL
Phendimetrazine
OMNICOL*
Chlorpheniramine
Dextromethorphan
Phenindamine
Phenylephrine
OMNIGESIC*
Acecarbromal
Acetaminophen
Bromisovalum
OMNIPEN
Ampicillin
OMNIPEN-N
Ampicillin
OMURETIC
Benzthiazide
ONCOVIN
Vincristine
ONDENA
Daunorubicin
ONE-A-DAY
Vitamins, Multiple
ONE-A-DAY PLUS IRON*
Iron
Vitamins, Multiple
ONE-A-DAY VITAMINS PLUS MINERALS*
Minerals, Multiple
Vitamins, Multiple
ONE-ALPHA
Alfacalcidol
ONSET
Isosorbide Dinitrate
OPERAND
Povidone-Iodine
OPERAND DOUCHE
Povidone-Iodine
OPERIDINE
Phenoperidine
OPHTHAINE
Proparacaine
OPHTHALGAN
Glycerin
OPHTHEL-S
Sulfacetamide
OPHTHETIC
Proparacaine
OPHTHOCHLOR
Chloramphenicol
OPHTHOCORT*
Choramphenicol
Hydrocortisone
Polymyxin B

OP-SULFA30
  Sulfacetamide
OPT-EASE
  Tetrahydrozoline
OPTEF
  Hydrocortisone
OPTICROM
  Cromolyn Sodium
OPTIGENE II
  Phenylephrine
OPTILETS-M-500
  Minerals, Multiple
  Vitamins, Multiple
OPTILETS-500
  Vitamins, Multiple
OPTIMINE
  Azatadine
OPTIMYD*
  Prednisolone
  Sulfacetamide
OPTINOXAN
  Methaqualone
OPTISED OPHTHALMIC*
  Phenylephrine
  Zinc Sulfate
OPTOCRYMAL
  Phenylephrine
OPTOMETHASONE
  Dexamethasone
OPTOPENTOLATE
  Cyclopentolate
OPTOPILO
  Pilocarpine
OPTOSULFEX
  Sulfacetamide
OPTOTROPINAL
  Atropine
OPTOZOLINE
  Naphazoline
OPTREX
  Witch Hazel
OPTYN
  Butacaine
OPV
  Poliovirus Vaccine,
    Live Oral
ORABASE HCA
  Cortisol
ORABASE WITH BENZOCAINE
  Benzocaine
ORABILEX
  Bunamiodyl
ORACAINE
  Meprylcaine
ORACIN
  Benzocaine
ORADEX-C*
  Benzocaine
  Cetylpyridinium
ORADRATE
  Chloral Hydrate
ORAFLEX
  Benoxaprofen
ORAGEST
  Medroxyprogesterone
ORAGRAFIN
  Ipodate
ORAHIST*
  Chlorpheniramine
  Phenylpropanolamine
ORA-JEL
  Benzocaine
ORA-LUTIN
  Ethisterone
ORAMIDE
  Tolbutamide
ORAMINIC*
  Atropine
  Chlorpheniramine
ORANIXON
  Mephenesin
ORAP
  Pimozide
ORAPAV TIMECELLES
  Papaverine
ORAPHEN-PD
  Acetaminophen
ORASONE
  Prednisone
ORATESTIN
  Fluoxymesterone
ORA-TESTRYL
  Fluoxymesterone
ORATRAST
  Barium
ORATROL
  Dichlorphenamide
ORAVIRON
  Methyltestosterone
ORAZINC

Zinc Sulfate
ORBENIN
Cloxacillin
ORBINAMON
Thiothixene
ORCHISTERONE-M
Methyltestosterone
ORCHISTERONE-P
Testosterone
ORDIMEL
Acetohexamide
ORENZYME*
Chymotrypsin
Trypsin
ORETIC
Hydrochlorothiazide
ORETICYL*
Deserpidine
Hydrochlorothiazide
ORETON
Testosterone
ORETON BUCCAL
Testosterone
ORETON METHYL
Methyltestosterone
ORETON PELLETS FOR SUBCUTANEOUS IMPLANTATION
Testosterone
ORETON PROPIONATE
Testosterone
OREXIN SOFTABS
Vitamins, Multiple
ORGANIDIN
Iodinated Glycerol
ORGATRAX
Hydroxyzine
ORIGINAL ECLIPSE SUNSCREEN*
Aminobenzoic Acid
Padimate
ORIMETEN
Aminoglutethimide
ORIMUNE
Poliovirus Vaccine, Live Oral
ORINASE
Tolbutamide
ORISUL
Sulfaphenazole
ORLEX H.C. OTIC*
Chloroxylenol
Hydrocortisone
ORLEX OTIC
Chloroxylenol
ORMAZINE
Chlorpromazine
ORNACOL*
Dextromethorphan
Phenylpropanolamine
ORNADE*
Chlorpheniramine
Isopropamide
Phenylpropanolamine
ORNADE 2 LIQUID FOR CHILDREN*
Chlorpheniramine
Phenylpropanolamine
ORNEX*
Acetaminophen
Phenylpropanolamine
OROBRONZE
Canthaxanthine
ORO-NAF
Sodium Fluoride
ORTEGA OTIC M*
Glycerin
Hydrocortisone
Neomycin
Polymyxin B
Propylene Glycol
ORTHO-CREME
Nonoxynol 9
ORTHO DIENESTROL CREAM
Dienestrol
ORTHO-NOVUM*
Mestranol
Norethindrone
ORTHO-NOVUM 10/11*
Ethinyl Estradiol
Norethindrone
ORTHO-NOVUM 7/7/7*
Ethinyl Estradiol
Norethindrone
ORTHOXICOL*
Dextromethorphan
Methoxyphenamine
ORTHOXINE
Methoxyphenamine
OR-TYL

Dicyclomine
ORUDIS
Ketoprofen
OS-CAL*
Calcium Carbonate
Ergocalciferol
OS-CAL FORTE*
Minerals, Multiple
Vitamins, Multiple
OS-CAL-GESIC*
Calcium Carbonate
Ergocalciferol
Salicylamide
OS-CAL PLUS*
Minerals, Multiple
Vitamins, Multiple
OS-CAL 500
Calcium Carbonate
OSMITROL
Mannitol
OSMOGLYN
Glycerin
OSTENSIN
Trimethidinium Methosulfate
OSTOFORTE
Cholecalciferol
OSTOGEN
Cholecalciferol
OSTREX TONIC
Vitamins, Multiple
OTALL EAR DROPS*
Chloroxylenol
Hydrocortisone
Pramoxine
OTETRYN
Oxytetracycline
OTIC DOMEBORO SOLUTION
Aluminum Acetate
OTIC-HC EAR DROPS*
Acetic Acid
Benzalkonium Chloride
Chloroxylenol
Hydrocortisone
Pramoxine
OTIC NEO-CORT-DOME*
Hydrocortisone
Neomycin
OTO*
Antipyrine
Benzocaine
OTOBIOTIC
Neomycin
OTOCORT EAR DROPS*
Antipyrine
Dibucaine
Hydrocortisone
Neomycin
Polymyxin B
OTO-PEDIAT*
Antipyrine
Benzocaine
OTOREID-HC*
Antipyrine
Dibucaine
Glycerin
Hydrocortisone
Neomycin
Polymyxin B
OTRIVIN
Xylometazoline
OVABAN
Megestrol
OVCON*
Ethinyl Estradiol
Norethindrone
OVEST
Conjugated Estrogens
OVOCYLIN
Estradiol
OVOL
Simethicone
OVOL 80
Simethicone
OVRAL*
Ethinyl Estradiol
Norgestrel
OVRETTE
Norgestrel
O-V STATIN
Nystatin
OVULEN*
Ethynodiol
Mestranol
OWS BLUE*
Chlorobutanol
Methylcellulose
OXAINE

Oxethazaine
OXALID
Oxyphenbutazone
OXAMYCIN
Cycloserine
OX BILE EXTRACT
Bile Salts
OXIPOR VHC LOTION FOR PSORIASIS*
Benzocaine
Coal Tar
Salicylic Acid
OXLOPAR
Oxytetracycline
OXOBID
Oxolinic Acid
OXOTHALEIN*
Cascara Sagrada
Phenolphthalein
OXSORALEN
Methoxsalen
OXUCIDE
Piperazine
OXYBUTAZONE
Oxyphenbutazone
OXYCHOLINE
Desoxycholic Acid
OXYDERM
Benzoyl Peroxide
OXYDESS II
Dextroamphetamine
OXYLONE
Fluorometholone
OXYMYCIN
Oxytetracycline
OXYSTAT
Dyphylline
OXY-TETRACHEL
Oxytetracycline
OXY WASH
Benzoyl Peroxide
OXYZAL WEST*
Benzalkonium Chloride
Oxyquinoline
OXY-10
Benzoyl Peroxide
OXY-5
Benzoyl Peroxide

P

PABAGEL
Aminobenzoic Acid
PABA GEL
Aminobenzoic Acid
PABAK
Potassium Aminobenzoate
PABALATE*
Sodium Aminobenzoate
Sodium Salicylate
PABALATE-SF*
Potassium Aminobenzoate
Potassium Salicylate
PABANOL
Aminobenzoic Acid
PABAPLUS
Aminobenzoic Acid
PABIRIN*
Aminobenzoic Acid
Aspirin
PABIZOL WITH PAREGORIC*
Aluminum Magnesium Silicate
Bismuth Subsalicylate
Paregoric
Phenyl Salicylate
Zinc Phenolsulfonate
PAC*
Aspirin
Caffeine
PACADYNE
Povidone-Iodine
PACATAL
Mepazine
P-A-C COMPOUND*
Aspirin
Caffeine
PAC COMPOUND WITH CODEINE*
Aspirin
Caffeine
Codeine
PACKER'S PINE TAR
Pine Tar
PAGITANE

Cycrimine
PAIN & FEVER
Acetaminophen
PALADAC
Vitamins, Multiple
PALADAC WITH MINERALS*
Minerals, Multiple
Vitamins, Multiple
PALAFER
Ferrous Fumarate
PALARON
Aminophylline
PALBAR NO. 2*
Atropine
Butabarbital
Hyoscyamine
Scopolamine
PALLACE
Megestrol
PALMIRON
Ferrous Fumarate
PALMIRON-C*
Ascorbic Acid
Ferrous Fumarate
PALOCILLIN
Penicillin G
PALOHEX
Inositol Niacinate
PALS
Vitamins, Multiple
PALS WITH IRON
Iron
Vitamins, Multiple
PALTET
Tetracycline
PALUDRINE
Chloroguanide
PAMA*
Aluminum Hydroxide
Magnesium Trisilicate
PAMELOR
Nortriptyline
PAMINE
Methscopolamine
PAMISYL
Aminosalicylic Acid
PAMISYL SODIUM
Aminosalicylate
PAMOVIN
Pyrvinium Pamoate
PAMPRIN*
Acetaminophen
Pamabrom
Pyrilamine
PANADOL
Acetaminophen
PANADOL WITH CODEINE*
Acetaminophen
Codeine
PANADYL*
Pheniramine
Phenylpropanolamine
Pyrilamine
PANAFIL OINTMENT*
Papain
Urea
PANAFIL-WHITE OINTMENT*
Papain
Urea
PANALGESIC*
Aspirin
Camphor
Menthol
Methyl Salicylate
PANAMIN
Acetaminophen
PANAZID
Isoniazid
PANAZYME DIGESTANT
Pepsin
PAN-CLORIDE
Potassium Chloride
PANCREASE
Pancrelipase
PANECTYL
Trimeprazine
PANELEX*
Acetaminophen
Carbromal
PANEX
Acetaminophen
PANHEMATIN
Hemin
PANHEPRIN
Heparin
PANITOL*
Acetaminophen

Butalbital
PANMYCIN
Tetracycline
PANODYNES ANALGESIC*
Acetaminophen
Aspirin
Caffeine
Salicylamide
PANOL
Dexpanthenol
PANOXYL
Benzoyl Peroxide
PANPARNIT
Caramiphen
PANRITIS*
Acetaminophen
Salicylamide
PANSCOL*
Lactic Acid
Phenol
Salicylic Acid
PANTERIC
Pancreatin
PANTHODERM
Panthenol
PANTOFENICOL
Chloramphenicol
PANTOPON
Opium
PANWARFIN
Warfarin
PANZYME*
Homatropine
Hyoscyamine
Pancreatin
Pepsin
Phenobarbital
Scopolamine
PAPACON
Papaverine
PAR*
Allantoin
Aminacrine
Sulfanilamide
PARACODIN
Drocode
PARACORT
Prednisone
PARACORTOL
Prednisolone
PARADIONE
Paramethadione
PARAFLEX
Chlorzoxazone
PARAFON FORTE*
Acetaminophen
Chlorzoxazone
PARALGIN
Acetaminophen
PARAMINYL
Pyrilamine
PARASAL
Aminosalicylate
PARASULE
Papaverine
PARA-THOR-MONE
Parathyroid
PARAZINE
Piperazine
PARBOCYL-REV
Sodium Salicylate
PAREDRINE
Hydroxyamphetamine
PARELIXIR*
Opium
Pectin
PARENOGEN
Fibrinogen
PARENZYME
Trypsin
PARENZYMOL
Trypsin
PAREPECTOLIN*
Kaolin
Paregoric
Pectin
PAREST
Methaqualone
PARFENAC
Bufexamac
PARFURAN
Nitrofurantoin
PARGEL*
Kaolin
Pectin
PARGESIC 65
Propoxyphene
PARKEMED
Mefenamic Acid
PARLODEL

Bromocriptine
PAR-MAG
Magnesium Oxide
PARMINE
Phentermine
PARNATE
Tranylcypromine
PAROIDIN
Parathyroid
PARPANIT
Caramiphen
PARSIDOL
Ethopropazine
PARSITAN
Ethopropazine
PARTIAL ECLIPSE SUNTAN*
Padimate
PARTUSISTEN
Fenoterol
PAR-VAG*
Allantoin
Aminacrine
Sulfanilamide
PAS DEPRESS
Hydroxyzine
PASDIUM
Aminosalicylate
PASEM SODIUM
Aminosalicylate
PASMIN
Dicyclomine
PATHIBAMATE*
Meprobamate
Tridihexethyl
PATHILON
Tridihexethyl
PATHOCIL
Dicloxacillin
PAVABID HP
Papaverine
PAVABID PLATEAU CAPS
Papaverine
PAVACAP UNICELLES
Papaverine
PAVACEN
Papaverine
PAVADUR
Papaverine
PAVADYL
Papaverine
PAVAGEN
Papaverine
PAVAKEY
Papaverine
PAVA-MEAD T.D.
Papaverine
PAVA PAR
Papaverine
PAVA RX
Papaverine
PAVATRAN TD
Papaverine
PAVATYM
Papaverine
PAVERAL
Codeine
PAVERIL
Dioxyline
PAVERINE SPANCAPS
Papaverine
PAVEROLAN LANACAPS
Papaverine
PAVERONE
Dioxyline
PAVULON
Pancuronium
PAXAREL
Acecarbromal
PAXEL
Diazepam
PAXIPAM
Halazepam
PAZO HEMORRHOID*
Benzocaine
Camphor
Ephedrine
PBZ
Tripelennamine
PBZ EXPECTORANT W/EPHEDRINE*
Ammonium Chloride
Ephedrine
Tripelennamine
PBZ LONTABS
Tripelennamine
PBZ-SR
Tripelennamine
PBZ WITH EPHEDRINE*
Ephedrine

Tripelennamine
PDM
Phendimetrazine
PECTAMOL
Oxeladin
PECTO-KALIN*
Kaolin
Paregoric
Pectin
PEDAMETH
Racemethionine
PEDIACOF*
Chlorpheniramine
Codeine
Phenylephrine
Potassium Iodide
PEDIAFLUR
Sodium Fluoride
PEDIALYTE
Electrolytes, Multiple
PEDIAMYCIN
Erythromycin
PEDIAPHEN
Acetaminophen
PEDIAQUILL*
Guaifenesin
Phenylephrine
PEDIAZOLE*
Erythromycin Ethylsuccinate
Sulfisoxazole
PEDI-BORO
Aluminum Acetate
PEDI-CORT V*
Hydrocortisone
Iodochlorhydroxyquin
PEDI-DENT
Sodium Fluoride
PEDI-VIT A
Vitamin A
PEDRIC
Acetaminophen
PEGANONE
Ethotoin
PEKTAMALT*
Kaolin
Pectin
PENALEV
Penicillin G
PENAMOX
Amoxicillin
PEN A ORAL
Ampicillin
PENAPAR
Penicillin V Potassium
PENAPAR VK
Penicillin V Potassium
PENBEC-V
Penicillin V Potassium
PENBRISTOL
Ampicillin
PENBRITIN
Ampicillin
PENBROCK
Ampicillin
PENCITABS
Penicillin G
PENETRA
Pentaerythritol Tetranitrate
PENIDURAL
Penicillin G
PENIORAL-500
Penicillin G
PENISEM
Penicillin G
PENISTAPH
Methicillin
PENNPHENO*
Pentaerythritol Tetranitrate
Phenobarbital
PENPLENUM
Hetacillin
PENSIVE
Meprobamate
PENSTAPHO
Oxacillin
PENSYN
Ampicillin
PENTAFIN
Pentaerythritol Tetranitrate
PENTALAX
Bisacodyl
PENTAMYCETIN

Chloramphenicol
PENTANCA
Pentobarbital
PENTAZIN
Pentazocine
PENTAZINE
Trifluoperazine
PENTAZYME*
Cellulose
Ox Bile Extract
Pancreatin
Pepsin
PENTESTAN
Pentaerythritol Tetranitrate
PENTHRANE
Methoxyflurane
PENTIDS
Penicillin G
PENTOGEN
Pentobarbital
PENTOSTAM
Stibogluconate
PENTOTHAL
Thiopental
PENTRAX TAR SHAMPOO
Coal Tar
PENTRAZOL
Pentylenetetrazol
PENTRITOL
Pentaerythritol Tetranitrate
PENTRIUM*
Chlordiazepoxide
Pentaerythritol Tetranitrate
PENTRYATE
Pentaerythritol Tetranitrate
PENTUSS*
Chlorpheniramine
Codeine
PENTYLAN WITH PHENOBARBITAL*
Pentaerythritol Tetranitrate
Phenobarbital
PEN-VEE
Penicillin V
PEN-VEE K
Penicillin V Potassium
PEN VK
Penicillin V Potassium
PEPTAVLON
Pentagastrin
PEPTO-BISMOL*
Bismuth Subsalicylate
Calcium Carbonate
PEPTO BISMOL LIQUID
Bismuth Subsalicylate
PEPTOL
Cimetidine
PERANDREN
Testosterone
PERAZIL
Chlorcyclizine
PERCHLORACAP
Potassium Perchlorate
PERCOBARB*
Aspirin
Caffeine
Hexobarbital
Oxycodone
PERCOCET*
Acetaminophen
Oxycodone
PERCOCET-DEMI*
Acetaminophen
Oxycodone
PERCOCET-5*
Acetaminophen
Oxycodone
PERCODAN*
Aspirin
Caffeine
Oxycodone
PERCODAN-DEMI*
Aspirin
Caffeine
Oxycodone
PERCOGESIC*
Acetaminophen
Phenyltoloxamine
PERCORTEN
Desoxycorticosterone

PERCORTEN ACETATE
  Desoxycorticosterone
PERCY MEDICINE*
  Bismuth Subnitrate
  Calcium Hydroxide
PERDIEM*
  Plantago Seed
  Senna
PERDIEM PLAIN
  Plantago Seed
PERDILATAL
  Nylidrin
PERGONAL
  Menotropins
PERIACTIN
  Cyproheptadine
PERI-COLACE*
  Casanthranol
  Docusate Sodium
PERI-CONATE*
  Casanthranol
  Docusate Sodium
PERIDIN-C*
  Ascorbic Acid
  Rutin
PERI-DOSS*
  Casanthranol
  Docusate Sodium
PERIFOAM*
  Allantoin
  Benzalkonium
    Chloride
  Lanolin
  Pramoxine
PERIHEMIN*
  Ascorbic Acid
  Cyanocobalamin
  Ferrous Fumarate
  Folic Acid
  Intrinsic Factor
PERIN
  Piperazine
PERIO CAL-D*
  Calcium Phosphate
  Ergocalciferol
PERIOLAV
  Carbamide Peroxide
PERISTIM FORTE
  Casanthranol
PERITINIC
  Vitamins, Multiple
PERITRATE
  Pentaerythritol
    Tetranitrate
PERITRATE WITH
    PHENOBARBITAL*
  Pentaerythritol
    Tetranitrate
  Phenobarbital
PERMAPEN
  Penicillin G
    Benzathine
PERMATHENE H2OFF*
  Ammonium Chloride
  Caffeine
PERMATHENE-12*
  Caffeine
  Phenylpropanolamine
PERMITIL
  Fluphenazine
PERNOX*
  Salicylic Acid
  Sulfur
PEROIDIN
  Potassium
    Perchlorate
PEROXYL
  Hydrogen Peroxide
PERSADOX
  Benzoyl Peroxide
PERSA-GEL
  Benzoyl Peroxide
PERSANTINE
  Dipyridamole
PERSISTIN*
  Aspirin
  Salsalate
PERSO-GEL
  Benzoyl Peroxide
PERTOFRANE
  Desipramine
PERTUSSIN
  Dextromethorphan
PERTUSSIN COUGH FOR
    CHILDREN*
  Dextromethorphan
  Guaifenesin
PERTUSSIN 8-HOUR COUGH
    FORMULA
  Dextromethorphan
PERVADIL
  Nylidrin

PETINIMID
  Ethosuximide
PETINUTIN
  Methsuximide
PETROGALAR*
  Cascara Sagrada
  Mineral Oil
  Phenolphthalein
PETRO-SYLLIUM NO. 1 PLAIN*
  Mineral Oil
  Plantago Seed
PETRO-SYLLIUM NO. 2 WITH PHENOLPHTHALEIN*
  Mineral Oil
  Phenolphthalein
  Plantago Seed
PEVARYL
  Econazole
PFIKLOR
  Potassium Chloride
PFI-LITHIUM
  Lithium Carbonate
PFIZER-E
  Erythromycin Stearate
PFIZER-E FILM COATED
  Erythromycin
PFIZERPEN-A
  Ampicillin
PFIZERPEN-AS
  Penicillin G Procaine
PFIZERPEN G
  Penicillin G
PFIZERPEN VK
  Penicillin V Potassium
P.G.A.
  Penicillin G
PHANODORN
  Cyclobarbital
PHARMACIN
  Aspirin
PHARMA-CORT
  Hydrocortisone
PHARMA C-500
  Ascorbic Acid
PHARMADINE
  Povidone-Iodine
PHARMALGEN
  Hymenopter Venom Extract
PHAZYME*
  Amylase
  Lipase
  Protease
  Simethicone
PHAZYME-PB*
  Amylase
  Lipase
  Phenobarbital
  Protease
  Simethicone
PHAZYME-95*
  Amylase
  Lipase
  Protease
  Simethicone
PHEDRAL*
  Ephedrine
  Phenobarbital
  Theophylline
PHEMEROL
  Benzethonium Chloride
PHEMITONE
  Mephobarbital
PHENACODEIN 002*
  Aspirin
  Caffeine
  Codeine
PHENACODEIN 003*
  Aspirin
  Caffeine
  Codeine
PHEN-AMIN
  Diphenhydramine
PHENANTOIN
  Mephenytoin
PHEN APAP*
  Acetaminophen
  Phenylpropanolamine
PHENAPHEN
  Acetaminophen
PHENAPHEN WITH CODEINE*
  Acetaminophen
  Codeine
PHENAPHEN-650 WITH CODEINE*

Acetaminophen
Codeine
PHENATAPP EXTEND*
Brompheniramine
Phenylephrine
Phenylpropanolamine
PHENATE*
Acetaminophen
Chlorpheniramine
Phenylpropanolamine
PHENAZINE
Perphenazine
PHENAZO
Phenazopyridine
PHENBUTAZONE
Phenylbutazone
PHENCEN
Promethazine
PHENDIMEAD
Phendimetrazine
PHENERGAN
Promethazine
PHENERGAN D*
Promethazine
Pseudoephedrine
PHENETRON
Chlorpheniramine
PHENETRON LANACAPS
Chlorpheniramine
PHENHIST ELIXIR*
Chlorpheniramine
Phenylpropanolamine
PHEN-LETS
Phenylpropanolamine
PHENO-BELLA*
Belladonna
Phenobarbital
PHENOJECT-50
Promethazine
PHENOLAX
Phenolphthalein
PHENONYL
Phenobarbital
PHENOPTIC
Phenylephrine
PHENO-SQUAR
Phenobarbital
PHENOXALID
Aconiazide
PHENOXENE
Chlorphenoxamine
PHENTERMYL
Phentermine
PHENTROL
Phentermine
PHENURONE
Phenacemide
PHENYGENINE
Phenylsemicarbazide
PHENYLGESIC*
Acetaminophen
Phenyltoloxamine
PHENYLZIN*
Phenylephrine
Zinc Sulfate
PHENY-PAS-TEBAMIN
Phenyl Aminosalicylate
PHENZINE
Phendimetrazine
PHERMINE
Phentermine
PHILLIP'S MILK OF MAGNESIA*
Magnesium Hydroxide
Magnesium Oxide
PHISOAC*
Resorcinol
Sulfur
PHISOCARE
Entsufon
PHISODAN*
Sodium Salicylate
Sulfur
PHISODERM
Entsufon
PHISOHEX
Hexachlorophene
PHISOLAN
Entsufon
PHISO SCRUB
Hexachlorophene
PHOS-FLUR
Sodium Fluoride
PHOS-FLUR ORAL RINSE/SUPPLEMENT
Sodium Fluoride
PHOS-PHAID*
Ammonium Biphosphate

Sodium Acid
Pyrophosphate
Sodium Biphosphate
PHOSPHALJEL
Aluminum Phosphate
PHOSPHOCOL P32
Chromic Phosphate
PHOSPHOLINE IODIDE
Echothiophate Iodide
PHOSPHO-SODA*
Sodium Biphosphate
Sodium Phosphate
PHOSPHOTAPE
Sodium Phosphate
PHRENILAN FORTE*
Aspirin
Butalbital
PHRENILIN*
Acetaminophen
Butabarbital
Caffeine
P-HV FORTE
Isoniazid
PHYLDROX
Aminophylline
PHYLLOCONTIN
Aminophylline
PHYSEPTONE
Methadone
PHYSPAN
Theophylline
PHYTADON
Meperidine
PHYTOFEROL
Vitamin E
PIGMEX
Monobenzone
PIL-DIGIS
Digitalis
PILOCAR*
Benzalkonium
Chloride
Pilocarpine
PILOCEL OPH
Pilocarpine
PILOMIOTIN
Pilocarpine
PILOPTIC
Pilocarpine
PILOVISC
Pilocarpine
PIMA
Potassium Iodide
PINCETS
Piperazine
PINEX
Potassium
Guaiacolsulfonate
PINEX WILD CHERRY
Ammonium Chloride
PINKAMIN
Cyanocobalamin
PINSIRUP
Piperazine
PIOXOL
Pemoline
PIPADONE
Dipipanone
PIPANOL
Trihexyphenidyl
PIPRACIL
Piperacillin
PIPTAL
Pipenzolate
PIPTEL
Pipenzolate
PIRACAPS
Tetracycline
PIRITON
Chlorpheniramine
PISEC
Sulfur
PITOCIN
Oxytocin
PITRESSIN
Vasopressin
PITRESSIN TANNATE IN
OIL
Vasopressin
PITREX
Tolnaftate
PITUITRIN
Pituitary, Posterior
PLACIDYL
Ethchlorvynol
PLANOFORM
Butamben
PLAQUENIL
Hydroxychloroquine
PLATINOL

Cisplatin
PLEASANT RELIEF
Bismuth
Subsalicylate
PLEGINE
Phendimetrazine
PLEOCIDE
Nithiamide
PLEXONAL*
Barbital
Butalbital
Dihydroergotamine
Phenobarbital
Scopolamine
PLIACIDE
Iodine
PLOVA*
Dextrose
Plantago Seed
PMB 200
Chlorotrianisene
PMB-400
Meprobamate
PNEUMOVAX
Polyvalent
Pneumococcal
Vaccine
PNEUMOVAX 23
Polyvalent
Pneumococcal
Vaccine
PNU-IMUNE
Polyvalent
Pneumococcal
Vaccine
PNU-IMUNE 23
Pneumococcal Vaccine
PODIASPRAY*
Chloroxylenol
Salicylic Acid
Undecylenic Acid
PODOBEN
Podophyllum Resin
POINT-TWO DENTAL RINSE
Sodium Fluoride
POLARAMIME
EXPECTORANT*
Dexchlorpheniramine
Guaifenesin
Pseudoephedrine
POLARAMINE
Dexchlorpheniramine
POLARONIL
Chlorpheniramine
POLYBRENE
Hexadimethrine
POLYCILLIN
Ampicillin
POLYCILLIN-N FOR
INJECTION
Ampicillin
POLYCILLIN-PRB*
Ampicillin
Probenecid
POLYCITRA*
Citric Acid
Potassium Citrate
Sodium Citrate
POLYCITRA-K*
Citric Acid
Potassium Citrate
POLYCITRA-LC--SUGAR-
FREE*
Citric Acid
Potassium Citrate
Sodium Citrate
POLYCYCLINE
Tetracycline
POLYDINE
Povidone-Iodine
POLY-HISTINE-D*
Pheniramine
Phenylpropanolamine
Phenyltoloxamine
Pyrilamine
Tripelennamine
POLY-HISTINE-D ELIXIR*
Pheniramine
Phenylpropanolamine
Phenyltoloxamine
Pyrilamine
Tripelennamine
POLY-HISTINE-DX*
Brompheniramine
Pseudoephedrine
POLY-HISTINE
EXPECTORANT PLAIN*
Brompheniramine
Phenylpropanolamine
Potassium
Guaiacolsulfonate

POLY-HISTINE EXPECTORANT WITH CODEINE*
  Brompheniramine
  Codeine
  Phenylpropanolamine
  Potassium Guaiacolsulfonate
POLYKOL
  Poloxamer 188
POLYMAGMA PLAIN*
  Aluminum
  Attapulgite
  Pectin
POLYMOX
  Amoxicillin
POLY-PRED DROPS*
  Neomycin
  Polymyxin B
  Prednisolone
POLYSPECTRIN OPHTHALMIC*
  Neomycin
  Polymyxin B
POLYSPORIN*
  Gramicidin
  Polymyxin B
POLYSPORIN OPHTHALMIC*
  Bacitracin
  Polymyxin B
POLYTAR*
  Coal Tar
  Crude Coal Tar
  Juniper Tar
  Pine Tar
POLY-VI-FLOR*
  Fluoride
  Vitamins, Multiple
POLY-VI-FLOR WITH IRON*
  Fluoride
  Iron
  Vitamins, Multiple
POLY-VI-SOL
  Vitamins, Multiple
POLY-VI-SOL WITH IRON*
  Iron
  Vitamins, Multiple
PONDERAL
  Fenfluramine
PONDERAX
  Fenfluramine
PONDIMIN
  Fenfluramine
PONECIL
  Ampicillin
PONSTAN
  Mefenamic Acid
PONSTEL
  Mefenamic Acid
PONTOCAINE
  Tetracaine
POQUIL
  Pyrvinium Pamoate
PORCELANE
  Hydroquinone
POSSIPIONE
  Paroxypropione
POSTACNE LOTION
  Sulfur
POTABA
  Potassium Aminobenzoate
POTAGE
  Potassium Chloride
POTASSIUM ROUGIER
  Potassium Gluconate
POTASSIUM TRIPLEX*
  Potassium Acetate
  Potassium Bicarbonate
  Potassium Citrate
POVAN
  Pyrvinium Pamoate
POYAMIN
  Cyanocobalamin
PRAGMATAR*
  Coal Tar
  Salicylic Acid
  Sulfur
PRAMET FA*
  Minerals, Multiple
  Vitamins, Multiple
PRAMILET FA*
  Minerals, Multiple
  Vitamins, Multiple
PRAMINIL
  Imipramine
PRAMOSONE
  Hydrocortisone
PRANONE
  Ethisterone
PRANTAL

Diphemanil
PRANTURON
Gonadotropin, Chorionic
PRAXITEN
Oxazepam
PREDATE-L.A.S.A.
Prednisolone
PREDATE-100
Prednisolone
PRE-DEP-40
Methylprednisolone
PRE-DEP-80
Methylprednisolone
PRED FORTE
Prednisolone
PRED MILD
Prednisolone
PREDNE-DOME
Prednisolone
PREDNICON
Prednisolone
PREDNIS
Prednisolone
PREDOXINE
Prednisolone
PREDULOSE
Prednisolone
PREFRIN
Phenylephrine
PREFRIN-A*
Phenylephrine
Pyrilamine
PREFRIN LIQUIFILM
Phenylephrine
PREFRIN Z
Phenylephrine
PREGNESIN
Gonadotropin, Chorionic
PREGNYL
Gonadotropin, Chorionic
PRELUDIN
Phenmetrazine
PRELU-2
Phendimetrazine
PRE-MAR
Ritodrine
PREMARIN
Estrogens, Conjugated
PREMARIN WITH M.T.*
Conjugated Estrogens
Methyltestosterone
PREMARIN W/ METHYLTESTOSTERONE*
Estrogens, Conjugated
Methyltestosterone
PRE-MENS FORTE*
Ammonium Chloride
Caffeine
PREMESYN PMS*
Acetaminophen
Pamabrom
Pyrilamine
PRENOMISER FORTE
Isoproterenol
PRE-PEN
Benzylpenicilloyl Polylysine
PRESALINE*
Acetaminophen
Aluminum Hydroxide
Aspirin
Salicylamide
PRESAMINE
Imipramine
PRE-SATE
Chlorphentermine
PRE-SERT*
Benzalkonium Chloride
Polyvinyl alcohol
PRESINOL
Methyldopa
PRESSIMMUNE
Antihuman Lymphocyte Globulin
PRESSONEX
Metaraminol
PRESSORAL
Metaraminol
PRESUN
Aminobenzoic Acid
PRESUN 15*
Aminobenzoic Acid
Oxybenzone
Padimate

PREVARYL
  Econazole
PREVENAUSE
  Dimenhydrinate
PRIADEL
  Lithium Carbonate
PRIAMIDE
  Isopropamide
PRIMACAINE
  Metabutoxycaine
PRIMADENT
  Sodium Fluoride
PRIMATENE M*
  Ephedrine
  Pyrilamine
  Theophylline
PRIMATENE MIST
  Epinephrine
PRIMATENE P*
  Ephedrine
  Phenobarbital
  Theophylline
PRIMOLINE
  Primidone
PRIMPERAN
  Metoclopramide
PRINADOL
  Phenazocine
PRINCIPEN
  Ampicillin
PRINCIPEN WITH PROBENECID*
  Ampicillin
  Probenecid
PRIN V/S
  Diethylstilbestrol
PRIODAX
  Iodoalphionic Acid
PRIODERM
  Malathion
PRISCOLINE
  Tolazoline
PRIVINE
  Naphazoline
PRO-ACTIDIL
  Triprolidine
PROAQUA
  Benzthiazide
PROBACON*
  Atropine
  Chlorpheniramine
  Phenylpropanolamine
PROBACON II*
  Chlorpheniramine
  Isopropamide
  Phenylpropanolamine
PROBAL
  Meprobamate
PROBALAN
  Probenecid
PROBAMPACIN*
  Ampicillin
  Probenecid
PRO-BANTHINE
  Propantheline
PRO-BANTHINE WITH PHENOBARBITAL*
  Phenobarbital
  Propantheline
PROBEC-T
  Vitamins, Multiple
PROBENICILLIN*
  Ampicillin
  Probenecid
PROBILAGOL
  Homatropine
PRO-BIOSAN 500 KIT*
  Ampicillin
  Probenecid
PRO-CAL-SOF
  Docusate Calcium
PROCAN SR
  Procainamide
PROCARDIA
  Nifedipine
PROCHLOR-ISO*
  Isopropamide
  Prochlorperazine
PROCHOLON
  Dehydrocholic Acid
PROCOLIN*
  Glycerin
  Phenol
  Procaine
PRO-CORT M
  Hydrocortisone
PROCTOCORT
  Hydrocortisone
PROCTODON*
  Cholecalciferol

Diperodon
Vitamin A
PROCTOFOAM-HC
Hydrocortisone
PROCTOFOAM/NON-STEROID
Pramoxine
PROCYCLID
Procyclidine
PROCYTOX
Cyclophosphamide
PRO-DAX
Phenylpropanolamine
PRO-DEPO
Hydroxyprogesterone
PRODEXIN
Dihydroxyaluminum Aminoacetate
PRODIEM*
Plantago Seed
Senna
PRODIEM PLAIN
Plantago Seed
PRODOXAN
Ethisterone
PROFAC-O
Progesterone
PROFASI
Gonadotropin, Chorionic
PROFENIL
Alverine
PROFERDEX
Iron Dextran
PROFILATE
Antihemophilic Factor
PROFILININE
Factor IV complex
PROGELAN
Progesterone
PROGESIC
Propoxyphene
PROGESTAB
Ethisterone
PROGESTAJECT-50
Progesterone
PROGESTASERT
Progesterone
PROGESTEROL
Progesterone
PROGESTILIN
Progesterone
PROGESTIN
Progesterone
PROGESTORAL
Ethisterone
PROGLYCEM
Diazoxide
PROGYNON
Estradiol
PROGYNON B
Estradiol
PROGYNOVA
Estradiol
PRO-ISO*
Isopropamide
Prochlorperazine
PROKETAZINE
Carphenazine
PROKLAR
Sulfamethizole
PROLACTIN
Bromocriptine
PROLADONE
Oxycodone
PROLAMINE
Phenylpropanolamine
PROLENS*
Benzalkonium Chloride
Methylcellulose
Polyvinyl Alcohol
PROLIXIN
Fluphenazine
PROLOID
Thyroglobulin
PROLOPA*
Benserazide
Levodopa
PROLOPRIM
Trimethoprim
PROLUTON
Progesterone
PROMABEC
Promazine
PROMACETIN
Acetosulfone
PROMACHEL
Chlorpromazine
PROMANI

Triclosan
PROMANYL
Promazine
PROMAPAR
Chlorpromazine
PROMAQUID
Fonazine
PROMATUSSIN DM*
Dextromethorphan
Promethazine
Pseudoephedrine
PROMAZ
Chlorpromazine
PROMAZETTES
Promazine
PROMETH 25
Promethazine
PROMIN
Glucosulfone
PROMINAL
Mephobarbital
PROMOSOL
Chlorpromazine
PROMPT*
Plantago Seed
Sennosides A and B
PROMWILL
Promazine
PRONAPEN
Penicillin G
PRONEMIA*
Ascorbic Acid
Cyanocobalamin
Ferrous Fumarate
Folic Acid
Intrinsic Factor
PRONESTYL
Procainamide
PRONESTYL SR
Procainamide
PRONIDIN
Phentermine
PRONTYLIN
Sulfanilamide
PROPACIL
Propylthiouracil
PROPADERM
Beclomethasone
PROPADERM C*
Beclomethasone
Clioquinol
PROPADRINE
Phenylpropanolamine
PROPANTHEL
Propantheline
PROPA P.H. ACNE
Benzoyl Peroxide
PROPASA
Aminosalicylic Acid
PROPINE
Dipivefrin
PROPLEX
Factor IV complex
PROPRADERM
Beclomethasone
PROPYL-THYRACIL
Propylthiouracil
PROREX
Promethazine
PROSED*
Atropine
Benzoic Acid
Hyoscyamine
Methenamine
Methylene Blue
Salicylate
PROSTAPHLIN
Oxacillin
PROSTIGMIN
Neostigmine
PROSTIGMIN BROMIDE
Neostigmine
PROSTIN
Carboprost
PROSTIN E2
Dinoprostone
PROSTIN VR
Alprostadil
PROTACTYL
Promazine
PROTALBA
Protoveratrine A
PROTAMINE, ZINC & ILETIN
Insulin Protamine Zinc
PRO-TAN
Promazine
PROTAPHANE, HUMAN
Insulin Isophane, Human

PROTAPHANE MC
  Insulin Isophane
PROTAPHANE NPH INSULIN
  Insulin [Suspension]
    Isophane
PROTERNOL
  Isoproterenol
PROTHAZINE
  Promethazine
PROTHAZINE
    EXPECTORANT*
  Phenylpropanolamine
  Potassium
    Guaiacolsulfonate
  Pseudoephedrine
PROTIVAR
  Oxandrolone
PROTONA
  Stanolone
PROTOPAM
  Pralidoxime
PROTOPHYLLINE
  Dyphylline
PROTOSTAT
  Metronidazole
PROVENTIL
  Albuterol
PROVERA
  Medroxyprogesterone
PROVIGAN
  Promethazine
PROVIODINE
  Povidone-Iodine
PROV-U-SEP
  Methenamine
    Mandelate
PROXAGESIC
  Propoxyphene
PROXIGEL
  Carbamide Peroxide
PROZINE
  Promazine
PRO-65
  Propoxyphene
PRULET
  Phenolphthalein
PRULET LIQUITAB
  Phenolphthalein
PRUNICODEINE*
  Codeine
  Terpin Hydrate
PSEUDO-BID*
  Guaifenesin
  Pseudoephedrine
PSEUDODINE*
  Pseudoephedrine
  Triprolidine
PSEUDOFRIN
  Pseudoephedrine
PSEUDO-HIST*
  Chlorpheniramine
  Pseudoephedrine
PSEUDO-HIST
    EXPECTORANT*
  Chlorpheniramine
  Guaifenesin
  Hydrocodone
  Pseudoephedrine
PSEUDO-MAL*
  Dexbrompheniramine
  Pseudoephedrine
PSICOPAX
  Lorazepam
PSI-IV
  Prednisolone
PSOREX MEDICATED
  Coal Tar
PSORIACIDE
  Anthralin
PSORIGEL
  Coal Tar
P&S SHAMPOO*
  Lactic Acid
  Salicylic Acid
PSYCHOZINE
  Chlorpromazine
PSYQUIL 25
  Triflupromazine
P.T.-300
  Papaverine
PUREBROM*
  Brompheniramine
  Phenylephrine
  Phenylpropanolamine
PURETANE
  Brompheniramine
PURETANE DC
    EXPECTORANT
  Brompheniramine
PURETANE EXPECTORANT

Brompheniramine
PURETAPP ELIXIR*
Brompheniramine
Phenylephrine
Phenylpropanolamine
PURETAPP PA*
Brompheniramine
Phenylephrine
Phenylpropanolamine
PURGE
Castor Oil
PURINETHOL
Mercaptopurine
PURINOL
Allopurinol
PURODIGIN
Digitoxin
P.V. CARBACHOL
Carbachol
P.V. CARPINE
Pilocarpine
PVF
Penicillin V Potassium
PVF K
Penicillin V Potassium
P.V.M. APPETITE CONTROL
Phenylpropanolamine
P.V.M. APPETITE SUPPRESSANT
Phenylpropanolamine
PVP-IODINE
Povidone-Iodine
P-V TUSSIN*
Guaifenesin
Hydrocodone
Phenindamine
PYCAZIDE
Isoniazid
PYELOSIL
Iodopyracet
PYLORA*
Atropine
Hyoscyamine
Phenobarbital
Scopolamine
PYMA
Pyrilamine
PYMAFED
Pyrilamine
PYOCIDIN*
Neomycin
Polymyxin B
PYOCIDIN-OTIC*
Hydrocortisone
Polymyxin B
PYOPEN
Carbenicillin
PYRACORT-D
Phenylephrine
PYRAMAL
Pyrilamine
PYRA-MALEATE
Pyrilamine
PYRATHYN
Methapyrilene
PYRIBENZAMINE
Tripelennamine
PYRIDIATE
Phenazopyridine
PYRIDIUM
Phenazopyridine
PYRIDIUM PLUS*
Butabarbital
Hyoscyamine
Phenazopyridine
PYRIZIDIN
Isoniazid
PYRIZIL
Tripelennamine
PYRONIL
Pyrrobutamine
PYR-PAM
Pyrvinium Pamoate
PYRRALAN EXPECTORANT*
Ammonium Chloride
Chlorpheniramine
Dextromethorphan
Ephedrine
PYRROXATE*
Aspirin
Chlorpheniramine
Methoxyphenamine
PZI
Insulin [Suspension] Protamine Zinc
P1E1*
Epinephrine
Pilocarpine

P2E1*
Epinephrine
Pilocarpine
P-200
Papaverine
P3E1*
Epinephrine
Pilocarpine
P4E1*
Epinephrine
Pilocarpine
P-50
Penicillin G
P6E1*
Epinephrine
Pilocarpine

Q

QIDAMP
Ampicillin
QM-260
Quinine
QUAALUDE
Methaqualone
QUAALUDE-300
Methaqualone
QUADRA-HIST*
Chlorpheniramine
Phenylephrine
Phenylpropanolamine
Phenyltoloxamine
QUADRINAL*
Ephedrine
Phenobarbital
Potassium Iodide
Theophylline
QUANTRIL
Benzquinamide
QUARZAN
Clidinium
QUELICIN
Succinylcholine
QUELIDRINE*
Ammonium Chloride
Chlorpheniramine
Dextromethorphan
Ephedrine
Ipecac Fluidextract
Phenylephrine
QUELTUSS*
Dextromethorphan
Guaifenesin
QUESTRAN
Cholestyramine Resin
QUIACTIN
Oxanamide
QUIAGEL*
Atropine
Hyoscyamine
Kaolin
Pectin
Scopolamine
QUIAGEL PG*
Atropine
Hyoscyamine
Kaolin
Opium
Pectin
Scopolamine
QUIBRON*
Guaifenesin
Theophylline
QUIBRON PLUS*
Butabarbital
Ephedrine
Guaifenesin
Theophylline
QUICK-PEP
Caffeine
QUIDE
Piperacetazine
QUIDPEN G
Penicillin G
QUIDTET
Tetracycline
QUIESS
Hydroxyzine
QUIETAL
Meprobamate
QUIET-NITE*
Chlorpheniramine
Dextromethorphan
Ephedrine
QUIET WORLD*
Acetaminophen
Aspirin
Pyrilamine
QUILENE

Pentapiperide
Methylsulfate
QUIMOTRASE
Chymotrypsin
QUINACHLOR
Chloroquine
QUINADOME
Iodoquinol
QUINAGLUTE
Quinidine
QUINAMBICIDE
Iodochlorhydroxyquin
QUINAMM
Quinine
QUINATE
Quinidine
QUINE
Quinine
QUINICARDINE
Quinidine
QUINIDEX EXTENTABS
Quinidine
QUIN III
Iodochlorhydroxyquin
QUINITE*
Aminophylline
Quinine
QUINNONE
Hydroquinone
QUINOBARB
Quinidine
Phenylethyl-
barbiturate
QUIN-O-CREME
Iodochlorhydroxyquin
QUINORA
Quinidine
QUINOXYL
Chiniofon
QUINSANA PLUS*
Undecylenic Acid
Zinc Undecylenate
QUINSANA PLUS
MEDICATED FOOT
POWDER
Undecylenic Acid
QUINTESS*
Activated Attapulgite
Attapulgite
QUINTRATE PB*
Pentaerythritol
Tetranitrate
Phenobarbital
QUIPHILE
Quinine
QUOTANE
Dimethisoquin
QUOTICIDINE
Dequalinium

R

RACET CREAM*
Clioquinol
Cortisol
RACET LCD CREAM*
Clioquinol
Coal Tar
Cortisol
RACET RESICORT
Hydrocortisone
RADECOL
Nicotinyl Alcohol
RADIOSTOL
Cholecalciferol
RAGUS*
Minerals, Multiple
Vitamins, Multiple
RAM
Dimenhydrinate
RASPBERIN
Salicylamide
RASTINON
Tolbutamide
RATE-20
Pentaerythritol
Tetranitrate
RATIO*
Calcium Carbonate
Magnesium Carbonate
RAUBASERP
Raubasine
RAUDIXIN
Rauwolfia Serpentina
RAULOYDIN
Reserpine
RAUNORMINE
Deserpidine
RAUPENA

Rauwolfia Serpentina
RAURESCIN
Rescinnamine
RAURINE
Reserpine
RAU-SED
Reserpine
RAUSERFIA
Rauwolfia Serpentina
RAUSERPA
Rauwolfia Serpentina
RAUSERPIN
Rauwolfia Serpentina
RAU-TAB
Alseroxylon
RAUTENSIN
Alseroxylon
RAUTINA
Rauwolfia Serpentina
RAUVAL
Rauwolfia Serpentina
RAUVERID
Rauwolfia Serpentina
RAUWILOID
Alseroxylon
RAUZIDE*
Bendroflumethiazide
Rauwolfia Serpentina
RAVOCAINE
Propoxycaine
RAWFOLA
Rauwolfia Serpentina
RAY-D
Vitamins, Multiple
RECOUP*
Ascorbic Acid
Ferrous Fumarate
RECTACORT*
Bismuth Subgallate
Hydrocortisone
RECTAGENE BALM*
Benzocaine
Bismuth Subgallate
Phenylephrine
Pyrilamine
Zinc Oxide
RECTALAD*
Docusate Potassium
Glycerin
RECTAL MEDICONE-HC SUPPOSITORIES*
Benzocaine
Hydrocortisone
Oxyquinoline
RECTAL MEDICONE SUPPOSITORIES*
Benzocaine
Oxyquinoline
RECTAL MEDICONE UNGUENT*
Benzocaine
Oxyquinoline
RECTO BARIUM
Barium
RECTOID
Hydrocortisone
RECTULES
Chloral Hydrate
REDEPTIN
Fluspirilene
REDISOL
Cyanocobalamin
REDOXON
Ascorbic Acid
REDPEN-VK
Penicillin V
RED PILLS
Ferrous Fumarate
REDUCIN
Oxyphenbutazone
REFOBACIN
Gentamicin
REFUSAL
Disulfiram
REGACILIUM
Plantago Seed
REGENON
Diethylpropion
REGIBON
Diethylpropion
REGITINE
Phentolamine
REGLAN
Metoclopramide
REGONOL
Pyridostigmine
REGRETOS
Levopropoxyphene
REGROTON*
Chlorthalidone
Reserpine
REGUL-AID

Docusate Sodium
REGULEX
Docusate Sodium
REGULEX-D*
Danthron
Docusate Sodium
REGULOID
Plantago Seed
REGULTON
Amezinium
REGUTOL
Docusate Sodium
REIDAMINE
Dimenhydrinate
RELA
Carisoprodol
RELASMA*
Aminophylline
Amobarbital
Ephedrine
RELAXADON*
Atropine
Hyoscyamine
Phenobarbital
Scopolamine
RELAXANT
Dantrolene
RELAXIL
Chlordiazepoxide
RELAX-U-CAPS
Methapyrilene
RELECORT
Hydrocortisone
RELEFACT TRH
Protirelin
RELEMINE*
Chlorpheniramine
Phenylephrine
Phenylpropanolamine
Pyrilamine
RELESERP-5
Reserpine
RELESPOR*
Bacitracin
Neomycin
Polymyxin B
RELETUSS*
Chlorpheniramine
Dextromethorphan
Guaifenesin
Phenylpropanolamine
REM*
Ammonium Chloride
Dextromethorphan
REMIN
Phenaglycodol
REMSED
Promethazine
RENACIDIN*
Citric Acid
Gluconic Acid
RENCAL
Phytate Sodium
RENELATE
Methenamine Mandelate
RENESE
Polythiazide
RENESE-R*
Polythiazide
Reserpine
RENOGRAFIN
Diatrizoate Meglumine
RENO-M-DIP
Diatrizoate Meglumine
RENO-M-30
Diatrizoate Meglumine
RENO-M-60
Meglumine
RENOQUID
Sulfacytine
RENOVIST*
Diatrizoate Meglumine
Diatrizoate Sodium
RENOVIST II*
Diatrizoate Meglumine
Diatrizoate Sodium
RENOVUE-DIP
Iodamide Meglumine
RENOVUE-65
Iodamide Meglumine
REOMAX
Ethacrynic Acid
REPAN*
Acetaminophen
Butalbital
Caffeine

REPEN-VK
  Penicillin V
    Potassium
REPOISE
  Butaperazine
REP-PRED 40
  Methylprednisolone
REP-PRED 80
  Methylprednisolone
RESAID T.D.*
  Chlorpheniramine
  Phenylpropanolamine
RESCISAN
  Rescinnamine
RESECTISOL
  Mannitol
RESERCEN
  Reserpine
RESERCRINE
  Reserpine
RESERFIA
  Reserpine
RESERJEN
  Reserpine
RESERPANCA
  Reserpine
RESERPOID
  Reserpine
RESISTAB
  Thonzylamine
RESISTOPEN
  Oxacillin
RESOLUTION HALF
    STRENGTH
  Phenylpropanolamine
RESOLUTION I
  Phenylpropanolamine
RESOLUTION II
  Phenylpropanolamine
RESOLVE
  Dyclonine
RESONIUM CALCIUM
  Calcium Polystyrene
    Sulfonate
RESPAIRE
  Acetylcysteine
RESPAIR-S.R.*
  Guaifenesin
  Pseudoephedrine
RESPID
  Theophylline
RESPINOL L.A.*
  Guaifenesin
  Phenylephrine
  Phenylpropanolamine
RESPIROL*
  Ephedrine
  Phenobarbital
  Theophylline
RESTORIL
  Temazepam
RESULIN*
  Resorcinol
  Sulfur
RESYL
  Guaifenesin
RETARDIN
  Diphenoxylate
RETET
  Tetracycline
RETIN-A
  Tretinoin
REVERIN
  Rolitetracycline
REVIMINE
  Dopamine
REVROCIN
  Erythromycin
REXOLATE
  Sodium
    Thiosalicylate
REZAMID*
  Resorcinol
  Sulfur
REZIPAS
  Aminosalicylic Acid
R-GENE
  Arginine
R-HCTZ-H*
  Hydralazine
  Hydrochlorothiazide
  Reserpine
RHEABAN
  Activated
    Attapulgite
RHEOMACRODEX
  Dextran 40
RHEOTRAN
  Dextran 40
RHINAFED-EX*

Chlorpheniramine
Pseudoephedrine
RHINALAR
Flunisolide
RHINDECON
Phenylpropanolamine
RHINEX*
Aspirin
Chlorpheniramine
Phenylephrine
RHINEX D-LAY*
Acetaminophen
Chlorpheniramine
Phenylpropanolamine
Salicylamide
RHINEX DM*
Chlorpheniramine
Dextromethorphan
Phenylephrine
RHINIDRIN*
Acetaminophen
Phenylpropanolamine
Phenyltoloxamine
RHINOCAPS*
Acetaminophen
Aspirin
Phenylpropanolamine
RHINOCYN-DM*
Chlorpheniramine
Dextromethorphan
Glycerin
Propylene Glycol
Pseudoephedrine
RHINOCYN-PD*
Chlorpheniramine
Glycerin
Propylene Glycol
Pseudoephedrine
RHINOGESIC*
Acetaminophen
Chlorpheniramine
Phenylephrine
Salicylamide
RHINOLAR*
Chlorpheniramine
Methscopolamine
Phenylpropanolamine
RHINOLAR-EX*
Chlorpheniramine
Phenylpropanolamine
RHINO-MEX
Naphazoline
RHINO-MEX-N
Naphazoline
RHINOSOL
Tuaminoheptane
RHINOSYN*
Chlorpheniramine
Glycerin
Propylene Glycol
Pseudoephedrine
RHINOSYN DM*
Dextromethorphan
Guaifenesin
RHINOSYN-X*
Dextromethorphan
Guaifenesin
Pseudoephedrine
RHINSPEC*
Acetaminophen
Guaifenesin
Phenylephrine
RHOCYA
Potassium Thiocyanate
RHODAVITE
Cyanocobalamin
RHO GAM
RH D Immune Globulin, Human
RHONAL
Aspirin
RHULICAINE*
Alcohol
Benzocaine
Isopropyl Alcohol
Menthol
Triclosan
RHULICORT
Hydrocortisone
RHULICREAM*
Benzocaine
Camphor
Menthol
Zirconium Oxide
RHULIGEL*
Alcohol
Benzyl Alcohol
Camphor
Menthol

RHULIHIST*
  Benzocaine
  Calamine
  Tripelennamine
RHULISPRAY*
  Benzocaine
  Benzyl Alcohol
  Calamine
  Camphor
  Isopropyl Alcohol
  Menthol
RHUS-ALL ANTIGEN*
  Oak Extract
  Posion Ivy Extract
  Sumac Extract
RHUS TOX ANTIGEN
  Poison Ivy Extract
RHUS TOX LOTION*
  Aluminum Acetate
  Phenol
RHYTHMIDINE
  Quinidine
RICIFRUIT
  Castor Oil
RID*
  Piperonyl Butoxide
  Pyrethrins
RID-A-PAIN*
  Acetaminophen
  Caffeine
  Salicylamide
RID-ITCH CREAM*
  Undecylenic Acid
  Zinc Undecylenate
RID-ITCH LIQUID*
  Benzoic Acid
  Chlorothymol
  Resorcinol
  Salicylic Acid
RID LIQUID
    PEDICULICIDE*
  Piperonyl Butoxide
  Pyrethrins
RIFADIN
  Rifampin
RIFAMATE*
  Isoniazid
  Rifampin
RIFOMYCIN
  Rifampin
RIG
  Rabies Immune
    Globulin
RIMACTANE
  Rifampin
RIMACTANE/INH DUAL
    PACK*
  Isoniazid
  Rifampin
RIMIFON
  Isoniazid
RIMSO-50
  Dimethyl Sulfoxide
RIOPAN
  Magaldrate
RIOPAN PLUS*
  Magaldrate
  Simethicone
RIOPLUS*
  Magaldrate
  Simethicone
RISORDAN
  Isosorbide Dinitrate
RITALIN
  Methylphenidate
RITALIN-SR
  Methylphenidate
RIVAL
  Diazepam
RIVOTRIL
  Clonazepam
RMS
  Morphine
ROAMPHED*
  Aminophylline
  Amobarbital
  Ephedrine
ROBALATE
  Dihydroxyaluminum
    Aminoacetate
ROBALYN
  Diphenhydramine
ROBAMATE
  Meprobamate
ROBAMOX
  Amoxicillin
ROBANTALINE
  Propantheline
ROBAXIN
  Methocarbamol

ROBAXISAL*
  Aspirin
  Methocarbamol
ROBAXISAL C-1/4*
  Aspirin
  Codeine
  Methocarbamol
ROBAXISAL C-1/8*
  Aspirin
  Codeine
  Methocarbamol
RO-BENECID
  Probenecid
ROBICILLIN VK
  Penicillin V
    Potassium
ROBIDEX
  Dextromethorphan
ROBIDONE
  Hydrocodone
ROBIDRINE
  Pseudoephedrine
ROBIGESIC
  Acetaminophen
ROBIMYCIN
  Erythromycin
ROBINUL
  Glycopyrrolate
ROBINUL FORTE
  Glycopyrrolate
ROBINUL-PH*
  Glycopyrrolate
  Phenobarbital
ROBINUL-PH FORTE*
  Glycopyrrolate
  Phenobarbital
ROBITET
  Tetracycline
ROBITUSSIN
  Guaifenesin
ROBITUSSIN A-C*
  Codeine
  Guaifenesin
ROBITUSSIN-CF*
  Dextromethorphan
  Guaifenesin
  Phenylpropanolamine
ROBITUSSIN DAC*
  Codeine
  Guaifenesin
  Pseudoephedrine
ROBITUSSIN-DM*
  Dextromethorphan
  Guaifenesin
ROBITUSSIN-DM COUGH
    CALMERS
  Dextromethorphan
ROBITUSSIN NIGHT
    RELIEF*
  Acetaminophen
  Dextromethorphan
  Phenylephrine
  Pyrilamine
ROBITUSSIN-PE*
  Guaifenesin
  Pseudoephedrine
ROCALTROL
  Calcitriol
ROCEPHIN
  Ceftriaxone
RO-CHLORO-SERP*
  Chlorothiazide
  Reserpine
RO-CHLOROZIDE
  Chlorothiazide
ROCYCLE-20
  Dicyclomine
RO-CYCLINE
  Tetracycline
ROCYCLO-10
  Dicyclomine
RODRYL
  Diphenhydramine
ROERIBEC
  Vitamins, Multiple
ROFACT
  Rifampin
ROFED SYRUP*
  Pseudoephedrine
  Triprolidine
ROGITINE
  Phentolamine
RO-HIST
  Tripelennamine
ROHYPNOL
  Flunitrazepam
ROIN
  Cinnarizine
ROLA-BENZ
  Benzthiazide

ROLAIDS
Dihydroxyaluminum Sodium Carbonate
ROLAPHENT
Phentermine
ROLATHIMIDE
Glutethimide
ROLAZID
Isoniazid
ROLAZINE
Hydralazine
ROLCALTROL
Calcitriol
ROLIDRIN
Nylidrin
ROLOX*
Aluminum Hydroxide
Magnesium Hydroxide
ROLSERP
Reserpine
ROMA-NOL
Iodine
ROMEX*
Chlorpheniramine
Dextromethorphan
Guaifenesin
Phenylephrine
ROMICIL
Oleandomycin
ROMILAR*
Chlorpheniramine
Dextromethorphan
Phenylephrine
ROMILAR
Dextromethorphan
ROMILAR CF*
Ammonium Chloride
Dextromethorphan
ROMILAR CHILDREN'S
Dextromethorphan
ROMILAR III*
Dextromethorphan
Phenylpropanolamine
RONDEC*
Carbinoxamine
Pseudoephedrine
RONDEC-DM*
Carbinoxamine
Dextromethorphan
Pseudoephedrine
RONDEC-TR*
Carbinoxamine
Pseudoephedrine
RONDOMYCIN
Methacycline
RONIACOL
Nicotinyl Alcohol
RO-NITRO
Nitroglycerin
ROPANTH
Propantheline
ROPLEDGE
Phendimetrazine
ROPRAMINE
Imipramine
ROPRES*
Reserpine
Trichlormethiazide
RO-PRIMIDONE
Primidone
RORASUL
Sulfasalazine
ROSOXOL
Sulfisoxazole
RO-SULFIRAM
Disulfiram
ROTANE EXPECTORANT*
Brompheniramine
Guaifenesin
Phenylpropanolamine
ROTAPP*
Brompheniramine
Phenylephrine
Phenylpropanolamine
ROTHAV-150
Ethaverine
ROUNOX
Acetaminophen
ROUNOX + CODEINE*
Acetaminophen
Codeine
ROUQUALONE "300"
Methaqualone
ROVAMYCINE
Spiramycin
ROVITE*
Minerals, Multiple
Vitamins, Multiple
ROXADYL
Rosoxacin

ROXANE
  Aluminum Hydroxide
ROXANOL
  Morphine
ROXINOID
  Reserpine
ROXSTAN
  Levothyroxine
ROYCHLOR
  Potassium Chloride
ROYDAN
  Danthron
ROYFLEX
  Trolamine Salicylate
ROYONATE
  Potassium Gluconate
ROZOLAMIDE
  Acetazolamide
RP-MYCIN
  Erythromycin
RUBION
  Cyanocobalamin
RUBRAMIN
  Cyanocobalamin
RUBRAMIN PC
  Cyanocobalamin
RUBRANOVA
  Hydroxocobalamin
RUC-DANE*
  Danthron
  Docusate Sodium
RUFEN
  Ibuprofen
RUHEXATAL WITH
    RESERPINE*
  Mannitol Hexanitrate
  Reserpine
RU-HY-T
  Rauwolfia Serpentina
RU-K-N*
  Belladonna Alkaloids
  Kaolin
  Paregoric
  Pectin
RU-LOR-N
  Drocode
RULOX*
  Aluminum Hydroxide
  Magnesium Hydroxide
RUM-K
  Potassium Iodide
RU-SPAS NO.2
  Homatropine
RU-TUSS*
  Atropine
  Chlorpheniramine
  Hyoscyamine
  Phenylephrine
  Phenylpropanolamine
  Scopolamine
RU-TUSS II*
  Chlorpheniramine
  Phenylpropanolamine
RU-VERT*
  Niacin
  Pentylenetetrazol
  Pheniramine
RVPABA LIP STICK*
  Aminobenzoic Acid
  Petrolatum
RYMED-TR*
  Guaifenesin
  Phenylephrine
  Phenylpropanolamine
RYNA-C LIQUID*
  Chlorpheniramine
  Codeine
  Pseudoephedrine
RYNACROM
  Cromolyn Sodium
RYNA-CX LIQUID*
  Codeine
  Guaifenesin
  Pseudoephedrine
RYNA LIQUID*
  Chlorpheniramine
  Pseudoephedrine
RYNATAN*
  Chlorpheniramine
  Phenylephrine
  Pyrilamine
RYNATUSS*
  Carbetapentane
  Chlorpheniramine
  Ephedrine
  Phenylephrine
RYNA-TUSSADINE
    EXPECTORANT*
  Chlorpheniramine
  Guaifenesin

Phenylephrine
Phenylpropanolamine
Pyrilamine
RYTHMODAN
Disopyramide
RYTMIL
Bisacodyl

S

SABOL
Benzalkonium Chloride
S-A-C*
Acetaminophen
Caffeine
Salicylamide
SAF TIP PHOSPHATE ENEMA*
Sodium Biphosphate
Sodium Phosphate
SALACID
Salicylic Acid
SAL-ADULT
Aspirin
SALAMIDE
Salicylamide
SALATIN WITH CODEINE*
Aspirin
Caffeine
Codeine
SALAZOPYRIN
Sulfasalazine
SAL-DEX*
Isopropyl Alcohol
Salicylic Acid
Undecylenic Acid
SALETO-D*
Acetaminophen
Caffeine
Phenylpropanolamine
Salicylamide
SAL-FAYNE*
Aspirin
Caffeine
SAL HEPATICA*
Citric Acid
Monosodium Phosphate
Sodium Bicarbonate
Sodium Citrate
SALIBAR JR.*
Aspirin
Phenobarbital
SALICRESIN
Mercufenol
SALICYLATE
Carbazochrome Salicylate
SALIGEL
Salicylic Acid
SALIMEPH*
Acetaminophen
Salicylamide
SALINEX
Sodium Chloride
SAL-INFANT
Aspirin
SALINIDOL
Salicylanilide
SALOCOL*
Acetaminophen
Aluminum Hydroxide
Aspirin
Salicylamide
SALONIL
Salicylic Acid
SALOXIUM
Salsalate
SALPHENYL*
Acetaminophen
Chlorpheniramine
Phenylephrine
Salicylamide
SALRIN
Salicylamide
SALURIC
Chlorothiazide
SALURON
Hydroflumethiazide
SALUTENSIN*
Hydroflumethiazide
Reserpine
SALUTENSIN-DEMI*
Hydroflumethiazide
Reserpine
SALYRGAN
Mersalyl
SANDIMMUNE
Cyclosporine

SANDOLANID
  Acetyldigitoxin
SANDOMIGRAN
  Pizotyline
SANDOPTAL
  Butalbital
SANDOSTENE
  Thenalidine
SANDRIL
  Reserpine
SANOMA
  Carisoprodol
SANOREX
  Mazindol
SANSERT
  Methysergide
SANTYL
  Collagenase
S-AQUA
  Benzthiazide
SARAKA
  Plantago Seed
SARATOGA*
  Boric Acid
  Eucalyptol
  Petrolatum
  Zinc Oxide
SARENIN
  Saralasin Acetate
SARO-C
  Ascorbic Acid
SARODANT
  Nitrofurantoin
SAROFLEX*
  Acetaminophen
  Chlorzoxazone
SAROLAX*
  Dehydrocholic Acid
  Docusate Sodium
  Phenolphthalein
SARONIL
  Meprobamate
SAROTEN
  Amitriptyline
SASTID A1*
  Salicylic Acid
  Sulfur
SASTID PLAIN*
  Salicylic Acid
  Sulfur
SASTID SOAP*
  Salicylic Acid
  Sulfur
SAS-500
  Sulfasalazine
SATRIC
  Metronidazole
SAVACORT-D
  Dexamethasone
SAVENTRINE
  Isoproterenol
SAVLON
  Cetrimide
SAVLON-HOSPITAL
    CONCENTRATE
  Cetrimide
SAXIN
  Saccharin
SCABANCA
  Benzyl Benzoate
SCABANE
  Lindane
SCABIDE*
  Benzocaine
  Benzyl Benzoate
SCABIOL
  Benzyl Benzoate
SCHOENFELD
  Docusate Sodium
SCLAVO TEST-PPD
  Tuberculin
SCLEREX*
  Minerals, Multiple
  Vitamins, Multiple
SCOLINE
  Succinylcholine
S-CORTILEAN
  Hydrocortisone
SCOTT'S EMULSION*
  Cholecalciferol
  Vitamin A
SCREEN-TEX
  Sulisobenzone
SCRIP-LAX*
  Carboxymethyl-
    cellulose
  Casanthranol
  Docusate Sodium
SCYAN
  Thiocyanate

SDM NO.22
  Pentaerythritol
    Tetranitrate
SDM NO.23
  Pentaerythritol
    Tetranitrate
SDM NO.35
  Pentaerythritol
    Tetranitrate
SEALE'S LOTION
  Sulfur
SEA LEGS
  Piprinhydrinate
SEBAQUIN
  Iodoquinol
SEBASORB*
  Attapulgite
  Salicyclic Acid
SEBAVEEN*
  Collodial Oatmeal
  Salicylic Acid
  Sulfur
SEBEX*
  Salicyclic Acid
  Sulfur
SEBIZON
  Sulfacetamide
SEBUCARE
  Salicylic Acid
SEBULEX*
  Salicylic Acid
  Sulfur
SEBULEX SCALP CARE
    LOTION
  Salicylic Acid
SEBUSAN
  Selenium Sulfide
SEBUTONE*
  Coal Tar
  Salicylic Acid
  Sulfur
SECOGEN
  Secobarbital
SECONAL
  Secobarbital
SECOTABS
  Secobarbital
SECROSTERON
  Dimethisterone
SECTRAL
  Acebutolol
SEDACANE*
  Acetaminophen
  Caffeine
  Calcium Gluconate
  Salicylamide
SEDACAPS
  Methapyrilene
SEDALONE
  Methaqualone
SEDAMYL
  Acecarbromal
SEDAPAP-10*
  Acetaminophen
  Butabarbital
SEDARIL
  Hydroxyzine
SEDATUSS
  Dextromethorphan
SEDATUSS EXPECTORANT
  Guaifenesin
SEDICIN
  Diphenhydramine
SEDIODAL-DM
  Dextromethorphan
SEDOLATAN
  Prenylamine
SEDONAL NATRIUM
  Secobarbital
SEDS*
  Atropine
  Hyoscyamine
  Phenobarbital
  Scopolamine
SED.TENS.SE
  Homatropine
SEDULON
  Dihyprylone
SEDURAL
  Phenazopyridine
SEFFIN
  Cephalothin
SEFFLIN
  Cephalothin
SEFRIL
  Cephradine
SEGONTIN
  Prenylamine
SEGURIL
  Furosemide

SELACRYN
Ticrynafen
SELDANE
Terfenadine
SELECTOMYCIN
Spiramycin
SELESTOJECT
Betamethasone
SELLYMIN
Sodium Bicarbonate
SELOKEN
Metoprolol
SELSUN
Selenium Sulfide
SELSUN BLUE
Selenium Sulfide
SELSUN SUSPENSION
Selenium Sulfide
SELTZ K
Potassium Citrate
SELVIGON
Pipazethate
SEMBRINA
Methyldopa
SEMETS*
Benzocaine
Cetylpyridinium
SEMICID
Nonoxynol
SEMIKON
Methapyrilene
SEMILENTE ILETIN
Insulin Zinc
[Suspension] Prompt
SEMILENTE INSULIN
Insulin Zinc
[Suspension] Prompt
SEMITARD
Insulin Zinc
[Suspension] Prompt
SEMOXYDRINE
Methamphetamine
SENEXON
Senna
SENOKAP DSS*
Docusate Sodium
Senna
SENOKOT
Senna
SENOKOT-S*
Docusate Sodium
Senna
SENOKOT WITH PLANTAGO SEED*
Plantago Seed
Senna
SENOLAX
Senna
SENSACORT
Hydrocortisone
SENSORCAINE
Bupivacaine
SEOTAL SODIUM
Secobarbital
SEPO
Benzocaine
SEPP ANTISEPTIC
Povidone-Iodine
SEPTAL*
Bacitracin
Neomycin
Polymyxin B
SEPTAN
Co-Trimoxazole
SEPTI-SOFT
Hexachlorophene
SEPTISOL
Hexachlorophene
SEPTRA
Co-Trimoxazole
SEPTRA DS
Co-Trimoxazole
SEPTRA IV
Co-Trimoxazole
SEQUESTRENE A
Edetic Acid
SERAL
Secobarbital
SER-AP-ES*
Hydralazine
Hydrochlorothiazide
Reserpine
SERATYL
Trolamine
SERAX
Oxazepam
SERC
Betahistine
SERENACE
Haloperidol

SERENACK
  Diazepam
SERENID-D
  Oxazepam
SERENIUM
  Ethoxazene
SERENSIL
  Ethchlorvynol
SERENTIL
  Mesoridazine
SEREPAX
  Oxazepam
SERESTA
  Oxazepam
SERFIN
  Reserpine
SERFOLIAR
  Rauwolfia Serpentina
SERGETYL
  Etymemazine
SERMAKA
  Flurandrenolide
SEROCICLINA
  Cycloserine
SEROMYCIN
  Cycloserine
SERPALAN
  Reserpine
SERPANRAY
  Reserpine
SERPASIL
  Reserpine
SERPASIL-APRESOLINE*
  Hydralazine
  Reserpine
SERPASIL-ESIDRIX*
  Hydrochlorothiazide
  Reserpine
SERPATE
  Reserpine
SERTAN
  Primidone
SERUTAN
  Plantago Seed
SERVISONE
  Prednisone
SETHADIL
  Sulfaethidole
SETONIL
  Diazepam
SETROL
  Oxyphencyclimine
SEXOVID
  Cyclofenil
SHI
  Insulin Human
SIBLIN
  Plantago Seed
SIDONNA*
  Atropine
  Butabarbital
  Hyoscyamine
  Scopolamine
  Simethicone
SIGNA SUL-A*
  Phenazopyridine
  Sulfamethizole
SIGTAB
  Vitamins, Multiple
SILAIN-GEL*
  Aluminum Hydroxide
  Magnesium Carbonate
  Magnesium Oxide
  Simethicone
SILENCE IS GOLDEN
  Dextromethorphan
SILEXIN*
  Dextromethorphan
  Guaifenesin
SILOPENTOL
  Oxeladin
SILVADENE
  Silver Sulfadiazine
SIMAAL GEL*
  Aluminum Hydroxide
  Magnesium Hydroxide
SIMECO*
  Aluminum Hydroxide
  Magnesium Hydroxide
  Simethicone
SIMPLENE
  Epinephrine
SIMPLOTAN
  Tinidazole
SIMRON
  Ferrous Gluconate
SIMRON PLUS
  Vitamins, Multiple
SINACON*
  Acetaminophen

Pseudoephedrine
SINALOST
Mechlorethamine
SINAN
Mephenesin
SINAPHEN-NASAL
Phenylephrine
SINAPILS*
Acetaminophen
Chlorpheniramine
Phenylpropanolamine
SINAREST*
Acetaminophen
Chlorpheniramine
Phenylpropanolamine
SINAREST NASAL SPRAY*
Acetaminophen
Chlorpheniramine
Phenylephrine
SINAXAR
Styramate
SINCOMEN
Spironolactone
SINE-AID*
Acetaminophen
Phenylpropanolamine
SINE-AID EXTRA STRENGTH*
Acetaminophen
Pseudoephedrine
SINEMET*
Carbidopa
Levodopa
SINE-OFF*
Aspirin
Chlorpheniramine
Phenylpropanolamine
SINE-OFF-ASPIRIN FORMULA*
Aspirin
Chlorpheniramine
Phenylpropanolamine
SINE-OFF ASPIRIN-FREE EXTRA STRENGTH*
Acetaminophen
Chlorpheniramine
Phenylpropanolamine
SINE-OFF EXTRA STRENGTH - NO DROWSINESS*
Acetaminophen
Phenylpropanolamine
SINE-OFF ONCE-A-DAY
Xylometazoline
SINEQUAN
Doxepin
SINEX
Phenylephrine
SINEX DECONGESTANT NASAL SPRAY*
Cetylpyridinium
Phenylephrine
SINEXIN*
Caffeine
Chlorpheniramine
Phenylephrine
Salicylamide
SINEX-L.A.
Xylometazoline
SINGLET*
Acetaminophen
Chlorpheniramine
Phenylephrine
SINGOSERP
Syrosingopine
SINO-COMP*
Acetaminophen
Chlorpheniramine
Phenylephrine
Salicylamide
SINOCON*
Chlorpheniramine
Phenylephrine
Phenylpropanolamine
Phenyltoloxamine
SINOGRAFIN*
Diatrizoate Meglumine
Iodipamide Meglumine
SINOMIN
Sulfamethoxazole
SINOVAN TIMED*
Chlorpheniramine
Methscopolamine
Phenylephrine
SINTHROME
Acenocoumarol
SINTROM
Acenocoumarol
SINUBID*

Acetaminophen
Phenylpropanolamine
Phenyltoloxamine
SINUFED
Pseudoephedrine
SINUGEN*
Acetaminophen
Phenylpropanolamine
Phenyltoloxamine
SINU-LETS*
Acetaminophen
Phenylpropanolamine
Phenyltoloxamine
SINULIN*
Acetaminophen
Chlorpheniramine
Phenylpropanolamine
Salicylamide
SINUREX*
Chlorpheniramine
Methapyrilene
Phenylpropanolamine
Salicylamide
SINUSOL-D*
Atropine
Chlorpheniramine
SINUS SPRAY
Xylometazoline
SINUSTAT*
Acetaminophen
Phenylpropanolamine
Phenyltoloxamine
SINUTAB*
Acetaminophen
Phenylpropanolamine
Phenyltoloxamine
SINUTAB EXTRA STRENGTH*
Acetaminophen
Chlorpheniramine
Phenylpropanolamine
SINUTAB II*
Acetaminophen
Phenylpropanolamine
SINUTAB LONG-LASTING DECONGESTANT SINUS SPRAY
Xylometazoline
SINUTAB NASAL SPRAY
Xylometazoline
SINUTREX*
Acetaminophen
Phenylpropanolamine
Phenyltoloxamine
SIQUIL
Triflupromazine
SK-AMITRIPTYLINE
Amitriptyline
SK-AMPICILLIN
Ampicillin
SK-AMPICILLIN-N
Ampicillin
SK-APAP
Acetaminophen
SK-APAP WITH CODEINE*
Acetaminophen
Codeine
SK-BAMATE
Meprobamate
SK-BISACODYL
Bisacodyl
SK-CHLORAL HYDRATE
Chloral Hydrate
SK-CHLOROTHIAZIDE
Chlorothiazide
SK-DEXAMETHASONE
Dexamethasone
SK-DIGOXIN
Digoxin
SK-DIPHENHYDRAMINE
Diphenhydramine
SK-DIPHENOXYLATE*
Atropine
Diphenoxylate
SKELAXIN
Metaxalone
SK-ERYTHROMYCIN
Erythromycin
SK-HYDROCHLOROTHIAZIDE
Hydrochlorothiazide
SKIODAN
Methiodal
SKLEROMEXE
Clofibrate
SK-LYGEN
Chlordiazepoxide
SK-NIACIN
Niacin
SKOPYL
Methscopolamine

SK-PENICILLIN G
  Penicillin G
SK-PENICILLIN VK
  Penicillin V
    Potassium
SK-PHENOBARBITAL
  Phenobarbital
SK-PRAMINE
  Imipramine
SK-PREDNISONE
  Prednisone
SK-PROBENECID
  Probenecid
SK-QUINIDINE
  Quinidine
SK-RESERPINE
  Reserpine
SK-SOXAZOLE
  Sulfisoxazole
SK-TETRACYCLINE
  Tetracycline
SK-TOLBUTAMIDE
  Tolbutamide
SK-TRIAMCINOLONE
  Triamcinolone
SK 65
  Propoxyphene
SK-65 APAP*
  Acetaminophen
  Propoxyphene
SK-65 COMPOUND*
  Aspirin
  Caffeine
  Propoxyphene
SLEEP-EZE
  Pyrilamine
SLEEPINAL
  Methapyrilene
SLIM LINE GUM
  Benzocaine
SLIM ONE*
  Caffeine
  Phenylpropanolamine
SLOAN'S LINIMENT*
  Methyl Salicylate
  Oil of Camphor
  Oil of Pine
  Turpentine Oil
SLO-BID
  Theophylline
SLO-PHYLLIN GG*
  Guaifenesin
  Theophylline
SLO-PHYLLIN GYROCAPS,
  Theophylline
SLO-PHYLLIN 80
  Theophylline
SLO-POT
  Potassium Chloride
SLO-POT 600
  Potassium Chloride
SLOW-FE
  Ferrous Sulfate
SLOW-K
  Potassium Chloride
SLOW-TRASICOR
  Oxprenolol
SMZ-TMP
  Trimethoprim
SOAKARE
  Benzalkonium
    Chloride
SOBELIN
  Clindamycin
SODA MINT
  Sodium Bicarbonate
SODASONE
  Prednisolone
SODESTRIN
  Conjugated Estrogens
SODESTRIN H
  Conjugated Estrogens
SODIUM EDECRIN
  Ethacrynate
SODIUM SULAMYD
  Sulfacetamide
SODIUM VERSENATE
  Edetate Calcium
    Disodium
SODIURETIC
  Bendroflumethiazide
SOF-LAX WAFERS*
  Docusate Sodium
  Plantago Seed
SOFRAMYCIN
  Framycetin
SOFRA-TULLE
  Framycetin
SOFT'N SOOTHE
  Benzocaine

SOFTRAN
  Buclizine
SOLACEN
  Tybamate
SOLAQUIN
  Hydroquinone
SOLARCAINE
  Benzocaine
SOLARCAINE LIP BALM
  Benzocaine
SOLATENE
  Beta Carotene
SOLAZINE
  Trifluoperazine
SOLBAR*
  Dioxybenzone
  Oxybenzone
SOLBRINE
  Dimenhydrinate
SOLFOTON
  Phenobarbital
SOLGANAL
  Aurothioglucose
SOLIUM
  Chlordiazepoxide
SOLOXSALEN
  Methoxsalen
SOLTICE*
  Dextromethorphan
  Guaifenesin
  Phenylpropanolamine
SOLTICE NASAL SPRAY
  Phenylephrine
SOLTICE QUICK RUB*
  Camphor
  Eucalyptol
  Menthol
  Methyl Salicylate
SOLU-BARB
  Phenobarbital
SOLU-B-FORTE(S-B-F) STERILE POWDER
  Vitamins, Multiple
SOLU-B STERILE
  Vitamin B Complex
SOLU-B WITH ASCORBIC ACID STERILE POWDER*
  Ascorbic Acid
  Vitamin B Complex
SOLU-CORTEF
  Hydrocortisone
SOLU-DIAZINE
  Sulfadiazine
SOLU-FLUR
  Sodium Fluoride
SOLU-MEDROL
  Methylprednisolone
SOLUREX-L.A.
  Dexamethasone
SOLUTHRICIN
  Tyrothricin
SOLVEX ATHLETE'S FOOT SPRAY*
  Chlorothymol
  Triclosan
  Undecylenic Acid
SOLVEX OINTMENT*
  Benzoic Acid
  Salicylic Acid
SOLVEX POWDER*
  Chlorothymol
  Hydroxyquinoline
  Salicylic Acid
  Sulfur
SOMA
  Carisoprodol
SOMA COMPOUND WITH CODEINE*
  Caffeine
  Carisoprodol
  Codeine
SOMBUCAPS
  Hexobarbital
SOMBULEX
  Hexobarbital
SOMIDE
  Glutethimide
SOMINEX (CANADA)
  Diphenhydramine
SOMINEX (USA)*
  Aminoxide Hydrobromide
  Methapyrilene
  Salicylamide
SOMINEX FORMULA 2
  Diphenhydramine
SOMNAFAC
  Methaqualone
SOMNALERT
  Hexobarbital
SOMNESIN

Meparfynol
SOMNICAPS
Methapyrilene
SOMNI SED
Chloral Hydrate
SOMNIUM
Diphenhydramine
SOMNOS
Chloral Hydrate
SOMNOTHANE
Halothane
SOMOPHYLLIN
Aminophylline
SOMOPHYLLIN-CRT
Theophylline
SOMOPHYLLIN-DF
Aminophylline
SOMOPHYLLIN-T
Theophylline
SONAZINE
Chlorpromazine
SONERYL
Butethal
SONILYN
Sulfachlorpyridazine
SOOTHE(CANADA)
Phenylephrine
SOOTHE EYE DROPS
Tetrahydrozoline
S.O.P.
Idoxuridine
SOPAMYCETIN
Chloramphenicol
SOPOR
Methaqualone
SOPRODOL*
Caffeine
Carisoprodol
Phenacetin
SOPRODOL
Carisoprodol
SOQUETTE*
Benzalkonium
Chloride
Polyvinyl Alcohol
SORADEN
Adenosine
SORATE
Isosorbide Dinitrate
SORBIDE
Isosorbide Dinitrate
SORBITAT
Isosorbide Dinitrate
SORBITRATE
Isosorbide Dinitrate
SORBITRATE SA
Isosorbide Dinitrate
SORBUTUSS*
Dextromethorphan
Guaifenesin
Ipecac Fluidextract
SORDINOL
Clopenthixol
SORMETAL
Edetate Calcium
Disodium
SORQUAD
Isosorbide Dinitrate
SOSEGON
Pentazocine
SOTRADECOL
Sodium Tetradecyl
Sulfate
SOVENTOL
Bamipine
SOY DOME CLEANSER
Hexachlorophene
SPACOLIN
Alverine
S-PAINACET*
Acetaminophen
Propoxyphene
S-PAIN-65
Propoxyphene
SPALIX*
Atropine
Hyoscyamine
Phenobarbital
Scopolamine
SPANCAP C
Vitamins, Multiple
SPANCAP NO.1
Dextroamphetamine
SPANESTRIN P
Estrone
SPAN-FF
Ferrous Fumarate
SPANTAC*
Chlorpheniramine
Phenylpropanolamine
SPANTROL*

Carboxymethyl-
cellulose
Phenylpropanolamine
SPANTUSS*
Chlorpheniramine
Dextromethorphan
Phenylephrine
SPARINE
Promazine
SPARTOCIN
Sparteine
SPASAID*
Atropine
Hyoscyamine
Phenobarbital
Scopolamine
SPASGESIC*
Acetaminophen
Chlorzoxazone
SPASLIN*
Atropine
Hyoscyamine
Phenobarbital
Scopolamine
SPASMALEX
Dihexyverine
SPASMAVERINE
Alverine
SPASMOBAN
Dicyclomine
SPASMOBAN-PH*
Dicyclomine
Phenobarbital
SPASMOJECT
Dicyclomine
SPASMOLIN*
Atropine
Hyoscyamine
Phenobarbital
Scopolamine
SPASMOPHEN*
Atropine
Hyoscyamine
Phenobarbital
Scopolamine
SPASMOREL*
Atropine
Hyoscyamine
Phenobarbital
Scopolamine
SPASQUID*
Atropine
Hyoscyamine
Phenobarbital
Scopolamine
SPASTOSED*
Calcium Carbonate
Magnesium Carbonate
SPASTYL WITH
PHENOBARBITAL*
Dicyclomine
Phenobarbital
SPAZOC
Isometheptene
S.P.C.*
Caffeine
Salicylamide
SPECTAZOLE
Econazole
SPECTRA-SORB UV 284
Sulisobenzone
SPECTROBID
Bacampicillin
SPECTROCIN*
Gramicidin
Neomycin
SPEC-T SORE THROAT
ANESTHETIC
Benzocaine
SPEC-T SORE THROAT/
COUGH SUPPRESSANT*
Benzocaine
Dextromethorphan
SPEC-T SORE THROAT/
DECONGESTANT*
Benzocaine
Phenylephrine
Phenylpropanolamine
SPENAXIN
Methocarbamol
SPENCORT
Triamcinolone
SPENIACOL
Nicotinyl Alcohol
Tartrate
SPENSOMIDE
Benzalkonium
Chloride
SPHERULIN
Coccidioidin

SPIROCID
  Acetarsone
SPONGIACAINE
  Benzocaine
SPONTIN
  Ristocetin
SPORILINE
  Tolnaftate
SPOROSTACIN*
  Benzalkonium
    Chloride
  Chlordantoin
SPRX
  Phendimetrazine
SPS
  Sodium Polystyrene
    Sulfonate
S-P-T
  Thyroid
SSKI
  Potassium Iodide
S.S.S. TONIC
  Vitamins, Multiple
STABILENE
  Ethyl Biscoumacetate
STABINOL
  Chlorpropamide
STABISOL
  Bismuth
    Subsalicylate
STADOL
  Butorphanol
STAMINE
  Pyrilamine
STANBACK*
  Aspirin
  Caffeine
  Salicylamide
STANCO
  Aspirin
STANDRYL
  Diphenhydramine
STANGYL
  Trimipramine
STAPHCILLIN
  Methicillin
STAPHOBRISTOL-250
  Cloxacillin
STAR-OTIC*
  Acetic Acid
  Aluminum Acetate
  Boric Acid
STATICIN*
  Alcohol
  Erythromycin
STATIMO
  Carbazochrome
    Salicylate
STATOBEX
  Phendimetrazine
STATROL OPHTHALMIC*
  Benzalkonium
    Chloride
  Neomycin
  Polymyxin B
S.T. DECONGEST*
  Brompheniramine
  Phenylephrine
  Phenylpropanolamine
STECLIN
  Tetracycline
STELAZINE
  Trifluoperazine
STEMETIL
  Prochlorperazine
STEMEX
  Paramethasone
STENEDIOL
  Methandriol
STENTAL
  Phenobarbital
STERA-FORM*
  Hydrocortisone
  Iodochlorhydroxyquin
  Pramoxine
STERAMINE OTIC*
  Acetic Acid
  Benzalkonium
    Chloride
  Hydrocortisone
  Pramoxine
STERANE
  Prednisolone
STERAPRED UNI-PAK
  Prednisone
STERINE
  Methenamine
    Mandelate
STERISIL
  Hexetidine

STERISOL
  Hexetidine
STEROGYL-15
  Ergocalciferol
STEROLONE
  Prednisolone
STEROSAN
  Chlorquinaldol
S.T. EXPECTORANT
  Guaifenesin
S-T FORTE*
  Guaifenesin
  Hydrocodone
  Pheniramine
  Phenylephrine
  Phenylpropanolamine
STIBILIUM
  Diethylstilbestrol
STIGMONENE
  Benzpyrinium
STILBESTROL
  Diethylstilbestrol
STILBETIN
  Diethylstilbestrol
STILPHOSTROL
  Diethylstilbestrol
STIMATE
  Desmopressin
STIM-TABS
  Caffeine
STIMUL
  Pemoline
STIMULAX*
  Cascara Sagrada
  Docusate Sodium
STIMULEXIN
  Doxapram
STINERVAL
  Phenelzine
STING-EZE*
  Benzocaine
  Camphor
  Diphenhydramine
  Eucalyptol
  Phenol
ST. JOSEPH ASPIRIN
  Aspirin
ST. JOSEPH ASPIRIN FOR CHILDREN CHEWABLE
  Aspirin
ST. JOSEPH COLD FOR CHILDREN*
  Aspirin
  Phenylpropanolamine
ST. JOSEPH COUGH FOR CHILDREN
  Dextromethorphan
ST. JOSEPH DECONGESTANT FOR CHILDREN
  Oxymetazoline
ST. JOSEPH NASAL SPRAY/DROPS
  Oxymetazoline
STOVAGINAL
  Acetarsone
STOVARSOL
  Acetarsone
STOXIL
  Idoxuridine
STREMA
  Quinine
STREPOCIDE
  Sulfanilamide
STREPOLIN
  Streptomycin
STREPTASE
  Streptokinase
STREPTODORNASE
  Streptokinase
STREPTOHYDRAZID
  Streptonicozid
STREPTOSOL 25%
  Streptomycin
STRESSCAPS
  Vitamins, Multiple
STRESS-PAM
  Diazepam
STRESSTABS 600
  Vitamins, Multiple
STRESSTABS 600 WITH IRON*
  Iron
  Vitamins, Multiple
STRESSTABS 600 WITH ZINC*
  Iron
  Vitamins, Multiple
  Zinc
STRIATRAN

Emylcamate
STRI-DEX B.P.
Benzoyl Peroxide
STRI-DEX MEDICATED PADS
Salicylic Acid
STROMBA
Stanozolol
STRYCIN
Streptomycin
STUART FORMULA
Vitamins, Multiple
STUART FORMULA LIQUID
Vitamins, Multiple
STUART HEMATINIC
Vitamins, Multiple
STUART HEMATINIC LIQUID
Vitamins, Multiple
STUARTINIC
Vitamins, Multiple
STUARTNATAL*
Minerals, Multiple
Vitamins, Multiple
STUART PRENATAL*
Minerals, Multiple
Vitamins, Multiple
STUART PRENATAL FORMULA
Vitamins, Multiple
STUART THERAPEUTIC MULTIVITAMIN
Vitamins, Multiple
STULAX
Docusate Sodium
STURGEON
Cinnarizine
STUTGERON
Cinnarizine
S.T. 37
Hexylresorcinol
SUAVITIL
Benactyzine
SUBLIMAZE
Fentanyl
SUB-QUIN
Procainamide
SUBTOSAN
Povidone
SUCARYL
Saccharin
SUCOSTRIN
Succinylcholine
SUCRAPHEN
Phenylephrine
SUCRETS
Hexylresorcinol
SUCRETS COUGH CONTROL FORMULA
Dextromethorphan
SUDADRINE
Pseudoephedrine
SUDAFED
Pseudoephedrine
SUDAFED COUGH*
Dextromethorphan
Guaifenesin
Pseudoephedrine
SUDAFED PLUS*
Chlorpheniramine
Pseudoephedrine
SUDAFED S.A.
Pseudoephedrine
SUDODRIN
Pseudoephedrine
SUDOPRIN
Acetaminophen
SUDO-60
Pseudoephedrine
SUDROMA
Chlorophyllin
SUFAMAL*
Allantoin
Aminacrine
Sulfanilamide
SUGRACILLIN
Penicillin G
SULADYNE
Phenazopyridine
SULAMYD SODIUM
Sulfacetamide
SUL-BLUE
Selenium Sulfide
SULCRATE
Sucralfate
SULDIAZO*
Phenazopyridine
Sulfisoxazole
SULESTREX
Estropipate

SULFABID
  Sulfaphenazole
SULFABUTIN
  Busulfan
SULFACEL-15
  Sulfacetamide
SULFACET
  Sulfur
SULFACET-R LOTION*
  Sulfacetamide
  Sulfur
SULFACTIN
  Dimercaprol
SULFACTOL
  Sodium Thiosulfate
SULFADETS
  Sulfadiazine
SULFADINE
  Sulfamethazine
SULFADRIN NASAL
    SUSPENSION*
  Phenylephrine
  Sulfathiazole
SULFADYNE
  Sulfasalazine
SULFALAR
  Sulfisoxazole
SULFAMETHIN
  Sulfisomidine
SULFAMUL
  Sulfathiazole
SULFAMYLON CREAM
  Mafenide
SULFASUXIDINE
  Succinyl-
    sulfathiazole
SULFATHALIDINE
  Phthalyl-
    sulfathiazole
SULFATRIN
  Co-Trimoxazole
SULFIZOLE
  Sulfisoxazole
SULFOIL
  Sulfur
SULFONAMIDES DUPLEX*
  Sulfadiazine
  Sulfamerazine
SULFORCIN*
  Resorcinol
  Sulfur
SULFOXYL LOTION*
  Benzoyl Peroxide
  Sulfur
SULFSTAT FORTE
  Sulfamethizole
SULFUNO
  Sulfamoxole
SULF-10
  Sulfacetamide
SULF-30
  Sulfacetamide
SULLA
  Sulfameter
SULMYCIN
  Gentamicin
SULPHETRONE
  Solasulfone
SUL-SPANSION
  Sulfaethidole
SULTRIN*
  Sulfabenzamide
  Sulfacetamide
  Sulfathiazole
SUMMIT*
  Acetaminophen
  Caffeine
SUMOX
  Amoxicillin
SUMYCIN
  Tetracycline
SUNBRELLA SUNSCREEN
  Aminobenzoic Acid
SUN DARE 15*
  Oxybenzone
  Padimate
SUNDOWN SUNBLOCK*
  Oxybenzone
  Padimate
SUNGARD
  Sulisobenzone
SUNGER SUNBLOCK*
  Oxybenzone
  Padimate
SUNRIL*
  Acetaminophen
  Pamabrom
  Pyrilamine
SUNSTICK
  Digalloyl Trioleate

SUNSWEPT
  Digalloyl Trioleate
SUNTAN
  Homosalate
SUPAC*
  Acetaminophen
  Aspirin
  Caffeine
  Calcium Gluconate
SUPASA
  Aspirin
SUPEN
  Ampicillin
SUPER A
  Vitamin A
SUPER ANAHIST*
  Acetaminophen
  Pseudoephedrine
SUPER ANAHIST NASAL SPRAY
  Phenylephrine
SUPER CALCICAPS
  Vitamins, Multiple
SUPER CARDIALINE
  Vitamin E
SUPERCITIN*
  Chlorpheniramine
  Dextromethorphan
SUPER D COD LIVER OIL
  Vitamins, Multiple
SUPER-DECON*
  Methapyrilene
  Phenylephrine
  Salicylamide
SUPER DOSS*
  Brewer's Yeast
  Docusate Sodium
SUPER D PERLES
  Vitamins, Multiple
SUPER HYDRAMIN
  Vitamins, Multiple
SUPER ODRINEX*
  Caffeine
  Phenylpropanolamine
SUPER PLENAMINS
  Vitamins, Multiple
SUPER SHADE*
  Oxybenzone
  Padimate
SUPERTAH*
  Coal Tar
  Zinc Oxide
SUPER TONIVEN
  Ascorbic Acid
SUPEUDOL
  Oxycodone
SUPPAP-120
  Acetaminophen
SUPRARENIN
  Epinephrine
SUPRES*
  Chlorothiazide
  Methyldopa
SURBEX
  Vitamins, Multiple
SURBEX-T
  Vitamins, Multiple
SURBEX WITH C*
  Ascorbic Acid
  Vitamins, Multiple
SURBEX 750 WITH IRON*
  Calcium
  Iron
  Vitamins, Multiple
SURBEX 750 WITH ZINC*
  Calcium
  Vitamins, Multiple
  Zinc
SURFACAINE
  Cyclomethycaine
SURFAK
  Docusate Calcium
SURGAM
  Tiaprofenic Acid
SURGI-CEN
  Hexachlorophene
SURGI-KLEEN*
  Lanolin
  Methylbenzethonium
SURGI-SEP
  Povidone-Iodine
SURITAL
  Thiamylal
SURMONTIL
  Trimipramine
SUSADRIN
  Nitroglycerin
SUSANO*
  Atropine
  Hyoscyamine

Phenobarbital
Scopolamine
SUSPEN
Penicillin V
Potassium
SUS-PHRINE
Epinephrine
SUSTAIRE
Theophylline
SUVREN
Captodiame
SUX-CERT
Succinylcholine
SUXINUTIN
Ethosuximide
SWEEN KARAYA POWDER
Parachlorometa-
xylenol
SWISS KRISS
Senna
SYCOTROL
Piperilate
SYLLACT*
Dextrose
Plantago Seed
SYLLACT
Plantago Seed
SYLLAMALT*
Malt Soup Extract
Plantago Seed
SYLLAMALT
EFFERVESCENT*
Dextrose
Malt Soup Extract
Plantago Seed
Sodium Bicarbonate
SYM-FER*
Ferrous Gluconate
SYMMETREL
Amantadine
SYMPTOM I
Dextromethorphan
SYMPTOM 2
Pseudoephedrine
SYMPTOM 3
Brompheniramine
SYNACORT
Hydrocortisone
SYNACTHEN DEPOT
Cosyntropin
SYNADONE
Fluocinolone
SYNADRIN
Prenylamine
SYNALAR
Fluocinolone
SYNALAR-HP
Fluocinolone
SYNALGOS*
Aspirin
Caffeine
Promethazine
SYNALGOS-DC*
Aspirin
Caffeine
Drocode
Promethazine
SYNAMOL
Fluocinolone
SYNANDRETS
Methyltestosterone
SYNANDROL F
Testosterone
SYNANDROTABS
Methyltestosterone
SYNASAL
Phenylephrine
SYNASTERNOL
Oxymetholone
SYNATAN
Dextroamphetamine
SYNCILLIN
Phenethicillin
SYNCORTIN
Desoxycorticosterone
SYNCURINE
Decamethonium
SYNDROX
Methamphetamine
SYNEMOL
Fluocinolone
SYNESTROL
Dienestrol
SYNGESTERONE
Progesterone
SYNGESTRETS
Progesterone
SYNGESTROTABS
Ethisterone
SYNKAVITE

Menadiol
SYNKAYVITE
Menadiol
SYNOPHYLATE
Theophylline
SYNOPHYLATE-GG*
Guaifenesin
Theophylline
SYNTARIS
Flunisolide
SYNTETREX
Rolitetracycline
SYNTETRIN
Rolitetracycline
SYNTHALOIDS*
Benzocaine
Calcium-Iodine Complex
SYNTHROID
Levothyroxine
SYNTICILLIN
Methicillin
SYNTOCINON
Oxytocin
SYNTROGEL*
Aluminum Hydroxide
Magnesium Carbonate
Magnesium Hydroxide
SYRACOL*
Dextromethorphan
Phenylpropanolamine
SYSTRAL
Chlorphenoxamine
SYTOBEX
Cyanocobalamin
SYTOBEX-H
Hydroxocobalamin
S45 ANTI-PAIN COMPOUND*
Acetaminophen
Caffeine
Salicylamide

T

TABLOID BRAND A.P.C. WITH CODEINE*
Aspirin
Caffeine
Codeine
TABLOID BRAND THIOGUANINE
Thioguanine
TABLUCYL
Plantago Seed
TABRON FILMSEAL*
Ferrous Fumarate
Vitamins, Multiple
TACARYL
Methdilazine
TACE
Chlorotrianisene
TACHYSTIN
Dihydrotachysterol
TAGAFED*
Pseudoephedrine
Triprolidine
TAGAMET
Cimetidine
TAGATAP*
Brompheniramine
Phenylephrine
Phenylpropanolamine
TAGATHEN
Chlorothen
TAKA-COMBEX KAPSEALS
Vitamins, Multiple
TALADREN
Ethacrynic Acid
TALAMO
Amobarbital
TALIMOL
Thalidomide
TALPHENO
Phenobarbital
TALWIN
Pentazocine
TALWIN COMPOUND*
Aspirin
Caffeine
Pentazocine
TALWIN NX*
Naloxone
Pentazocine
TALWIN 50
Pentazocine
TAMATE
Meprobamate
TAMBOCOR

Flecainide
TAMINE*
Brompheniramine
Phenylephrine
Phenylpropanolamine
TANDEARIL
Oxyphenbutazone
TANDERIL
Oxyphenbutazone
TAO
Troleandomycin
TAPAR
Acetaminophen
TAPAZOLE
Methimazole
TARACTAN
Chlorprothixene
TARASAN
Chlorprothixene
TARBONIS
Coal Tar
TAR DISTILLATE "DOAK"
Coal Tar
TAR-DOAK LOTION*
Coal Tar
Iodochlorhydroxyquin
Resorcinol
Salicylic Acid
Sulfur
TARDOCILLIN
Penicillin G
TARGEL
Coal Tar
TARGEL S.A.
Coal Tar
TARLENE*
Coal Tar
Propylene Glycol
Salicylic Acid
TARODYL
Glycopyrrolate
TARSUM*
Coal Tar
Salicylic Acid
TAVEGIL
Clemastine
TAVIST
Clemastine
TAVIST-D*
Clemastine
Phenylpropanolamine
TAVOR
Lorazepam
TAZONE
Phenylbutazone
T-CAPS
Tetracycline
T.D. ALERMINE
Chlorpheniramine
T-DRYL
Diphenhydramine
TEAR-EFRIN
Phenylephrine
TEARISOL
Methylcellulose
TEARS NATURALE
Methylcellulose
TEARS PLUS*
Chlorobutanol
Polyvinyl Alcohol
Povidone
TEBRAZID
Pyrazinamide
TEDRAL*
Ephedrine
Phenobarbital
Theophylline
TEDRAL ELIXIR*
Alcohol
Ephedrine
Phenobarbital
Theophylline
TEDRAL EXPECTORANT*
Ephedrine
Guaifenesin
Phenobarbital
Theophylline
TEDRAL SA*
Ephedrine
Phenobarbital
Theophylline
TEDRAL-25*
Butabarbital
Ephedrine
Theophylline
TEEBACIN
Aminosalicylate
TEEBACONIN
Isoniazid
TEEJEL
Choline Salicylate
TEENAC

Sulfur
TEEN 10 LOTION
Benzoyl Peroxide
TEEN 5 LOTION
Benzoyl Peroxide
TEEN 5 WASH
Benzoyl Peroxide
TEETHING
Benzocaine
TEGA-C
Vitamins, Multiple
TEGA CAINE
Benzocaine
TEGA-E
Vitamins, Multiple
TEGA-SPAN
Niacin
TEGA-VERT*
Dimenhydrinate
Niacin
TEGISON
Etretinate
TEGMIDE
Trimethobenzamide
TEGOPEN
Cloxacillin
TEGRETOL
Carbamazepine
TEGRIN FOR PSORIASIS*
Allantoin
Crude Coal Tar Extract
TELDRIN
Chlorpheniramine
TELEPAQUE
Iopanoic Acid
TELMID
Dithiazanine
TELMIN
Mebendazole
TELODRON
Chlorpheniramine
TEMARIL
Trimeprazine
TEMEGESIC
Buprenorphine
TEMENTIL
Prochlorperazine
TEMESTA
Lorazepam
TEMLO
Acetaminophen
TEMPOSIL
Calcium Carbimide
TEMPRA
Acetaminophen
TEMSERIN
Timolol
TENATHAN
Bethanidine
TENICRIDINE
Quinacrine
TENLAP
Acetaminophen
TENOL
Acetaminophen
TENORETIC*
Atenolol
Chlorthalidone
TENORMIN
Atenolol
TENSILEST
Pentolinium
TENSILON
Edrophonium
TENSIUM
Diazepam
TENUATE
Diethylpropion
TENUATE DOSPAN
Diethylpropion
T.E.P.*
Ephedrine
Phenobarbital
Theophylline
TEPANIL
Diethylpropion
TEPANIL TEN-TAB
Diethylpropion
TEPICYCLINE
Tetracycline
TERAMINE
Phentermine
TERFLUZINE
Trifluoperazine
TERIDAX
Iophenoxic Acid
TERRA-CORTRIL*
Hydrocortisone
Oxytetracycline
TERRA-CORTRIL SPRAY WITH POLYMYXIN B*

Hydrocortisone
Oxytetracycline
Polymyxin B
TERRAMYCIN
Oxytetracycline
TERRAMYCIN OINTMENT*
Oxytetracycline
Polymyxin B
TERRAMYCIN OPHTHALMIC*
Oxytetracycline
Polymyxin B
TERRAMYCIN OPHTHALMIC OINTMENT*
Oxytetracycline
Polymyxin B
TERRAMYCIN OTIC OINTMENT*
Oxytetracycline
Polymyxin B
TERRAMYCIN TOPICAL OINTMENT*
Oxytetracycline
Polymyxin B
TERRAMYCIN VAGINAL*
Oxytetracycline
Polymyxin B
TERRAMYCIN WITH POLYMYXIN B*
Oxytetracycline
Polymyxin B
TERRASTATIN*
Nystatin
Oxytetracycline
TERSASEPTIC
Triclosan
TERSA-TAR
Coal Tar
TERTROXIN
Liothyronine
TESLAC
Testolactone
TESSALON
Benzonatate
TESTAFORM
Methyltestosterone
TESTAQUA
Testosterone
TESTATE
Testosterone
TESTAVAL 90/4*
Estradiol
Testosterone
TESTAVOL S
Vitamin A
TEST-ESTRIN*
Estradiol
Testosterone
TESTEX
Testosterone
TESTOJECT-E.P.
Testosterone
TESTOJECT-50
Testosterone
TESTONE
Testosterone
TESTORA
Methyltestosterone
TESTOSTEROID
Testosterone
TESTOSTROVAL P.A.
Testosterone
TEST P.S.P.
Phenol-sulfonphthalein
TESTRED
Methyltestosterone
TESTRONE
Testosterone
TET-CONN-G
Tetanus Immune Globulin, Human
TETRABIOTIC
Tetracycline
TETRA-C
Tetracycline
TETRACAPS
Tetracycline
TETRACHEL
Tetracycline
TETRACON
Tetrahydrozoline
TETRACRINE
Tetracycline
TETRACYN
Tetracycline
TETRALAN-250
Tetracycline
TETRALEAN
Tetracycline
TETRAM

Tetracycline
TETRAMINE
Oxytetracycline
TETRASINE
Tetrahydrozoline
TETRASTATIN*
Nystatin
Tetracycline
TETRAZOTYL
Rolitetracycline
TETREX
Tetracycline
TETROSOL
Tetracycline
TEXACORT
Hydrocortisone
THALAZOL
Phthalylsulfa-
thiazole
THALFED*
Ephedrine
Phenobarbital
Theophylline
THALITONE
Chlorthalidone
THAM
Tromethamine
THANTIS
Meralein
THECORD*
Ephedrine
Phenobarbital
Theophylline
THEELIN
Estrone
THEELOL
Estriol
THENFADIL
Thenyldiamine
THENYLENE
Methapyrilene
THEOBID DURCAP
Theophylline
THEOBID JR. DURCAPS
Theophylline
THEOBRON SR
Theophylline
THEOCALCIN
Theobromine
THEOCAP
Theophylline
THEOCLEAR
Theophylline
THEOCLEAR L.A.
Theophylline
THEOCYNE
Theophylline
THEODRIN PEDIATRIC
SUSPENSION*
Ephedrine
Phenobarbital
Potassium Iodide
Theophylline
THEO-DUR
Theophylline
THEO-DUR SPRINKLE
Theophylline
THEOFEDRAL*
Ephedrine
Phenobarbital
Theophylline
THEOGEN
Estrone
THEO-GUAIA*
Guaifenesin
Theophylline
THEOLAIR
Theophylline
THEOLAIR-PLUS 250*
Guaifenesin
Theophylline
THEOLAMINE
Aminophylline
THEOLIXIR
Theophylline
THEON
Theophylline
THEO-ORGANIDIN*
Iodinated Glycerol
Theophylline
THEOPHEDRIZINE*
Ephedrine
Hydroxyzine
Theophylline
THEOPHENYLLIN*
Ephedrine
Phenobarbital
Theophylline
THEOPHYL CHEWABLE
Theophylline

THEOPHYL-SR
  Theophylline
THEOPHYL-225
  Theophylline
THEORAL*
  Ephedrine
  Phenobarbital
  Theophylline
THEO-SLY-R*
  Mersalyl
  Theophylline
THEOSPAN
  Theophylline
THEOSPAN SR
  Theophylline
THEOSPAN 80
  Theophylline
THEOSTAT
  Theophylline
THEOTABS*
  Ephedrine
  Phenobarbital
  Theophylline
THEOVENT LONG-ACTING
  Theophylline
THEOZINE*
  Ephedrine
  Hydroxyzine
  Theophylline
THEO-24
  Theophylline
THEPHORIN
  Phenindamine
THERABID
  Vitamins, Multiple
THERAC*
  Salicylic Acid
  Sulfur
THERACEBRIN
  Vitamins, Multiple
THERA-COMBEX H-P*
  Ascorbic Acid
  Cyanocobalamin
  Niacinamide
  Panthenol
  Pyridoxine
  Riboflavin
  Thiamine
THERA-COMBEX H-P
    KAPSEALS
  Vitamins, Multiple
THERA-COMBEX KAPSEALS
  Vitamins, Multiple
THERA-COMPLEX H-P*
  Ascorbic Acid
  Vitamin B Complex
THERACORT*
  Hydrocortisone
  Salicylic Acid
  Sulfur
THERA-FLUR
  Sodium Fluoride
THERAGRAN
  Vitamins, Multiple
THERAGRAN LIQUID
  Vitamins, Multiple
THERAGRAN-M*
  Minerals, Multiple
  Vitamins, Multiple
THERALAX
  Bisacodyl
THERALENE
  Trimeprazine
THERANAC SCRUB
  Benzalkonium
    Chloride
THERAPADS*
  Alcohol
  Salicylic Acid
THERAPAV
  Papaverine
THERAPEUTIC VITAMINS
  Vitamins, Multiple
THERAPEUTIC VITAMINS
    AND MINERALS*
  Minerals, Multiple
  Vitamins, Multiple
THERA-SPANCAP
  Vitamins, Multiple
THERATUSS
  Pipazethate
THERON
  Vitamins, Multiple
THESODATE
  Theobromine
THEX FORTE*
  Ascorbic Acid
  Vitamin B Complex
THIACIDE*
  Methenamine
    Mandelate

Potassium Phosphate
THIANAL
Hydrochlorothiazide
THIASERP*
Hydrochlorothiazide
Reserpine
THILOPEMAL
Ethosuximide
THIOCOL
Potassium Guaiacolsulfonate
THIOCYL
Sodium Thiosalicylate
THIODYNE
Sodium Thiosalicylate
THIOMERIN
Mercaptomerin
THIORIL
Thioridazine
THIOSAL
Sodium Thiosalicylate
THIOSULFIL
Sulfamethizole
THIOSULFIL-A*
Phenazopyridine
Sulfamethizole
THIOSULFIL-A FORTE*
Phenazopyridine
Sulfamethizole
THIOSULFIL DUO-PAK*
Phenazopyridine
Sulfamethizole
THIOSULFIL FORTE
Sulfamethizole
THISUL
Sodium Thiosalicylate
THIURETIC
Hydrochlorothiazide
THORAZINE
Chlorpromazine
THORAZINE SPANSULES
Chlorpromazine
T.H.P.
Trihexyphenidyl
THROAT DISCS THROAT LOZENGES
Capsicum
THROMBOLYSIN
Fibrinolysin, Human
THROMBOSTAT
Thrombin
THRU PENETRATING LIQUID*
Benzocaine
Isopropyl Alcohol
Salicylamide
TH SAL
Sodium Thiosalicylate
THUMZ
Denatonium Benzoate
THYLOGEN
Pyrilamine
THYLOKAY
Menadiol
THYLOQUINONE
Menadione
THYLOX MEDICATED SOAP
Sulfur
THYPINONE
Protirelin
THYRACTIN
Thyroglobulin
THYRAR
Thyroid
THYREOSTAT
Methylthiouracil
THYROCRINE
Thyroid
THYROID STRONG*
Liothyronine
Thyroxine
THYROLAR
Liotrix
THYRONOL
Thyroid
THYROPROTEIN
Thyroglobulin
THYRO-TERIC
Thyroid
THYROTRON
Thyrotropin
THYTROPAR
Thyrotropin
TIA-DOCE INJECTABLE UNIVIAL*

Cyanocobalamin
Thiamine
TICAR
Ticarcillin
TICLID
Ticlopidine
TICLODIX
Ticlopidine
TICLODONE
Ticlopidine
TIG
Tetanus Immune Globulin
TIGAN
Trimethobenzamide
TIMCACOR
Timolol
TIMED COLD*
Chlorpheniramine
Pheniramine
Phenylpropanolamine
TIMOLIDE*
Hydrochlorothiazide
Timolol
TIMOPTIC
Timolol
TIMOPTOL
Timolol
TIMOVAN
Prothipendyl
TINACTIN
Tolnaftate
TINADERM
Tolnaftate
TINDAL
Acetophenazine
TING*
Benzoic Acid
Zinc Stearate
TINVER*
Isopropyl Alcohol
Salicylic Acid
Sodium Thiosulfate
TIREND
Caffeine
TISIN
Isoniazid
TISMA*
Acetaminophen
Caffeine
Sodium Salicylamide
TISOMYCIN
Cycloserine
TITRALAC
Calcium Carbonate
TIVRIN
Acetaminophen
TOBREX
Tobramycin
TOCINE
Sparteine
TOCLASE
Carbetapentane
TOCLONOL EXPECTORANT*
Carbetapentane
Terpin Hydrate
TOCLONOL WITH CODEINE*
Carbetapentane
Terpin Hydrate
TOCOPHEREX
Vitamin E
TOCOSAMINE
Sparteine
TOFAXIN
Vitamin E
TOFRANIL
Imipramine
TOFRANIL-PM
Imipramine
TOKOLS
Vitamin E
TOLBUTONE
Tolbutamide
TOLECTIN
Tolmetin
TOLECTIN DS
Tolmetin
TOLERON
Ferrous Fumarate
TOLIFER
Ferrous Fumarate
TOLINASE
Tolazamide
TOLLERCLIN
Demeclocycline
TOLNATE
Prothipendyl
TOLSERAM
Mephenesin
TOLSEROL

Mephenesin
TOLU-SED*
Codeine
Guaifenesin
TOLU-SED DM*
Dextromethorphan
Guaifenesin
TOLYSPAZ
Mephenesin
TOLZOL
Tolazoline
TONEBEC
Vitamins, Multiple
TONECOL*
Chlorpheniramine
Dextromethorphan
Guaifenesin
Phenylephrine
TONELAX
Danthron
TONOCAID
Tocainide
TONOCARD
Tocainide
TONOFTAL
Tolnaftate
TONOGARD
Tocainide
TOPCAINE
Benzocaine
TOPEX ACNE CLEARING MEDICATION
Benzoyl Peroxide
TOPIC BENZYL ALCOHOL GEL
Benzyl Alcohol
TOPICORT
Desoximetasone
TOPICYCLINE
Tetracycline
TOPILIDON
Lidocaine
TOPISOLON
Desoximetasone
TOPITRACIN
Bacitracin
TOPSYN GEL
Fluocinonide
TORA
Phentermine
TORECAN
Thiethylperazine
TORESTEN
Thiethylperazine
TORNALATE
Bitolterol
TORONTO INSULIN
Insulin Regular
TORYN
Caramiphen
TOSMILEN
Demecarium
TOSSECOL*
Ephedrine
Pheniramine
Phenylpropanolamine
Pyrilamine
TOSTRAM
Itramin Tosylate
TOTACILLIN
Ampicillin
TOTAL ECLIPSE SUNSCREEN*
Oxybenzone
Padimate
TOTAPEN
Ampicillin
T.P.I.*
Acetaminophen
Chlorpheniramine
Phenylephrine
Phenylpropanolamine
TRAC*
Atropine
Benzoic Acid
Hyoscyamine
Methenamine
Methylene Blue
Phenyl Salicylate
TRACILON
Triamcinolone
TRACRIUM
Atracurium
TRAISICOR
Oxprenolol
TRAL
Hexocyclium
TRALGON
Acetaminophen
TRALMAG*

Aluminum Hydroxide
Dihydroxyaluminum
Aminoacetate
Magnesium Hydroxide
TRAMACIN
Triamcinolone
TRANCIN
Fluphenazine
TRANCOPAL
Chlormezanone
TRANDATE
Labetalol
TRANIMUL
Diazepam
TRANITE
Pentaerythritol
Tetranitrate
TRANMEP
Meprobamate
TRANQIUM
Methapyrilene
TRANQUIL*
Acetaminophen
Methapyrilene
Sodium Salicylate
TRANQUILINE
Meprobamate
TRANSACT
Sulfur
TRANSBILIX
Meglumine
TRANSCYCLINE
Rolitetracycline
TRANSDERM-NITRO
Nitroglycerin
TRANSDERM-SCOP
Scopolamine
TRANSIBYL
Dehydrocholic Acid
TRANSPOISE
Mephenoxalone
TRANXENE
Clorazepate
TRANXILENE AZENE
Clorazepate
TRANZINE
Chlorpromazine
TRASENTINE
Adiphenine
TRASICOR
Oxprenolol
TRASYLOL
Aprotinin
TRATES
Nitroglycerin
TRAVAD
Barium
TRAVAMINE
Dimenhydrinate
TRAV-AREX
Dimenhydrinate
TRAVASE
Sutilains
TRAVASE OINTMENT
Protease
TRAVENOL
Sorbitol
TRECATOR
Ethionamide
TRECATOR-SC
Ethionamide
TRELMAR
Meprobamate
TREMARIL
Methixene
TREMIN
Trihexyphenidyl
TREMONIL
Methixene
TRENDAR*
Acetaminophen
Pamabrom
TRENTAL
Pentoxifylline
TREPIDONE
Mephenoxalone
TRESCATYL
Ethionamide
TRESORTIL
Methocarbamol
TREST
Methixene
TREXAN
Naltrexone
TRIACET CREAM
Triamcinolone
TRIACIN*
Pseudoephedrine
Triprolidine
TRIADERM

Triamcinolone
TRIADOR
Methaqualone
TRIAFED*
Pseudoephedrine
Triprolidine
TRIALKA
Calcium Carbonate
TRIAMALONE
Triamcinolone
TRIAMINIC*
Pheniramine
Phenylpropanolamine
Pyrilamine
TRIAMINIC ALLERGY*
Chlorpheniramine
Phenylpropanolamine
TRIAMINIC-DM COUGH FORMULA*
Dextromethorphan
Phenylpropanolamine
TRIAMINIC EXPECTORANT*
Guaifenesin
Pheniramine
Phenylpropanolamine
Pyrilamine
TRIAMINIC EXPECTORANT WITH CODEINE*
Codeine
Guaifenesin
Pheniramine
Phenylpropanolamine
Pyrilamine
TRIAMINICIN*
Aspirin
Chlorpheniramine
Phenylpropanolamine
TRIAMINICIN ALLERGY*
Chlorpheniramine
Phenylpropanolamine
TRIAMINICIN CHEWABLES*
Chlorpheniramine
Phenylpropanolamine
TRIAMINICIN NASAL SPRAY*
Phenylephrine
Phenylpropanolamine
TRIAMINICOL*
Ammonium Chloride
Dextromethorphan
Pheniramine
Phenylpropanolamine
Pyrilamine
TRIAMINICOL DECONGESTANT COUGH*
Ammonium Chloride
Dextromethorphan
Pheniramine
Phenylpropanolamine
Pyrilamine
TRIAPHEN-10
Aspirin
TRIAPRIN*
Acetaminophen
Pentobarbital
Salicylamide
TRIAVIL*
Amitriptyline
Perphenazine
TRIAZINE
Trifluoperazine
TRIAZURE
Azaribine
TRIBURON
Triclobisonium
TRICANDIL
Mepartricin
TRICHAZOL
Metronidazole
TRICHLOREX
Trichlormethiazide
TRICHOTINE
Sodium Borate
TRICILONE NNG*
Gramicidin
Neomycin
Nystatin
Triamcinolone
TRICLOS
Triclofos
TRICODENE C-V*
Codeine
Pyrilamine
Terpin Hydrate
TRICODENE DM
Dextromethorphan
TRICODENE FORTE*
Chlorpheniramine
Dextromethorphan

Phenylpropanolamine
TRICODENE NN*
Ammonium Chloride
Chlorpheniramine
Dextromethorphan
Phenylpropanolamine
TRICODENE PEDIATRIC*
Dextromethorphan
Phenylpropanolamine
TRI-CONE*
Amylase
Lipase
Prolase
Simethicone
TRI-CONE PLUS*
Amylase
Hyoscyamine
Lipase
Simethicone
TRIDATE BOWEL KIT*
Bisacodyl
Magnesium Citrate
TRIDESILON
Desonide
TRIDIL
Nitroglycerin
TRIDIONE
Trimethadione
TRIFED*
Pseudoephedrine
Triprolidine
TRI-FED*
Pseudoephedrine
Triprolidine
TRIFLURIN
Trifluoperazine
TRIGESIC*
Acetaminophen
Aspirin
Caffeine
TRIGOT
Ergoloid Mesylates
TRIHEMIC 600*
Ascorbic Acid
Cyanocobalamin
Docusate Sodium
Ferrous Fumarate
Folic Acid
Intrinsic Factor
Vitamin E
TRIHEXANE
Trihexyphenidyl
TRIHEXIDYL
Trihexyphenidyl
TRIHEXY-2
Trihexyphenidyl
TRIHISTA-PHEN*
Chlorpheniramine
Pheniramine
Phenylpropanolamine
Pyrilamine
TRI-IMMUNOL*
Diphtheria Toxoid
Pertussis Vaccine
Tetanus Toxoid
TRIKACIDE
Metronidazole
TRIKAMON
Metronidazole
TRIKETOL
Dehydrocholic Acid
TRILAFON
Perphenazine
TRILAX*
Dehydrocholic Acid
Docusate Sodium
Phenolphthalein
TRILCIN
Fluorometholone
TRILENE
Trichloroethylene
TRILISATE
Choline Magnesium
Trisalicylate
TRILIUM
Chlordiazepoxide
TRIMACORT
Triamcinolone
TRIMAGEL*
Aluminum Hydroxide
Magnesium
Trisilicate
TRIMAX
Magnesium
Trisilicate
TRI-MEDEX*
Guaifenesin
Phenylpropanolamine
TRIMEDONE
Trimethadione

TRIMELARSAN
Melarsonyl
TRIMETHOPRIM-SULFA
Co-Trimoxazole
TRIMETON
Pheniramine
TRIMINICOL COUGH SYRUP*
Ammonium Chloride
Dextromethorphan
Pheniramine
Phenylpropanolamine
Pyrilamine
TRIMO-SAN
Phenylmercuric Acetate
TRIMOX
Amoxicillin
TRIMPEX
Trimethoprim
TRIMSTAT
Phendimetrazine
TRIMTABS
Phendimetrazine
TRIMYSTEN
Clotrimazole
TRIND*
Chlorpheniramine
Phenylpropanolamine
TRIND DM*
Chlorpheniramine
Dextromethorphan
Phenylpropanolamine
TRI-NEFRIN*
Chlorpheniramine
Methapyrilene
Phenylpropanolamine
TRI-NORINYL*
Ethinyl Estradiol
Norethindrone
TRINSICON*
Ascorbic Acid
Cobalamin
Ferrous Fumarate
Folic Acid
Intrinsic Factor
TRINSICON M*
Ascorbic Acid
Cobalamin
Ferrous Fumarate
Intrinsic Factor
TRIOGEN*
Diphtheria Toxoid
Pertussis Vaccine
Tetanus Toxoid
TRI-PAVASULE
Papaverine
TRIPAZINE
Trifluoperazine
TRIPHASIL*
Ethinyl Estradiol
Norgestrel
TRIPHED*
Pseudoephedrine
Triprolidine
TRI-PHEN*
Brompheniramine
Phenylephrine
Phenylpropanolamine
TRI-PHEN-CHLOR*
Chlorpheniramine
Phenylephrine
Phenylpropanolamine
Phenyltoloxamine
TRIPHENYL EXPECTORANT*
Guaifenesin
Phenylpropanolamine
TRIPHOSPHODINE
Adenosine
TRIPLE ANTIBIOTIC*
Bacitracin
Neomycin
Polymyxin B
TRIPODRINE*
Pseudoephedrine
Triprolidine
TRIPOSED*
Pseudoephedrine
Triprolidine
TRIPTIL
Protriptyline
TRIPTONE
Scopolamine
TRIS AMINO
Tromethamine
TRISERP
Reserpine
TRI-SIL
Magnesium Trisilicate
TRI-SOF*

Carboxymethyl cellulose
Casanthranol
Docusate Sodium

TRISOGEL*
Aluminum Hydroxide
Magnesium Trisilicate

TRISOMIN
Magnesium Trisilicate

TRISORALEN
Trioxsalen

TRI-STATIN*
Gramicidin
Neomycin
Nystatin
Triamcinolone

TRITEN
Dimethindene

TRITHEON
Nithiamide

TRI-TINIC*
Ascorbic Acid
Cyanocobalamin
Ferrous Fumarate
Folic Acid

TRI-TUMINE
Tripelennamine

TRI-VI-FLOR*
Ascorbic Acid
Cholecalciferol
Fluoride
Vitamin A

TRI-VI-FLOR W/IRON DROPS*
Ascorbic Acid
Cholecalciferol
Fluoride
Iron
Vitamin A

TRI-VI-SOL*
Ascorbic Acid
Cholecalciferol
Vitamin A

TRI-VI-SOL CHEWABLE
Vitamins, Multiple

TRI-VI-SOL WITH IRON*
Ascorbic Acid
Cholecalciferol
Iron
Vitamin A

TRI-VI-SOL WITH IRON DROPS*
Iron
Vitamins, Multiple

TRIXYL
Trihexyphenidyl

TROBICIN
Spectinomycin

TROBICIN STERILE POWDER
Spectinomycin

TROCAINE
Benzocaine

TROCINATE
Thiphenamil

TROFAN
Tryptophan

TROKETTES*
Benzocaine
Cetalkonium
Cetylpyridinium

TROMBOVAR
Sodium Tetradecyl Sulfate

TROMEXAN
Ethyl Biscoumacetate

TRONOLANE
Pramoxine

TRONOTHANE
Pramoxine

TROPH-IRON*
Cyanocobalamin
Ferric Pyrophosphate
Thiamine

TROPH-IRON LIQUID*
Cyanocobalamin
Iron
Thiamine

TROPHITE*
Cyanocobalamin
Thiamine

TROSINONE
Ethisterone

TROUTMAN'S
Dextromethorphan

TRUPHYLLINE
Aminophylline

TRUXAL

Chlorprothixene
TRYMEGEN
Chlorpheniramine
TRYMEX
Triamcinolone
TRYPAFLAVIN
Acriflavine
TRYPTACIN
Tryptophan
TRYPTAR
Trypsin
TRYPTIZOL
Amitriptyline
T-STAT
Erythromycin
TUALONE-300
Methaqualone
TUAMINE
Tuaminoheptane
TUAZOLE
Methaqualone
TUBADIL
Tubocurarine
TUBARINE
Tubocurarine
TUBERSOL
Tuberculin
TUBEX
Corticotropin
TUCILLIN
Penicillin G
TUCKS CREAM
Witch Hazel
TUCKS OINTMENT
Witch Hazel
TUCKS PADS*
Benzalkonium Chloride
Glycerin
Witch Hazel
TUDECON*
Chlorpheniramine
Phenylephrine
Phenylpropanolamine
Phenyltoloxamine
TUINAL*
Amobarbital
Secobarbital
TUINAL PULVULES*
Amobarbital
Secobarbital
TUISEC
Secobarbital
TULOIDIN
Thyroid
TUMS
Calcium Carbonate
TUO-BARB*
Amobarbital
Secobarbital
TURBINAIRE DECADRON PHOSPHATE
Dexamethasone
TUSAL
Sodium Thiosalicylate
TUS-ORAMINIC*
Atropine
Chlorpheniramine
Dextromethorphan
Phenylpropanolamine
TUSS-ADE*
Atropine
Caramiphen
Chlorpheniramine
Phenylpropanolamine
TUSSAGESIC*
Dextromethorphan
Pheniramine
Phenylpropanolamine
Pyrilamine
Terpin Hydrate
TUSS ALLERGINE*
Caramiphen
Chlorpheniramine
Phenylpropanolamine
TUSSAMINIC*
Dextromethorphan
Pheniramine
Phenylpropanolamine
Pyrilamine
Terpin Hydrate
TUSSANCA
Guaifenesin
TUSSANIL SYRUP*
Chlorpheniramine
Phenylephrine
Phenylpropanolamine
Pyrilamine
TUSSAR DM*

Chlorpheniramine
Dextromethorphan
Phenylephrine
TUSSAR-SF*
Carbetapentane
Chlorpheniramine
Codeine
Guaifenesin
TUSSAR-2*
Carbetapentane
Chlorpheniramine
Codeine
Guaifenesin
TUSSCAPINE
Noscapine
TUSSCIDEN EXPECTORANT
Guaifenesin
TUSSEND*
Hydrocodone
Pseudoephedrine
TUSSEND EXPECTORANT*
Guaifenesin
Hydrocodone
Pseudoephedrine
TUSSETS
Ethyl Dibunate
TUSSIMOL
Oxeladin
TUSSIONEX*
Hydrocodone
Phenyltoloxamine
TUSSI-ORGANIDIN*
Chlorpheniramine
Codeine
Iodinated Glycerol
TUSSI-ORGANIDIN DM*
Chlorpheniramine
Dextromethorphan
Iodinated Glycerol
TUSS-ORNADE*
Caramiphen
Phenylpropanolamine
TUSSORPHAN
Dextromethorphan
TUSSTAT
Diphenhydramine
TUZON*
Acetaminophen
Chlorzoxazone
TWILIGHT*
Methapyrilene
Salicylamide
TWIN-K*
Potassium Citrate
Potassium Gluconate
TWISTON
Rotoxamine
TWISTON R-A
Rotoxamine
TWO-DYNE*
Acetaminophen
Butalbital
Caffeine
TYBATRAN
Tybamate
TYJODIN
Liothyronine
TYLAPRIN ELIXIR
Acetaminophen
TYLENOL
Acetaminophen
TYLENOL #1*
Acetaminophen
Codeine
TYLENOL #2*
Acetaminophen
Codeine
TYLENOL #3*
Acetaminophen
Codeine
TYLENOL #4*
Acetaminophen
Codeine
TYLENOL EXTRA STRENGTH
Acetaminophen
TYLENOL MAXIMUM STRENGTH SINUS MEDICATION*
Acetaminophen
Pseudoephedrine
TYLENOL NO.1 FORTE*
Acetaminophen
Codeine
TYLENOL WITH CODEINE*
Acetaminophen
Codeine
TYLOSTERONE*
Diethylstilbestrol
Methyltestosterone
TYLOX*

Acetaminophen
Oxycodone
TYMCAPS
Chlorpheniramine
TYMPAGESIC*
Antipyrine
Benzocaine
Phenylephrine
TYMTRAN
Ceruletide
TYRIMIDE
Isopropamide
TYRODERM
Tyrothricin
TYROHIST
Phenylephrine
TYVID
Isoniazid
TYZINE
Tetrahydrozoline
T-125
Tetracycline
T-250
Tetracycline
T-4-L*
Benzoic Acid
Salicylic Acid

U

UAA*
Atropine
Benzoic Acid
Hyoscyamine
Methenamine
Methylene Blue
Phenylsalicylate
UDOLAC
Dapsone
ULACORT
Prednisolone
ULCERBAN
Sucralfate
ULCORT
Hydrocortisone
ULO
Chlophedianol
ULONE
Chlorphedianol
ULTANDREN
Fluoxymesterone
UL-TAR
Coal Tar
ULTIMOX
Amoxicillin
ULTRACAINE
Lidocaine
ULTRACEF
Cefadroxil
ULTRA CLEAR MEDICATED SHAMPOO
Coal Tar
ULTRA DERM*
Glycerin
Lanolin
Mineral Oil
Petrolatum
Propylene Glycol
ULTRA-DERM BATH OIL*
Lanolin
Mineral Oil
ULTRALENTE
Insulin Zinc [Suspension] Extended
ULTRALENTE ILETIN
Insulin Zinc [Suspension] Extended
ULTRALENTE INSULIN
Insulin Zinc [Suspension] Extended
ULTRA MIDE
Urea
ULTRAMYCIN
Minocycline
ULTRAN
Phenaglycodol
ULTRA PAQUE
Barium
ULTRATARD
Insulin Zinc [Suspension] Extended
ULTRATEARS
Methylcellulose
UNACAINE

Metabutethamine
UNDOGUENT*
Undecylenic Acid
Zinc Undecylenate
UNGUENTINE
Benzocaine
UNGUENTINE PLUS*
Lidocaine
Parachlorometa-xylenol
Phenol
UNGUENTUM BOSSI*
Ammoniated Mercury
Coal Tar
Methenamine Sulfosalicylate
UNICAP
Vitamins, Multiple
UNICAP CHEWABLE
Vitamins, Multiple
UNICAP M
Vitamins, Multiple
UNICAP PLUS IRON*
Iron
Vitamins, Multiple
UNICAP SENIOR
Vitamins, Multiple
UNICAP T
Vitamins, Multiple
UNICORT
Hydrocortisone
UNIDIGIN
Digitoxin
UNIGEN
Estrone
UNIGESIC-A*
Aspirin
Propoxyphene
UNIK-PAK
Barium
UNILAX*
Danthron
Docusate Sodium
UNIPEN
Nafcillin
UNIPHYL
Theophylline
UNIPHYL 400
Theophylline
UNIPRES*
Hydralazine
Hydrochlorothiazide
Reserpine
UNISOIL
Castor Oil
UNISOL*
Boric Acid
Sodium Borate
Sodium Chloride
UNISOM
Doxylamine
UNISUL
Sulfamethizole
UNITENSEN
Cryptenamine
UNITROL
Phenylpropanolamine
UNIVOL*
Aluminum
Magnesium
UNPROCO*
Dextromethorphan
Guaifenesin
UPNOS
Diethylaminobarbital
URACEL
Sodium Salicylate
URACID
Racemethionine
URALGIC*
Atropine
Benzoic Acid
Hyoscyamine
Methenamine
Methylene Blue
Phenyl Salicylate
URAMINE*
Atropine
Benzoic Acid
Hyoscyamine
Methenamine
Methylene Blue
Phenyl Salicylate
URANAP
Racemethionine
URAZIDE
Benzthiazide
URBASON
Methylprednisolone
UREAPHIL

Urea
URECHOLINE
Bethanechol
UREKENE
Valproic Acid
UREMIDE*
Phenazopyridine
Sulfamethizole
UREMOL
Urea
UREMOL HC*
Hydrocortisone
Urea
URESE
Benzthiazide
URETEX
Urea
UREX
Methenamine
Hippurate
URICOSID
Probenecid
URIDON
Chlorthalidone
URIDONE
Anisindione
URIFON
Sulfamethizole
URI-PAK*
Phenazopyridine
Sulfamethizole
URISEC
Urea
URISED*
Atropine
Benzoic Acid
Hyoscyamine
Methenamine
Methylene Blue
Salicylate
URISEDAMINE*
Hyoscyamine
Methenamine
Mandelate
URISEP*
Atropine
Benzoic Acid
Hyoscyamine
Methenamine
Methylene Blue
Phenyl Salicylate
URISPAS
Flavoxate
URITAB*
Atropine
Benzoic Acid
Hyoscyamine
Methenamine
Methylene Blue
Phenyl Salicylate
URITABS W.O.*
Atropine
Benzoic Acid
Hyoscyamine
Methenamine
Phenyl Salicylate
URI-TET
Oxytetracycline
URITHOL*
Atropine
Benzoic Acid
Hyoscyamine
Methenamine
Methylene Blue
Phenyl Salicylate
URITOL
Furosemide
URITONE
Methenamine
UROBAK
Sulfamethoxazole
UROBIOTIC-250*
Oxytetracycline
Phenazopyridine
UROBLUE*
Atropine
Benzoic Acid
Hyoscyamine
Methenamine
Methylene Blue
Phenyl Salicylate
URODINE
Phenazopyridine
URO-GANTANOL*
Phenazopyridine
Sulfamethoxazole
UROKON SODIUM
Sodium Acetrizoate
URO-KP-NEUTRAL*
Potassium Phosphate

Sodium Phosphate
UROLAX
Bethanechol
UROLENE BLUE
Methylene Blue
UROLUCOSIL
Sulfamethizole
URO-MAG
Magnesium Oxide
URO-PHOSPHATE*
Methenamine
Sodium Acid Phosphate
UROQID-ACID*
Methenamine Mandelate
Sodium Phosphate
UROQID-ACID NO.2*
Methenamine Mandelate
Sodium Phosphate
UROSCREEN
Triphenyltetrazolium
UROSET
Potassium Oxyquinoline Sulfate
UROSTAT-FORTE*
Atropine
Benzoic Acid
Hyoscyamine
Methenamine
Methylene Blue
Phenyl Salicylate
UROTOIN
Nitrofurantoin
UROTROPIN
Methenamine
UROVIST
Diatrizoate Meglumine
UROVIST SODIUM 300
Diatrizoate Sodium
UROZIDE
Hydrochlorothiazide
URSINUS*
Carbaspirin Calcium
Pheniramine
Phenylpropanolamine
Pyrilamine
UTERACON
Oxytocin
UTIBID
Oxolinic Acid
UTICILLIN-K
Penicillin V Potassium
UTICILLIN-VK
Penicillin V Potassium
UTICORT
Betamethasone
UTRASUL
Sulfamethizole
UVAL
Sulisobenzone
UVINOL MS-40
Sulisobenzone

V

VACON
Phenylephrine
VACUETTS ADULT*
Sodium Acid Pyrophosphate
Sodium Bicarbonate
Sodium Biphosphate
VAGACREME*
Allantoin
Aminacrine
Sulfanilamide
VAGESTROL
Diethylstilbestrol
VAGIDINE*
Allantoin
Aminacrine
Sulfanilamide
VAGILIA CREAM/ SUPPOSITORIES*
Aminacrine
Sulfisoxazole
VAGI-NIL*
Allantoin
Aminacrine
Sulfanilamide
VAGITROL CREAM/ SUPPOSITORIES*
Aminacrine

Sulfanilamide
VAGOSPASMYL
Adiphenine
VALADOL
Acetaminophen
VALAX*
Danthron
Docusate Sodium
VALDRENE
Diphenhydramine
VALERGEN-10
Estradiol
VALIHIST*
Acetaminophen
Chlorpheniramine
Phenylephrine
VALISONE
Betamethasone
VALISONE-G
Betamethasone
VALISONE SCALP LOTION
Betamethasone
VALIUM
Diazepam
VALLERGAN
Trimeprazine
VALLESTRIL
Methallenestril
VALMID
Ethinamate
VALMIDATE
Ethinamate
VALOID
Cyclizine
VALORIN
Acetaminophen
VALPIN
Anisotropine
VALPIN 50
Anisotropine
VALPIN 50-PB*
Anisotropine
Phenobarbital
VALRELEASE
Diazepam
VALSYN
Furaltadone
VANATAL*
Atropine
Hyoscyamine
Phenobarbital
Scopolamine
VANAY
Triacetin
VANCENASE NASAL INHALER
Beclomethasone
VANCERIL
Beclomethasone
VANCERIL ORAL INHALER
Beclomethasone
VANCIDE ZP
Pyrithione Zinc
VANCOCIN
Vancomycin
VANDID
Ethamivan
VANOBID
Candicidin
VANODONNAL*
Atropine
Hyoscyamine
Phenobarbital
Scopolamine
VANOXIDE*
Benzoyl Peroxide
Chlorhydroxyquinoline
VANQUIN
Pyrvinium Pamoate
VANQUISH CAPLET*
Acetaminophen
Aspirin
Caffeine
VANSEB*
Salicylic Acid
Sulfur
VANSEB-T*
Coal Tar
Salicylic Acid
Sulfur
VANSIL
Oxamniquine
VAPO-ISO
Isoproterenol
VAPONEFRIN
Epinephrine
VAPO-N-ISO
Isoproterenol
VARIDASE*

Streptodornase
Streptokinase
VASAL GRANUCAPS
Papaverine
VASCUALS
Vitamin E
VASITOL
Pentaerythritol Tetranitrate
VASOCAP
Papaverine
VASO CLEAR
Naphazoline
VASOCON
Naphazoline
VASOCON A*
Antazoline
Naphazoline
VASOCON REGULAR
Naphazoline
VASODIATOL
Pentaerythritol Tetranitrate
VASODILAN
Isoxsuprine
VASOLAN
Verapamil
VASOMED
Trolnitrate
VASOMINIC TD*
Pheniramine
Phenylpropanolamine
Pyrilamine
VASOPRINE
Isoxsuprine
VASOROME KOWA
Oxandrolone
VASOSPAN
Papaverine
VASOSULF*
Phenylephrine
Sulfacetamide
VASOXYL
Methoxamine
VASO-80 UNICELLES
Pentaerythritol Tetranitrate
VASTRAN
Vitamins, Multiple
VATRAN
Diazepam
VA-TRO-NOL
Ephedrine
VATRONOL NOSE DROPS*
Camphor
Ephedrine
Eucalyptol
Menthol
Salicylate
V-CIL-K
Penicillin V Potassium
V-CILLIN
Penicillin V
V-CILLIN-K
Penicillin V Potassium
VC-K 500
Penicillin V Potassium
VECTRIN
Minocycline
VEETIDS '125'
Penicillin V Potassium
VEETIDS '250'
Penicillin V Potassium
VEETIDS '500'
Penicillin V Potassium
VEGOLYSEN
Hexamethonium
VEGOLYSEN-T
Hexamethonium
VELACYCLINE
Rolitetracycline
VELBAN
Vinblastine
VELBE
Vinblastine
VELOSEF
Cephradine
VELTANE
Brompheniramine
VELTAP*
Brompheniramine
Phenylephrine
Phenylpropanolamine
VELVELAN

Urea
VENOMIL
Hymenopter Venom Extract
VENTAIRE
Protokylol
VENTHERA
Vitamins, Multiple
VENTOLIN
Albuterol
VENTUSSIN
Benzonatate
VEPESID
Etoposide
VERACILLIN
Dicloxacillin
VERACTIL
Methotrimeprazine
VERAPEN-K
Hetacillin
VERATRITE
Alkavervir
VERAZINC
Zinc Sulfate
VERB T.D.
Caffeine
VERCYTE
Pipobroman
VERDEFAM CREAM*
Copper Undecylenate
Propionic Acid
Salicylic Acid
Sodium Caprylate
Undecylenic Acid
VERDEFAM SOLUTION*
Copper Undecylenate
Propionic Acid
Salicylic Acid
Sodium Caprylate
Undecylenic Acid
VEREQUAD*
Ephedrine
Guaifenesin
Phenobarbital
Theophylline
VERGITRYL
Alkavervir
VERGO*
Ascorbic Acid
Calcium Pantothenate
VERILOID
Alkavervir
VERMISOL
Piperazine
VERMIZINE
Piperazine
VERMOX
Mebendazole
VERM-X
Piperazine
VERNACEL OPHTHALMIC*
Pheniramine
Phenylephrine
VERNATE*
Atropine
Chlorpheniramine
VERNITEST
Quinaldine Blue
VERONAL
Barbital
VEROPHEN
Promazine
VEROXIL
Piperazine
VERQUAD*
Ephedrine
Guaifenesin
Phenobarbital
Theophylline
VERSACAINE
Chloroprocaine
VERSAPEN
Hetacillin
VERSAPEN-K
Hetacillin
VERSENATE
Edetate Calcium Disodium
VERSENE ACID
Edetic Acid
VERSTAT*
Niacin
Pentylenetetrazol
Pheniramine
VERSTRAN
Prazepam
VERSUS
Bendazac
VERTEX*
Niacin

Pheniramine
VERTIBAN
Dimenhydrinate
VERTOLAN
Sulfamethazine
VERTROL
Meclizine
VESICHOLINE
Bethanechol
VESIPAQUE
Phenobutiodil
VESPRIN
Triflupromazine
VG*
Minerals, Multiple
Vitamins, Multiple
V-GAN-25
Promethazine
VIADERM-F.A.
Fluocinolone
VIADERM-N
Nystatin
VIADERM-TA
Triamcinolone
VIADRIL
Hydroxydione Sodium Succinate
VI-ALPHA
Vitamin A
VI-AQUA
Vitamins, Multiple
VIA-QUIL
Chlordiazepoxide
VIBALT
Cyanocobalamin
VIBAZINE
Buclizine
VIBELAN
Vitamin B Complex
VIBRAMYCIN
Doxycycline
VIBRA-TABS
Doxycycline
VICKS COUGH*
Dextromethorphan
Guaifenesin
VICKS COUGH DROPS
Menthol
VICKS COUGH SILENCER
Dextromethorphan
VICKS FORMULA 44 COUGH CONTROL DISCS*
Benzocaine
Dextromethorphan
Menthol
VICKS FORMULA 44 COUGH MIXTURE*
Dextromethorphan
Doxylamine
Sodium Citrate
VICKS FORMULA 44D DECONGESTANT COUGH MIXTURE*
Alcohol
Dextromethorphan
Guaifenesin
Phenylpropanolamine
VICKS INHALER*
Camphor
Desoxyephedrine
Methyl Salicylate
VICKS MEDI-TRATING*
Benzocaine
Cetylpyridinium
VICKS NYQUIL NIGHTTIME COLDS MEDICINE*
Acetaminophen
Alcohol
Dextromethorphan
Doxylamine
Ephedrine
VICKS SINEX DECONGESTANT NASAL SPRAY*
Camphor
Cetylpyridinium
Eucalyptol
Menthol
Phenylephrine
Salicylate
VICKS SINEX LONG-ACTING DECONGESTANT NASAL SPRAY
Xylometazoline
VICKS THROAT LOZENGES*
Benzocaine
Camphor
Cetylpyridinium
Eucalyptus Oil
Menthol

VICKS VAPORUB*
  Camphor
  Cedar Leaf Oil
  Eucalyptus Oil
  Menthol
  Nutmeg Oil
  Spirits of
    Turpentine
  Thymol
VICKS VAPOSTEAM*
  Camphor
  Eucalyptus Oil
  Menthol
  Tincture of Benzoin
VICKS VATRONOL NOSE
    DROPS*
  Camphor
  Ephedrine
  Eucalyptol
  Menthol
  Salicylate
VICODIN
  Hydrocodone
VICON
  Vitamins, Multiple
VICON-C*
  Minerals, Multiple
  Vitamins, Multiple
VICON PLUS
  Vitamins, Multiple
VICOPRIN*
  Aspirin
  Hydrocodone
VI-DAYLIN ADC DROPS*
  Ascorbic Acid
  Cholecalciferol
  Vitamin A
VI-DAYLIN CHEWABLE
  Vitamins, Multiple
VI-DAYLIN DROPS
  Vitamins, Multiple
VI-DAYLIN/F + IRON*
  Ferrous Sulfate
  Sodium Fluoride
  Vitamins, Multiple
VI-DAYLIN/F ADC + IRON
    DROPS*
  Ascorbic Acid
  Cholecalciferol
  Ferrous Sulfate
  Sodium Fluoride
  Vitamin A
VI-DAYLIN/F ADC DROPS*
  Ascorbic Acid
  Cholecalciferol
  Sodium Fluoride
  Vitamin A
VI-DAYLIN/F DROPS*
  Sodium Fluoride
  Vitamins, Multiple
VI-DAYLIN LIQUID
  Vitamins, Multiple
VI-DAYLIN PLUS IRON*
  Iron
  Vitamins, Multiple
VI-DAYLIN PLUS IRON
    ADC DROPS*
  Ascorbic Acid
  Cholecalciferol
  Ferrous Sulfate
  Vitamin A
VI-DAYLIN W/FLUORIDE
    CHEWABLE*
  Sodium Fluoride
  Vitamins, Multiple
VIGRAN
  Vitamins, Multiple
VIGRAN CHEWABLE
  Vitamins, Multiple
VIGRAN PLUS IRON*
  Iron
  Vitamins, Multiple
VI-MAGNA
  Vitamins, Multiple
VIMICON
  Cyproheptadine
VINACTANE-P
  Viomycin
VINETHENE
  Vinyl Ether
VINOTHIAM
  Thiamine
VIO-A
  Vitamin A
VIOBAMATE
  Meprobamate
VIO-BEC
  Vitamins, Multiple
VIOCIN
  Viomycin

VIOFORM
Iodochlorhydroxyquin
VIOFORM-HYDROCORTISONE*
Hydrocortisone
Iodochlorhydroxyquin
VIO-GERIC
Vitamins, Multiple
VIO HYDROSONE*
Hydrocortisone
Iodochlorhydroxyquin
Pramoxine
VIOKASE
Pancreatin
VIOPAN-T*
Minerals, Multiple
Vitamins, Multiple
VIOPRAMOSONE*
Hydrocortisone
Iodochlorhydroxyquin
Pramoxine
VIOSERP
Reserpine
VIO-SERPINE
Reserpine
VIO-THENE
Oxyphencyclimine
VI-PENTA F CHEWABLES*
Sodium Fluoride
Vitamins, Multiple
VI-PENTA F INFANT DROPS*
Sodium Fluoride
Vitamins, Multiple
VI-PENTA F MULTIVITAMIN DROPS*
Sodium Fluoride
Vitamins, Multiple
VI-PENTA INFANT DROPS
Vitamins, Multiple
VI-PENTA MULTIVITAMIN DROPS
Vitamins, Multiple
VIRA-A
Vidarabine
VIRANOL*
Lactic Acid
Salicylic Acid
VIRILON
Methyltestosterone
VIROFRAL
Amantadine
VIROMED*
Acetaminophen
Aspirin
Chlorpheniramine
Pseudoephedrine
VIROPTIC
Trifluridine
VIROSTERONE
Testosterone
VISADRON
Phenylephrine
VISALENS WETTING*
Benzalkonium Chloride
Methylcellulose
Polyvinyl Alcohol
VISAMMIN
Khellin
VISCEPHEN*
Dicyclomine
Phenobarbital
VISCEROL
Dicyclomine
VISCULOSE
Methylcellulose
VISINE EYE DROPS
Tetrahydrozoline
VISKEN
Pindolol
VISTACON
Hydroxyzine
VISTAJECT
Hydroxyzine
VISTARIL
Hydroxyzine
VISTRAX*
Hydroxyzine
Oxyphencyclimine
VISUDRISONE
Medrysone
VISUTENSIL
Guanethidine
VI-SYNERAL ONE-CAPS
Vitamins, Multiple
VITA-C
Ascorbic Acid
VITACEE

Ascorbic Acid
VITACREST
Vitamins, Multiple
VITA-E
Vitamin E
VITAGETT
Vitamins, Multiple
VITA-KAPS
Vitamins, Multiple
VITA-KAPS-M
Vitamins, Multiple
VITALONE
Methaqualone
VITA-METRAZOL*
Niacinamide
Pentylenetetrazol
Pyridoxine
Riboflavin
Thiamine
VITAMIN A ACID GEL
Tretinoin
VITA-SLIM
Phenylpropanolamine
VITERRA
Vitamins, Multiple
VITERRA C
Ascorbic Acid
VITERRA HIGH POTENCY
Vitamins, Multiple
VITRON-C*
Ascorbic Acid
Ferrous Fumarate
VITRON-C-PLUS*
Ascorbic Acid
Cyanocobalamin
Ferrous Fumarate
Folic Acid
VI-TWEL
Cyanocobalamin
VIVACTIL
Protriptyline
VIVALAN
Viloxazine
VIVARIN
Caffeine
VIVIDYL
Nortriptyline
VIVOL
Diazepam
VI-ZAC*
Ascorbic Acid
Vitamin A
Vitamin E
Zinc Phosphate
VI-ZAC
Vitamins, Multiple
V-LAX
Plantago Seed
VLEMASQUE*
Calcium Polysulfide
Calcium Thiosulfate
VLEM-DOME*
Calcium Polysulfide
Calcium Thiosulfate
VLEMINCKX*
Calcium Pentasulfide
Calcium Thiosulfate
VM PREPARATION
Vitamins, Multiple
VOIDS
Chlorophyllin
VOLAXIN*
Phenyltoloxamine
Salicylamide
VOLITAL
Pemoline
VOLTAREN
Diclofenac
VONTIL
Thioproperazine
VONTROL
Diphenidol
VORANIL
Clortermine
VOSOL HC OTIC SOLUTION*
Acetic Acid
Hydrocortisone
VOSOL OTIC SOLUTION
Acetic Acid
VOXIN-PG*
Guaifenesin
Phenylpropanolamine
VYTONE*
Hydrocortisone
Iodoquinol

W

WAMPOCAP

Niacin
WANS*
Pentobarbital
Pyrilamine
WARCOUMIN
Warfarin
WARFILONE
Warfarin
WARNERIN
Warfarin
WART-AID*
Ascorbic Acid
Calcium Pantothenate
WART-OFF
Salicylic Acid
WATKINS ANTISEPTIC
Cetylpyridinium
WEHAMINE
Dimenhydrinate
WEHDRYL
Diphenhydramine
WEHGEN
Estrone
WEHVERT
Meclizine
WEIGHTROL
Phendimetrazine
WEL-K
Potassium Tartrate
WELLBUTRIN
Bupropion
WELLCORTIN
Hydrocortisone
WELLCOVORIN
Leucovorin
WESCOHEX
Hexachlorophene
WESMATIC FORTE*
Chlorpheniramine
Ephedrine
Guaifenesin
Phenobarbital
Theophylline
WESPRIN BUFFERED
Aspirin
WESTADONE
Methadone
WESTAPP*
Brompheniramine
Phenylephrine
Phenylpropanolamine
WESTCORT
Hydrocortisone
WESTHROID 1/4
Thyroid
WESTRIM LA
Phenylpropanolamine
WET-N-SOAK*
Benzalkonium Chloride
Polyvinyl Alcohol
WETTING SOLUTION*
Benzalkonium Chloride
Polyvinyl Alcohol
WEXAPHOS
Dexamethasone
WHITFIELD'S*
Benzoic Acid
Salicylic Acid
WHITSPHILL*
Benzoic Acid
Salicylic Acid
WIGRAINE*
Belladonna Alkaloids
Caffeine
Ergotamine
WILLCOTRIN
Cyanocobalamin
WILLNESTROL
Dienestrol
WILPOWR
Phentermine
WINCILLIN-VK
Penicillin V Potassium
WINGEL*
Aluminum Hydroxide
Magnesium Hydroxide
WIN-KINASE
Urokinase
WINOXIN
Digoxin
WINPRED
Prednisone
WINSTROL
Stanozolol
WINTODON
Glycobiarsol
WINTOMYLON

Nalidixic Acid
WINTRACIN
Tetracycline
WIN-V-K
Penicillin V
Potassium
WOLFINA
Rauwolfia Serpentina
WOODWARD'S K.P.*
Kaolin
Pectin
W-T ANTICHOLINERGIC
Oxyphencyclimine
WYACORT
Methylprednisolone
WYAMINE
Mephentermine
WYAMYCIN
Erythromycin
WYANOIDS HC RECTAL SUPPOSITORIES*
Belladonna Alkaloids
Bismuth Oxyiodide
Boric Acid
Ephedrine
Hydrocortisone
Zinc Oxide
WYANOIDS HEMORRHOIDAL SUPPOSITORIES*
Belladonna Alkaloids
Bismuth Oxyiodide
Boric Acid
Ephedrine
Zinc Oxide
WYCILLIN
Penicillin G
WYCILLIN AND PROBENECID*
Penicillin G
Probenecid
WYDASE
Hyaluronidase
WYETH*
Diphtheria Toxoid
Tetanus Toxoid
WYGESIC*
Acetaminophen
Propoxyphene
WYMOX
Amoxicillin
WYOVIN
Dicyclomine
WYTENSIN
Guanabenz
WYVAC
Human Diploid Cell Rabies Vaccine

X

XAMETINA
Trimethobenzamide
XANAX
Alprazolam
XENAGOL
Phenazocine
XERA BP
Benzoyl Peroxide
XERAC
Sulfur
XERAC BP 10
Benzoyl Peroxide
X-OTAG
Orphenadrine
X-PREP
Senna
XSEB SHAMPOO
Salicylic Acid
XSEB-T SHAMPOO*
Coal Tar
Salicylic Acid
XYLOCAINE
Lidocaine
XYLOCAINE ENDOTRACHEAL AEROSOL
Lidocaine
XYLOCAINE JELLY
Lidocaine
XYLOCAINE OINTMENT
Lidocaine
XYLOCAINE TOPICAL SPRAY
Lidocaine
XYLOCAINE VISCOUS
Lidocaine
XYLOCARD
Lidocaine
XYLONEST
Prilocaine

Y

YATREN
  Chiniofon
YODOXIN
  Iodoquinol
YOMESAN
  Niclosamide
YUTOPAR
  Ritodrine

Z

ZACTANE
  Ethoheptazine
ZACTIRIN*
  Aspirin
  Ethoheptazine
ZADITEN
  Ketotifen
ZAMANIL
  Oxyphencyclimine
ZANCHOL
  Florantyrone
ZANOSAR
  Streptozocin
ZANTAC
  Ranitidine
ZARONTIN
  Ethosuximide
ZAROXOLYN
  Metolazone
ZARUMIN*
  Potassium
    Salicylate
  Salicylamide
Z-BEC
  Vitamins, Multiple
ZEM-HISTINE
  Pyrilamine
ZEMO*
  Bismuth Subnitrate
  Menthol
  Methyl Salicylate
  Triclosan
ZENADRIN
  Prednisone
ZENTINIC*
  Ferrous Fumarate
  Folic Acid
  Vitamins, Multiple
ZENTROL CHEWABLE*
  Ascorbic Acid
  Ferrous Fumarate
  Vitamin B Complex
ZENTRON LIQUID*
  Ascorbic Acid
  Ferrous Sulfate
  Vitamin B Complex
ZEPHIRAN CHLORIDE
  Benzalkonium
    Chloride
ZEPHREX*
  Guaifenesin
  Pseudoephedrine
ZEPHREX-LA*
  Guaifenesin
  Pseudoephedrine
ZEPINE
  Reserpine
ZEROXIN
  Benzoyl Peroxide
ZETAR
  Coal Tar
ZETAR EMULSION
  Coal Tar
ZETAR SHAMPOO*
  Chloroxylenol
  Coal Tar
ZETTYN
  Cetalkonium
ZIDE
  Hydrochlorothiazide
ZINACEF
  Cefuroxime
ZINCAPS
  Vitamins, Multiple
ZINCFRIN
  Phenylephrine
ZINCFRIN-A*
  Antazoline
  Naphazoline
  Zinc Sulfate
ZINCOFAX
  Zinc Oxide
ZINC OMADINE
  Pyrithione Zinc
ZINCON
  Pyrithione Zinc
ZINCON DANDRUFF
    SHAMPOO

Pyrithione Zinc
ZINC SULFIDE COMPOUND LOTION
Sulfur
ZINC-220
Zinc Sulfate
ZINTINIC*
Ascorbic Acid
Ferrous Fumarate
Folic Acid
Vitamin B Complex
ZIPAN-25 & -50
Promethazine
ZIRADRYL LOTION*
Alcohol
Diphenhydramine
Zinc Oxide
ZN-PLUS
Zinc
ZOLYSE
Chymotrypsin
ZOMAX
Zomepirac
ZONULYN
Chymotrypsin
ZORANE*
Ethinyl Estradiol
Norethindrone
ZORPRIN
Aspirin
ZOVIRAX
Acyclovir
ZOXAPHEN*
Acetaminophen
Chlorzoxazone
Z-PRO-C*
Ascorbic Acid
Zinc Sulfate
ZP 11 MEDICATED SHAMPOO
Pyrithione Zinc
ZYLATE
Benzyl Benzoate
ZYLOPRIM
Allopurinol
ZYLORIC
Allopurinol
ZYMACAP
Vitamins, Multiple
ZYMALIXIR
Vitamins, Multiple
ZYMASYRUP
Vitamins, Multiple
ZYMENOL
Mineral Oil
ZYNOL
Sulfinpyrazone
ZYPAN*
Ammonium Chloride
Betaine
Pancreatin
Pepsin
1-SEDRIN PLAIN
Ephedrine
2/G
Guaifenesin
2/G-DM*
Dextromethorphan
Guaifenesin
2-PAM
Pralidoxime
20/20 EYE DROPS
Naphazoline
217*
Aspirin
Caffeine
217 MEP*
Aspirin
Caffeine
Meprobamate
217 STRONG*
Aspirin
Caffeine
222*
Aspirin
Caffeine
Codeine
282*
Aspirin
Caffeine
Codeine
282 MEP*
Aspirin
Caffeine
Codeine
Meprobamate
292*
Aspirin
Caffeine
Codeine
293*
Aspirin
Caffeine

Codeine
294*
Aspirin
Caffeine
Codeine
4-WAY*
Naphazoline
Phenylephrine
Phenylpropanolamine
4-WAY COLD*
Aspirin
Phenylephrine
4-WAY LONG ACTING NASAL SPRAY
Xylometazoline
4-WAY NASAL SPRAY*
Naphazoline
Phenylephrine
Pyrilamine
642
Propoxyphene
692*
Aspirin
Caffeine
Propoxyphene
812*
Aspirin
Caffeine

Part II

Generic Names of Active Ingredients and Corresponding Brand Names

A

ACEBUTOLOL
Sectral
ACECARBROMAL
Abasin
Acetyl Adalin
Omnigesic*
Paxarel
Sedamyl
ACECLIDINE
Glaucostat
ACEFYLLINE
Dynaphylline
Etaphylline
Etophylate
ACENOCOUMAROL
Sinthrome
Sintrom
ACETAMINOPHEN
Acenol
Acephen Acetaminophen Rectal Suppositories
Aceta
Acetaco*
Aceta-Gesic*
Acetamin
Acetaminophen With Codeine Elixir*
Actamin
Advanced Formula Dristan*
Akes-N-Pain*
Al-Ay*
Alba-Temp Suppositories
Allerest Sinus Pain Formula*
Alumadrine*
Amaphen*
Amphenol
Anacin-3
Anaphen*
Anatuss*
Anodynos*
Anodynos Forte*
Anoquan*
Anuphen Suppositories
Apamide
APAP*
Arthralgen*
Aspirin Free Anacin-3*
Aspirin Free Dristan*
Atasol
Atasol Forte
Atasol-15*
Atasol-30*
Atasol-8*
Bancap*
Bancap HC*
Bancap With Codeine*
Banesin*
Bayapap
Bowman Cold Tablets*
Bromo-Seltzer*
Butigetic*
Calpol
Campain
Capital
Capital With Codeine*
Capron*
Cardui*
Catazol
Cenaid*
Chexit*
Childrens Co Tylenol*
Childrens Panadol
Chlorofon-F*
Chlorzoxazone w/APAP*
Clistin-D*
Coastaldyne*

Codalan*
Codimal*
Coldrine*
Colrex*
Comtrex*
Conacetol
Conex Plus*
Congespirin Chewable Cold Tablets for Children*
Contac Jr. Childrens' Cold Medicine*
Contac Severe Cold Formula*
Contac Severe Cold Formula Night Strength*
Coryza Brengle*
Co Tylenol*
Co Tylenol Cold Formula for Children*
CoTylenol Liquid Cold Formula*
Covangesic*
Dapa
Dapase
Darvocet-N*
Darvocet-N 100*
Datril
Datril 500
Daycare*
Deconex*
Dialog*
Dilone*
Dolacet*
Dolanex
Dolene-AP-65*
Dolor*
Drinophen*
Dristan Advanced Formula*
Dristan Ultra*
Dristan Ultra Coughs Formula*
D-Sinus*
Duadacin*
Dularin
Duoprin*
Duradyne*
Duradyne-Forte*
Dynosal*
Emagrin Forte*
Empracet
Empracet with Codeine Phosphate No. 3*
Empracet with Codeine Phosphate No. 4*
Empracet-30*
Endecon*
Esgic*
Euphenex*
Ex-Apap*
Excedrin*
Excedrin P.M.*
Exdol
Febrinol
Febrogesic
Femcaps*
Fendol*
Fendon
Flexaphen*
Gaysal*
Gaysal-S*
Gemnisyn*
G-2*
G-3*
Halenol Extra Strength
Hasacode*
Headway*
Histosal*
Hi-Temp
Hot Lemon*
Intensin*
Isobutal*
Kolephrin*
Liquiprin
Liquiprin Suspension
Liquix-C*
Lobac*
Maxigesic*
Maximum Cramp Relief*
Meadache*
Medache*
Medigesic Plus*
Mersyndol with Codeine*
Midran Decongestant*
Midrin*
Miflex*
Migralam*

Minotal*
Myocalm*
Myocalm Revised II*
Myoforte*
Naldegesic*
Napap
ND-Gesic*
Nebs
Neopap Supprettes
Neorhiban*
Neo-Synephrine Compound*
Nilain*
Nilprin
Norcet*
Norel Plus*
Nyquil Nighttime Colds Medicine*
NyQuil*
Omex*
Omnigesic*
Oraphen-PD
Ornex*
Pain & Fever
Pamprin*
Panadol
Panadol with Codeine*
Panamin
Panelex*
Panex
Panitol*
Panodynes Analgesic*
Panritis*
Parafon Forte*
Paralgin
Pediaphen
Pedric
Percocet*
Percocet-Demi*
Percocet-5*
Percogesic*
Phen APAP*
Phenaphen
Phenaphen with Codeine*
Phenaphen-650 with Codeine*
Phenate*
Phenylgesic*
Phrenilin*
Premesyn PMS*
Presaline*
Quiet World*
Repan*
Rhinex D-Lay*
Rhinidrin*
Rhinocaps*
Rhinogesic*
Rhinspec*
Rid-A-Pain*
Robigesic
Robitussin Night Relief*
Rounox
Rounox + Codeine*
S-A-C*
Saleto-D*
Salimeph*
Salocol*
Salphenyl*
Saroflex*
Sedacane*
Sedapap-10*
Sinacon*
Sinapils*
Sinarest*
Sinarest Nasal Spray*
Sine-Aid*
Sine-Aid Extra Strength*
Sine-Off Aspirin-Free Extra Strength*
Sine-Off Extra Strength - No Drowsiness*
Singlet*
Sino-Comp*
Sinubid*
Sinugen*
Sinulin*
Sinustat*
Sinutab*
Sinutab Extra Strength*
Sinutab II*
Sinutrex*
Sinu-Lets*
SK-APAP
SK-APAP with Codeine*
SK-65 APAP*
S-Painacet*
Spasgesic*

Sudoprin
Summit*
Sunril*
Supac*
Super Anahist*
Suppap-120
S45 Anti-Pain Compound*
Tapar
Temlo
Tempra
Tenlap
Tenol
Tisma*
Tivrin
T.P.I.*
Tralgon
Tranquil*
Trendar*
Triaprin*
Trigesic*
Tuzon*
Two-Dyne*
Tylaprin Elixir
Tylenol
Tylenol #1*
Tylenol #2*
Tylenol #3*
Tylenol #4*
Tylenol with Codeine*
Tylenol Extra Strength
Tylenol Maximum Strength Sinus Medication*
Tylenol No.1 Forte*
Tylox*
Valadol
Valihist*
Valorin
Vanquish Caplet*
Vicks Nyquil Nighttime Colds Medicine*
Viromed*
Wygesic*
Zoxaphen*

ACETARSONE
Gynoplix
Kharophene
Spirocid
Stovaginal
Stovarsol

ACETAZOLAMIDE
Acetazolam
Ak-Zol
Diamox
Diamox Sequels
Hydrazol
Oedemin
Rozolamide

ACETIC ACID
Aci-Jel*
Benzodyne Drops*
Dureze Otic Drops*
Fungotic*
New Freshness
Otic-HC Ear Drops*
Star-Otic*
Steramine Otic*
VoSol HC Otic Solution*
VoSol Otic Solution

ACETIC ACID, GLACIAL
Compound W*

ACETOHEXAMIDE
Dimelin
Dimelor
Dymelor
Ordimel

ACETOHYDROXAMIC ACID
Lithostat

ACETOPHENAZINE
Tindal

ACETOSULFONE
Promacetin

ACETYLCHOLINE
Acecoline
Miochol

ACETYLCYSTEINE
Airbron
Mucomyst
NAC
Respaire

ACETYLDIGITOXIN
Acylanid
Sandolanid

ACIDOPHILLUS
DoFus

ACONIAZIDE

Phenoxalid
ACRIFLAVINE
Euflavine
Trypaflavin
ACRISORCIN
Akrinol
ACTIVATED ATTAPULGITE
Quintess*
Rheaban
ACYCLOVIR
Zovirax
ADENOSINE
Adeno
Adenotriphos
Cobalasine
My-B-Den
Soraden
Triphosphodine
ADIPHENINE
Trasentine
Vagospasmyl
ADRENAL CORTEX EXTRACT
Adrenalex
Eschatin
ALBUTEROL
Proventil
Ventolin
ALCOHOL
Accurbron*
Bactalin*
Castellanis Paint*
Childrens Co Tylenol*
Comtrex*
Corlin Infant Drops*
Drysol*
Geravite Elixir*
Gerix Elixir*
Heet Analgesic
Liniment*
Hill-Shade Lotion*
Hydromax Syrup*
I.L.X. B12 Elixir*
Isogen Compound
Elixir*
Isuprel Compound
Elixir*
Medi-Quik*
Neo-Castaderm*
Rhulicaine*
Rhuligel*
Staticin*
Tedral Elixir*
Therapads*
Vicks Formula 44D
Decongestant Cough
Mixture*
Vicks Nyquil
Nighttime Colds
Medicine*
Ziradryl Lotion*
ALDOSTERONE
Aldocortin
Electrocortin
ALFACALCIDOL
One-Alpha
ALFADOLONE
Alfathesin*
ALFAXALONE
Alfathesin*
ALGINIC ACID
Algemol*
ALKAVERVIR
Veratrite
Vergitryl
Veriloid
ALLANTOIN
AAS*
Alphosyl-HC Lotion &
Cream*
Alphosyl Lotion &
Cream*
Amide-VC*
Andoin*
A.T.S.*
AVC Cream*
AVC Suppositories*
Benegyn*
Cantri Vaginal Cream*
Cervex Vaginal Cream*
Cutemol*
DeHavac*
Domerine*
Femguard*
HTO Stainless Manzan
Hemorrhoidal
Tissue Ointment*
Nil*
Par*
Par-Vag*
Perifoam*

Sufamal*
Tegrin For Psoriasis*
Vagacreme*
Vagidine*
Vagi-Nil*

ALLOBARBITAL
Dial
Dialog*

ALLOPURINOL
Alloprin
Bloxanth
Foligan
Lopurin
Purinol
Zyloprim
Zyloric

ALLYLESTRENOL
Gestanin
Gestanon

ALPHAPRODINE
Nisentil

ALPRAZOLAM
Xanax

ALPROSTADIL
Prostin VR

ALSEROXYLON
Rautensin
Rauwiloid
Rau-Tab

ALUMINUM
Buffergel*
Chemdrox*
Chemgastric*
Chemlox*
Neosorb Plus*
Neutralca-S*
Neutralox*
Polymagma Plain*
Univol*

ALUMINUM ACETATE
Acid Mantle
Bluboro*
Burdeo*
Buro-Sol
Dermaphill*
Domeboro
Florida Foam Improved*
Otic Domeboro Solution
Pedi-Boro
Rhus Tox Lotion*
Star-Otic*

ALUMINUM CARBONATE
Basaljel*

ALUMINUM CHLORIDE
Drysol*

ALUMINUM CHLOROHYDRATE
Medrol Acne Lotion*
Neomedrol Acne Lotion*

ALUMINUM HYDROXIDE
A-H Gel
Albicon*
Alcid
Aldrox
Algemol*
Algenic Alka Improved Tablets*
Almacone*
AlternaGel
Aludrox*
Alumid Suspension*
Alurex*
Alurex No.2
Aluscop*
Alu-Cap
Al-U-Creme
Alu-Tab
Amphojel
Amphojel 65*
A.M.T.*
Antacid Powder*
Arthritis Pain Formula*
Ascriptin*
Ascriptin A/D*
Azolid-A*
B-A*
Banacid*
Basaljel*
Basaljel Extra Strength
Buffets*
Cama*
Camalox*
Chemgel Antacid
Cope*
Creamalin*
Delcid*

Dewitt's Antacid Powder*
Dialume
Di-Gel*
Diovol*
Diovol Ex*
Escot*
Estomul-M*
Flacid*
Fluagel
Gaviscon Antacid*
Gaviscon-2 Antacid*
Gaysal*
Gaysal-S*
Gelumina*
Gelusil*
Gelusil Extra Strength Liquid*
Gelusil II*
Gelusil M*
Glycogel*
Kessadrox*
Kolantyl*
Kudrox*
Liquid Antacid*
Maalox*
Maalox #1*
Maalox #2*
Maalox Plus*
Magmalin*
Magnatril*
Magna Gel*
Maxamag Suspension*
Mygel*
Mylanta*
Mylanta II*
Mylanta-2 Extra Strength*
Nephrox Suspension*
Neutracomp*
Noraiac*
Noralac*
Nutrajel
Pama*
Presaline*
Rolox*
Roxane
Rulox*
Salocol*
Silain-Gel*
Simaal Gel*
Simeco*
Syntrogel*
Tralmag*
Trimagel*
Trisogel*
WinGel*

ALUMINUM MAGNESIUM SILICATE
Pabizol with Paregoric*

ALUMINUM OXIDE
Brasivol
Epi-Clear Scrub Cleanser
Magnesia and Alumina Oral Suspension*
Nutramag*

ALUMINUM PHOSPHATE
Phosphaljel

ALVERINE
Kalmadol
Profenil
Spacolin
Spasmaverine

AMANTADINE
Symmetrel
Virofral

AMBENONIUM
Mysuran
Mytelase

AMBUPHYLLINE
Butaphyllamine
Buthoid

AMCINONIDE
Cyclocort

AMDINOCILLIN
Coactin

AMEZINIUM
Regulton

AMIKACIN
Amikin

AMILORIDE
Midamor
Moduret*
Moduretic*

AMINACRINE
AAS*
Acriflex
Amide-VC*

AVC Cream*
AVC Suppositories*
Benegyn*
Cantri Vaginal Cream*
Cervex Vaginal Cream*
DeHavac*
Femguard*
Flavedrin Mild*
Monacrin
Nil*
Par*
Par-Vag*
Sufamal*
Vagacreme*
Vagidine*
Vagilia Cream/
Suppositories*
Vagitrol Cream/
Suppositories*
Vagi-Nil*

AMINOACETIC ACID
Calcilac*
Co-Gel Liquitabs*
Glycate*
Glycolixir

AMINOBENZOIC ACID
Block-Aid*
Hill-Shade Lotion*
Neocylate*
Original Eclipse
Sunscreen*
Pabagel
Paba Gel
Pabanol
Pabaplus
Pabirin*
PreSun
PreSun 15*
RVPaba Lip Stick*
Sunbrella Sunscreen

AMINOCAPROIC ACID
Amicar
Capromol
Epsamon
Epsikapron

AMINOGLUTETHIMIDE
Cytadren
Orimeten

AMINOPENTAMIDE
Centrine

AMINOPHYLLINE
Amesec*
Aminodur Dura-Tabs
Aminophyl
Amodrine*
Amoline
Amphylline
Asthmacon*
Chemphyl*
Corophyllin
Corphyllin
Ethophylline
Lixaminol
Mini-Lix
Mudrane*
Mudrane GG*
Mudrane GG-2*
Mudrane-2*
Palaron
Phyldrox
Phyllocontin
Quinite*
Relasma*
Roamphed*
Somophyllin
Somophyllin-DF
Theolamine
Truphylline

AMINOPROMAZINE
Lispamol
Lorusil

AMINOSALICYLATE
D.A.S.
Pamisyl Sodium
Parasal
Pasdium
Pasem Sodium
Teebacin

AMINOSALICYLIC ACID
Di-Isopacin*
Double Isopacin*
Inapasade-SQ*
Nemasol
Pamisyl
Propasa
Rezipas

AMINOXIDE HYDROBROMIDE
Nite Rest*
Sominex (USA)*

AMIODARONE

Atlansil
Cordarone
AMIPHENAZOLE
Amphisol
Daptazole
Fenamizol
AMITRIPTYLINE
Amiline
Amitid
Amitril
Deprex
Elatrol
Elavil
Endep
Etrafon*
Etrafon-A*
Etrafon Forte*
Laroxyl
Levate
Limbitrol*
Mareline
Meravil
Novotriptyn
Saroten
SK-Amitriptyline
Triavil*
Tryptizol
AMMONIA
Blistex*
AMMONIATED MERCURY
Unguentum Bossi*
AMMONIUM BIPHOSPHATE
Phos-pHaid*
AMMONIUM CHLORIDE
Ambenyl Expectorant*
Amchlor
Ammoneric
Amonidrin*
Baby Cough
Bayaminicol*
Benylin DM*
Chlor-Trimeton Expectorant*
Chlor-Trimeton Expectorant with Codeine*
Colrex Expectorant*
Coricidin Antitussive*
Co-Salt*
Dewitt's Baby Cough*
Dextrotussin*
DM-4 Children's Cough Control*
DM-8*
Efricon*
Endotussin-NN*
Endotussin-NN Pediatric*
Histadyl EC*
Histivite-D*
Kiddies Pediatric*
Kophane Cough & Cold Formula*
N-N Cough*
Noratuss*
PBZ Expectorant w/ Ephedrine*
Permathene H2Off*
Pinex Wild Cherry
Pre-Mens Forte*
Pyrralan Expectorant*
Quelidrine*
Rem*
Romilar CF*
Triaminicol*
Triaminicol Decongestant Cough*
Tricodene NN*
Triminicol Cough Syrup*
Zypan*
AMOBARBITAL
Amesec*
Amytal
Amytalily
Amytal & Aspirin*
Asthmacon*
Bi-Secogen*
Chemphyl*
Dexamyl*
Dormytal
Duo-Barb*
Eunoctal
Intrased
Isobec
Novamo-Secobarb*
Relasma*
Roamphed*

Talamo
Tuinal*
Tuinal Pulvules*
Tuo-Barb*
AMODIAQUINE
Camoquin
Flavoquin
AMOLANONE
Amethone
AMOXAPINE
Asendin
AMOXICILLIN
Amoxil
AmoxiCan
Augmentin*
Larotid
Moxacin
Moxilean
Novamoxin
Penamox
Polymox
Robamox
Sumox
Trimox
Ultimox
Wymox
AMPHECLORAL
Acutran
AMPHETAMINE
Benzedrine
Biphetamine*
Delcobese
Obetrol*
AMPHOTERICIN B
Fungizone
Mysteclin-F*
AMPICILLIN
Acillin
Alpen
Amcap
Amcill
Ampen
Ampicin
Ampicin-PRB*
Ampilean
Amplin
Binotal
Biosan
D-Amp
Fomnipen
Novoampicillin
Omnipen
Omnipen-N
Pen A Oral
Penbristol
Penbritin
Penbrock
Pensyn
Pfizerpen-A
Polycillin
Polycillin-N for Injection
Polycillin-PRB*
Ponecil
Principen
Principen with Probenecid*
Probampacin*
Probenicillin*
Pro-Biosan 500 Kit*
Qidamp
SK-Ampicillin
SK-Ampicillin-N
Supen
Totacillin
Totapen
AMRINONE
Inocor
Inocor IV
AMYLASE
Bilezyme*
Converzyme*
Digolase*
Enzymacol*
Festal*
Festalan*
Kutrase*
Ku-Zyme*
Phazyme*
Phazyme-PB*
Phazyme-95*
Tri-Cone*
Tri-Cone Plus*
ANGIOTENSIN AMIDE
Hypertensin
ANILERIDINE
Apodol
Leritine
ANISINDIONE
Miradon

Uridone
ANISOTROPINE
Valpin
Valpin 50
Valpin 50-PB*
ANTAZOLINE
Albalon-A*
Antastan
Antistine
Antistine-Privine*
Histostab
Vasocon A*
Zincfrin-A*
ANTHRALIN
Anthera
Anthra-Derm
Anthra-Derm Oil
Cignolin
Drithocreme
Lasan Pomade
Lasan Unguent
Psoriacide
ANTI-INHIBITOR COAGULANT COMPLEX
Autoplex
Feiba Immuno
ANTIHEMOPHILIC FACTOR
Actif VIII
Factorate
Hemofil
Humafac
Koate
Profilate
ANTIHUMAN LYMPHOCYTE GLOBULIN
Pressimmune
ANTIPYRINE
Auralgan*
Aurasol*
Auricrine*
Auromid*
Collyrium*
Collyrium Drops*
Eardro*
Felsol Powder
Larylgan Throat Spray*
Neo-Hydro*
Oto*
Otocort Ear Drops*
Oto-Pediat*
Otoreid-HC*
Tympagesic*
ANTIRABIES SERUM EQUINE
ARS
APRIDINE
Fiboran
APRINDINE
Fibocil
APROBARBITAL
Alurate
APROTININ
Trasylol
ARGININE
Modumate
R-Gene
ASCORBIC ACID
A.C.N.*
Adenex
Alba-Ce
Ascorbicap
Ascoril
AVP Natal*
Becotin-T*
Becotin With Vitamin C*
Bejectal with Vitamin C*
Bejex*
Berocca*
Berocca-C*
Best C Caps
Cantaxin Forte
Cebione
Cecon
Ceebate
Cee-500 T.D.
Cefera*
Cemill
Cenolate
Cerebro-Nicin*
Cetane
Cetane-Caps TD
Cetane Timed
Cevalin
Cevex
Ce-Vi-Sol
Ce-Vi-Sol Drops
Chromagen*
Citra*

C-Level
C-Long
Cortiforte*
C-Ron*
C-Ron Forte*
C-Ron Freckles*
Cytoferin*
Dequasine*
Dextrotussin*
Erivit C
Fe-O.D.*
Ferancee*
Ferancee-HP*
Fergon with C Caplets*
Ferosorb-C*
Fero-Folic-500*
Ferrobid*
Flavorcee
Formatrix*
Fumaral Elixir and Spancaps*
I.L.X. B12*
Irolong*
Iron with C*
Jay C
Kamu Jay
K-Forte Potassium Supplement with Vitamin C Chewable*
Magacin*
Mol-Iron with Vitamin C*
Natrascorb
Niarb Super*
Niferex with Vitamin C*
Nor-Lief*
Palmiron-C*
Peridin-C*
Perihemin*
Pharma C-500
Pronemia*
Recoup*
Redoxon
Saro-C
Solu-B with Ascorbic Acid Sterile Powder*
Super Toniven
Surbex with C*
Thera-Combex H-P*
Thera-Complex H-P*
Thex Forte*
Trinsicon*
Trinsicon M*
TriHemic 600*
Tri-Tinic*
Tri-Vi-Flor*
Tri-Vi-Flor w/Iron Drops*
Tri-Vi-Sol*
Tri-Vi-Sol with Iron*
Vergo*
Vi-Daylin ADC Drops*
Vi-Daylin/F ADC + Iron Drops*
Vi-Daylin/F ADC Drops*
Vi-Daylin Plus Iron ADC Drops*
Vitacee
Vita-C
Viterra C
Vitron-C*
Vitron-C-Plus*
Vi-Zac*
Wart-Aid*
Zentrol Chewable*
Zentron Liquid*
Zintinic*
Z-Pro-C*

ASPARAGINASE
Crasnitin
Elspar
Kidrolase

ASPIRIN
Acetal
Acetonyl
Acetophen
Acetyl-Sal
Alka-Seltzer Effervescent Pain Reliever and Antacid*
Alka-Seltzer Plus*
Amytal & Aspirin*
Anacin*
Ancasal
Ancasal Compound No.1*

Ancasal Compound
No.2*
Ancasal Compound
No.3*
Anexsia with Codeine*
Anodynos*
Ansemco #2*
Apac*
Apa-Deine*
APAP*
APC*
APC with Codeine*
Apectol*
APF
Arthritis Pain
Formula*
Arthritis Strength
Bufferin*
ASA
A.S.A. and Codeine
Compound*
A.S.A. Compound*
A.S.A. Enseals
Ascodeen-30*
Ascriptin*
Ascriptin A/D*
Asperbuf
Aspergum
Asphac-G*
Asphal-G*
Astrin
Axotal*
B-A*
Bayer Aspirin
Bayer Children's
Aspirin
Bayer Children's
Cold*
Bayer Decongestant*
Bayer Timed-Release
Arthritic Pain
Bayer Timed-Release
Aspirin
BC*
BC Powder*
BC Tablets*
Buffadyne*
Buffadyne-Lemmon*
Buffaprin*
Bufferin*
Bufferin with
Codeine No. 3*
Buffets*
Buffex
Buffinol*
Buff-A Comp*
Buf-Tabs
Cafacetin*
Cama*
Capron*
Catasal
Children's 217*
Codasa*
Codophen-R*
Cope*
Coricidin*
Coricidin "D"*
Coricidin Demilets*
Coricidin Medilets*
Coryphen
Coryphen-Codeine*
Cosprin
CP2 Tablets*
C3*
C4*
Darvon with A.S.A.*
Darvon Compound-65*
Darvon-N Compound*
Darvon-N With ASA*
DasiKon*
Dasin*
Dolcin*
Dolene Compound-65*
Dolor*
Drinophen*
Dristan*
Duradyne*
Duragesic*
Dynosal*
Easprin
Ecotrin
Emagrin*
Empirin Compound*
Empirin With
Codeine*
Emprazil*
Emprazil-C*
Encaprin
Enteric Coated ASA
Entrophen

Entrophen with
  Codeine*
Equagesic*
Ex-Apap*
Excedrin*
Fiorinal*
Fiorinal-C1/2*
Fiorinal-C1/4*
Fiorinal With
  Codeine*
Fizrin Powder
Gemnisyn*
Goody's Headache
  Powder*
Hipirin
Measurin
Meprogesic*
Methocarbamol w/ASA*
Micrainin*
Midol*
Momentum*
Monacet with Codeine*
Neoline
Neopirine Co. with
  Codeine*
Neopirine Co. No.35*
Neopirine No.25
Nilain*
Norgeis Forte*
Norgesic*
Norgesic Forte*
Novasen
Nova-Phase
Nova-Phase with
  Pheno*
Novopropoxyn
  Compound*
Pabirin*
PAC*
P-A-C Compound*
PAC Compound with
  Codeine*
Panalgesic*
Panodynes Analgesic*
Percobarb*
Percodan*
Percodan-Demi*
Persistin*
Pharmacin
Phenacodein 002*
Phenacodein 003*
Phrenilan Forte*
Presaline*
Pyrroxate*
Quiet World*
Rhinex*
Rhinocaps*
Rhonal
Robaxisal*
Robaxisal C-1/4*
Robaxisal C-1/8*
Sal-Adult
Salatin with Codeine*
Sal-Fayne*
Salibar Jr.*
Sal-Infant
Salocol*
Sine-Off*
Sine-Off-Aspirin
  Formula*
SK-65 Compound*
Stanback*
Stanco
St. Joseph Aspirin
St. Joseph Aspirin
  for Children
  Chewable
St. Joseph Cold for
  Children*
Supac*
Supasa
Synalgos*
Synalgos-DC*
Tabloid Brand A.P.C.
  with Codeine*
Talwin Compound*
Triaminicin*
Triaphen-10
Trigesic*
Unigesic-A*
Vanquish Caplet*
Vicoprin*
Viromed*
Wesprin Buffered
Zactirin*
Zorprin
217*
217 MEP*
217 Strong*
222*
282*
282 MEP*

292*
293*
294*
4-Way Cold*
692*
812*
ATENOLOL
Tenoretic*
Tenormin
ATRACURIUM
Tracrium
ATROPINE
Aid-Tuss*
Alised*
Antrocol*
Arco-Lase Plus*
Atrobarb*
Atrobarbital*
Atropine with Demerol*
Atropisol
Atrosed*
Barbidonna*
Bellaphen*
Bellastal*
Bilagog*
Bufopto Atropine Solution
Butabell HMB*
Chlorofed Injection*
Comhist*
Dasikon*
Dasin*
Dehist*
Diaction*
Di-Atro*
Digestamic*
Diphenatol*
Dolsed*
Donnagel*
Donnagel-PG*
Donnamor Elixir*
Donnatal*
Donnatal Extentabs*
Donnazyme*
Donphen*
Elmotil*
Enoxa*
Femcaps*
Festalan*
Hasp*
Histaject*
Hybephen*
Hyosophen*
Isopto Atropine
Kinesed*
Lofene*
Loflo*
Lomotil*
Lonox*
Lo-Trol*
Low Quel*
Malatal*
Murocoll
Mydrapred Ophthalmic*
Nasahist II*
N.D.-Stat*
Neoquess Tablets*
Nogest*
Norel Plus Injection*
Nor-Mil*
Omnibel*
Optotropinal
Oraminic*
Palbar No. 2*
Probacon*
Prosed*
Pylora*
Quiagel*
Quiagel PG*
Relaxadon*
Ru-Tuss*
Seds*
Sidonna*
Sinusol-D*
SK-Diphenoxylate*
Spalix*
Spasaid*
Spaslin*
Spasmolin*
Spasmophen*
Spasmorel*
Spasquid*
Susano*
Trac*
Tus-Oraminic*
Tuss-Ade*
UAA*
Uralgic*
Uramine*
Urised*
Urisep*

Uritab*
Uritabs W.O.*
Urithol*
Uroblue*
Urostat-Forte*
Vanatal*
Vanodonnal*
Vernate*

ATTAPULGITE
Diarkote*
Diar-Aid*
Polymagma Plain*
Quintess*
Sebasorb*

AUROTHIOGLUCOSE
Solganal

AUROTHIOGLYCANIDE
Lauron

AZACYCLONOL
Frenquel

AZAPETINE
Ilidar

AZARIBINE
Triazure

AZATADINE
Idulian
Optimine

AZATHIOPRINE
Imuran
Imuril

AZLOCILLIN
Azlin

AZTREONAM
Azactam

AZURESIN
Diagnex Blue

B

BACAMPICILLIN
Spectrobid

BACITRACIN
Alba-3 Ointment*
Baciguent Ointment
Baciguent Ophthalmic*
Bacimycin*
Bacitin
BPN Ointment*
Clinicydin*
Cortisporin Ointment*
Cortisporin Ointment Ophthalmic*
Epimycin "A"*
Mity-Mycin*
Mycitracin*
N.B.P.*
Neomixin*
Neosporin*
Neo-Polycin*
Neo-Thrycex*
Novantrone*
Polysporin Ophthalmic*
Relespor*
Septal*
Topitracin
Triple Antibiotic*

BACLOFEN
Lioresal
Lioresal DS

BAMIPINE
Soventol

BARBITAL
Embinal
Hypnodol
Medinal
Plexonal*
Veronal

BARIUM
Barodense
Baroflave
Baroloid
Barosperse
Barotrast
Colonatrast
Esophotrast
Fleet Barobag
Fleet Oral
Gel-Unix
Oratrast
Recto Barium
Travad
Ultra Paque
Unik-Pak

BASIC FUCHSIN
Castellanis Paint*

BECLOMETHASONE

Aldecin Inhaler
Beclovent Inhaler
Beconase
Becotide Inhaler
Propaderm
Propaderm C*
Propraderm
Vancenase Nasal Inhaler
Vanceril
Vanceril Oral Inhaler

BEESWAX
Blistex*

BELLADONNA
Allerprop*
Belladenal*
Belladenal-S*
Bellergal*
Bellergal-S*
Bellermine-O.D.*
Chardonna-2*
Maldex*
Pheno-Bella*

BELLADONNA ALKALOIDS
Amogel PG*
Diarkote*
Kaodonna*
Kaodonna-PG*
Kaomead with Belladonna*
Ru-K-N*
Wigraine*
Wyanoids HC Rectal Suppositories*
Wyanoids Hemorrhoidal Suppositories*

BELLADONNA EXTRACT
Amobell*
Belap
Bellkatai*
Bellophen*
Butibel*

BEMEGRIDE
Megimide
Mikedimide

BENACTYZINE
Actozine
Deprol*
Levol
Suavitil

BENDAZAC
Versus

BENDROFLUMETHIAZIDE
Aprinox
Benuron
Berkozide
Bristuron
Centyl
Corzide*
Naturetin
Neo-Naclex
Rauzide*
Sodiuretic

BENOXAPROFEN
Oraflex

BENOXINATE
Dorsacaine
Fluress*
Novesine

BENSERAZIDE
Prolopa*

BENTIROMIDE
Chymex

BENTONITE
Buf Acne-Cleansing Bar*
Calamine*

BENZALKONIUM CHLORIDE
Akne Drying*
Almocarpine*
Aqua-Flow*
Bactine*
Bactine Antiseptic Anesthetic*
Benzachlor-50
Benzodyne Drops*
Cleaning & Soaking*
Comfort Drops*
Contique Dual Wet*
Di-Delamine*
Drapolex Cream
Dureze Otic Drops*
Florida Foam Improved*
Fungotic*
Genoptic*
Germicin
Germ-i-Tol
Hyamine 3500
Hy-flow*

Ice-O-Derm Gel
Ionax
Ivy-Chex*
Lavoptik Eye Wash*
Lensine Extra Strength*
Lens-Mate*
Liquifilm Wetting*
Locon*
Mediconet*
Medi-Quik*
Mercurochrome*
Mercurochrome II*
Methopto*
Mydrapred Ophthalmic*
Nonsul Jelly
Otic-HC Ear Drops*
Oxyzal West*
Perifoam*
Pilocar*
Pre-sert*
Prolens*
Sabol
Soakare
Soquette*
Spensomide
Sporostacin*
Statrol Ophthalmic*
Steramine Otic*
Theranac Scrub
Tucks Pads*
Visalens Wetting*
Wetting Solution*
Wet-N-Soak*
Zephiran Chloride

BENZETHONIUM CHLORIDE
Hyamine 1622
Phemerol

BENZOCAINE
Aero Caine
Aero Therm
Americaine
Americaine-Otic*
Anbesol Antiseptic Anesthetic*
Anesthesin
Auralgan*
Aurasol*
Auricrine*
Auromid*
Axon*
Ayds Appetite Suppressant
Baby Orajel
Baby Teething Lotion
Benzocol
Benzodent*
Bicozene Creme*
Boil-Ease*
Boyol*
Burntame
Calamatum*
Cepacol Troches*
Cetacaine Topical Anesthetic*
Chiggerex
Children's Chloraseptic Lozenges
Colrex Troches
Col-vi-nol
Conex Lozenge*
Dalidyne*
Dentition
Dentocaine
Dermacoat
Derma Medicone-HC Ointment*
Derma Medicone Ointment*
Dermoplast Aerosol Spray*
Eardro*
Foille
Fung-O-Spray*
Ger-o-Foam*
Hold*
HTO Stainless Manzan Hemorrhoidal Tissue Ointment*
Hurricaine
Isodettes Super*
Ivarest*
Kank-A*
Lanacane Medicated Creme*
Lanazets*
Listerine Cough Control

Medicone Dressing Cream*
Mycinettes*
Mycinettes Sugar Free*
Numzident*
Num-zit jel*
Orabase with Benzocaine
Oracin
Oradex-C*
Ora-Jel
Oto*
Oto-Pediat*
Oxipor VHC Lotion for Psoriasis*
Pazo Hemorrhoid*
Rectagene Balm*
Rectal Medicone-HC Suppositories*
Rectal Medicone Suppositories*
Rectal Medicone Unguent*
Rhulicaine*
Rhulicream*
Rhulihist*
Rhulispray*
Scabide*
Semets*
Sepo
Slim Line Gum
Soft'N Soothe
Solarcaine
Solarcaine Lip Balm
Spec-T Sore Throat Anesthetic
Spec-T Sore Throat/ Cough Suppressant*
Spec-T Sore Throat/ Decongestant*
Spongiacaine
Sting-Eze*
Synthaloids*
Teething
Tega Caine
Thru Penetrating Liquid*
Topcaine
Trocaine
Trokettes*
Tympagesic*
Unguentine
Vicks Formula 44 Cough Control Discs*
Vicks Medi-Trating*
Vicks Throat Lozenges*

BENZOIC ACID
Blis-To-Sol*
Cystex*
Dolsed*
Mazon*
Medicated Foot Powder*
NP-27 Cream*
NP-27 Liquid*
NP-27 Powder*
Prosed*
Rid-Itch Liquid*
Solvex Ointment*
Ting*
Trac*
T-4-L*
UAA*
Uralgic*
Uramine*
Urised*
Urisep*
Uritab*
Uritabs W.O.*
Urithol*
Uroblue*
Urostat-Forte*
Whitfield's*
Whitsphill*

BENZOIN COMPOUND
Kank-A*

BENZONATATE
Tessalon
Ventussin

BENZOQUINONIUM
Mytolon

BENZOXIQUINE
Barcone

BENZOYL PEROXIDE
Acetoxyl
Ben-Aqua-5
Benoxyl

Benzac
Benzagel
Benzamycin*
BP-5
Buf-Oxal
Clearasil BP
Clear By Design
Cuticura Medicated Acne
Dermodex 5 & 10 Gel
Dermoxyl
Desquam-X
Dry and Clear
Eloxyl
Epi-Clear*
Fostex BPO 5%
Loroxide Acne Lotion*
Loroxide-HC Lotion*
Oxyderm
Oxy Wash
Oxy-10
Oxy-5
Panoxyl
Persadox
Persa-Gel
Perso-Gel
Propa P.H. Acne
Stri-Dex B.P.
Sulfoxyl Lotion*
Teen 10 Lotion
Teen 5 Lotion
Teen 5 Wash
Topex Acne Clearing Medication
Vanoxide*
Xerac BP 10
Xera BP
Zeroxin

BENZPHETAMINE
Didrex

BENZPYRINIUM
Stigmonene

BENZQUINAMIDE
Emete-Con
Quantril

BENZTHIAZIDE
Aquastat
Aquatag
Benzide
Exna-R*
ExNa
Hydrex
Marazide
Naclex
Omuretic
Proaqua
Rola-Benz
S-Aqua
Urazide
Urese

BENZTROPINE
Bensylate
Cogentin

BENZYL ALCOHOL
Dalidyne*
Hemocyte Injection*
Rhuligel*
Rhulispray*
Topic Benzyl Alcohol Gel

BENZYL BENZOATE
Anugard-HC*
Anusol*
Anusol-HC*
Anusol Ointment*
Benylate
Scabanca
Scabide*
Scabiol
Zylate

BENZYLPENICILLOYL POLYLYSINE
Pre-Pen

BEPHENIUM
Alcopara

BETA CAROTENE
Solatene

BETAHISTINE
Serc

BETAINE
Dizyme*
Keff*
Normacid*
Zypan*

BETAINE CITRATE
Citrate de Betaine

BETAMETHASONE
Beben
Benisone
Betacort

Betaderm
Betatrex
Beta-Val
Betnelan
Betnesol
Betnovate
Celestan
Celestoderm
Celestoderm-V
Celestone
Cel-U-Jec
Diprosone
Flurobate Gel
Selestoject
Uticort
Valisone
Valisone-G
Valisone Scalp Lotion

BETAZOLE
Histalog

BETHANECHOL
Duvoid
Mictrol
Myotonachol
Urecholine
Urolax
Vesicholine

BETHANIDINE
Bethanid
Esbaloid
Esbatal
Tenathan

BIALAMICOL
Camoform

BILE SALTS
Amlax*
Bilron*
Donnazyme*
Entozyme*
Enzymacol*
Enzypan*
Festal*
Kanulase*
Ox Bile Extract

BIOTIN
Hepp-Iron Drops*

BIPERIDEN
Akineton

BISACODYL
Barium Enema Prep Kit*
Bicol
Biscolax
Bisco-Lax
Castor Oil
Cenalax
Deficol
Dulcodos*
Dulcolax
Erilax
Evac-Q-Kwik*
Fleet Bisacodyl Enema
Fleet Prep Kit*
Fleet Prep Kit 2*
Fleet Prep Kit 3*
Fleet Prep Kit 4*
Fleet Prep Kit 5*
Fleet Prep Kit 6*
Kit 1*
Laco
Nuvac
Pentalax
Rytmil
SK-Bisacodyl
Theralax
Tridate Bowel Kit*

BISMUTH ALUMINATE
Escot*
Noraiac*
Noralac*

BISMUTH DIPROPYLACETATE
Neo-Laryngobis

BISMUTH OXYIODIDE
Wyanoids HC Rectal Suppositories*
Wyanoids Hemorrhoidal Suppositories*

BISMUTH RESORCINOL
Anugard-HC*
Anusol*
Anusol-HC*
Anusol Suppositories*

BISMUTH SODIUM TRIGLYCOLLAMATE
Bistrimate

BISMUTH SUBCARBONATE
Emeroid*

BISMUTH SUBGALLATE

Amogel*
Anugard-HC*
Anusol*
Anusol-HC*
Anusol Suppositories*
Bisilad*
Devrom
Dia-Eze*
Digestalin*
Inodor
Rectacort*
Rectagene Balm*

BISMUTH SUBNITRATE
Anti-Acid No.1*
Percy Medicine*
Zemo*

BISMUTH SUBSALICYLATE
Bismol
Bi-Sub-Sal
Corrective Mixture*
Corrective Mixture with Paregoric*
Infantol Pink*
Kaodene*
Pabizol with Paregoric*
Pepto-Bismol*
Pepto Bismol Liquid
Pleasant Relief
Stabisol

BITHIONOL
Actamer
Bitin
Lorothidol

BITOLTEROL
Tornalate

BLEOMYCIN
Blenoxane

BORIC ACID
Aci-Jel*
Antibiopto Ophthalmic*
Auro
Aurocaine*
Auro-Dri*
Blinx*
Bluboro*
Bo-Car-Al
Boil n Soak*
Borofax
Borosorb
Borowas
Burdeo*
Collyrium*
Collyrium Drops*
Florida Foam Improved*
Lauro*
Lowila Cake*
Mydrapred Ophthalmic*
Neo-Castaderm*
Saratoga*
Star-Otic*
Unisol*
Wyanoids HC Rectal Suppositories*
Wyanoids Hemorrhoidal Suppositories*

BRETYLIUM
Bretylate
Bretylin
Bretylol
Darenthin

BREWER'S YEAST
Super Doss*

BROMELAINS
Ananase-50

BROMHEXINE
Bisolvon

BROMINDIONE
Circladin
Halinone

BROMISOVALUM
Bromural
Isoval
Omnigesic*

BROMOCRIPTINE
Parlodel
Prolactin

BROMODIPHENHYDRAMINE
Ambenyl Expectorant*
Ambodryl
Deserol

BROMPHENIRAMINE
Brocon Chewable*
Brocon C.R.*
Bromfed*
Bromophen*
Bromphen*
Cordamine*
Dimalix*
Dimetane

Dimetane
  Decongestant*
Dimetane Expectorant*
Dimetane Expectorant-
  DC*
Dimetane Extentabs*
Dimetapp with
  Codeine*
Dimetapp Elixir*
Dimetapp Extentabs*
Dimotane
Histatapp Elixir*
Histatapp T.D.*
Ilvin
Midatane Expectorant*
Midatap*
Multi-Symptom*
Normatane*
Normatane
  Expectorant*
Phenatapp Extend*
Poly-Histine-DX*
Poly-Histine
  Expectorant with
  Codeine*
Poly-Histine
  Expectorant Plain*
Purebrom*
Puretane
Puretane DC
  Expectorant
Puretane Expectorant
Puretapp Elixir*
Puretapp PA*
Rotane Expectorant*
Rotapp*
S.T. Decongest*
Symptom 3
Tagatap*
Tamine*
Tri-Phen*
Veltane
Veltap*
Westapp*

BUCLIZINE
  Bucladin-S
  Equivert
  Softran
  Vibazine

BUFEXAMAC
  Droxaryl
  Feximac
  Norfemac
  Parfenac

BUMETANIDE
  Bumex

BUNAMIODYL
  Orabilex

BUPIVACAINE
  Marcaine
  Sensorcaine

BUPRENORPHINE
  Buprenex
  Temegesic

BUPROPION
  Wellbutrin

BUSPIRONE
  Buspar

BUSULFAN
  Mielucin
  Myleran
  Sulfabutin

BUTABARBITAL
  Bubartal TT
  Buta-Barb
  Butabell HMB*
  Butibel*
  Buticaps
  Butigetic*
  Butiserpazide*
  Butisol
  Covap*
  Day-Barb
  Dolonil*
  Gaysal*
  G-2*
  G-3*
  Intasedol
  Mebutal
  Minotal*
  Neo-Barb
  Neurosedine
  Omnibel*
  Palbar No. 2*
  Phrenilin*
  Pyridium Plus*
  Quibron Plus*
  Sedapap-10*
  Sidonna*
  Tedral-25*

BUTACAINE
  Butyn

Optyn
BUTALBITAL
Amaphen*
Anaphen*
Anoquan*
Apectol*
Axotal*
Buff-A Comp*
Esgic*
Fiorinal*
Fiorinal-C1/2*
Fiorinal-C1/4*
Fiorinal With Codeine*
Isobutal*
Medigesic Plus*
Panitol*
Phrenilan Forte*
Plexonal*
Repan*
Sandoptal
Two-Dyne*
BUTAMBEN
Butesin
Planoform
BUTAPERAZINE
Repoise
BUTETHAL
Neonal
Soneryl
BUTETHAMINE
Monocaine
BUTORPHANOL
Stadol

C

CAFFEINE
Akes-N-Pain*
Al-Ay*
Amaphen*
Amostat
Anacin*
Anaphen*
Anexsia with Codeine*
Anodynos*
Anoquan*
Anorexin One-Span*
Ansemco #2*
Apac*
Apa-Deine*
APAP*
APC*
APC with Codeine*
Apectol*
A.S.A. and Codeine Compound*
A.S.A. Compound*
Asphac-G*
Asphal-G*
Aspirin Free Anacin-3*
Atasol-15*
Atasol-30*
Atasol-8*
BC Powder*
BC Tablets*
Bio Slim T*
Bowman Cold Tablets*
Bromo-Seltzer*
Buffadyne*
Buffadyne-Lemmon*
Buffets*
Buff-A Comp*
Butigetic*
Cafacetin*
Cafamine T.D.*
Cafergot*
Cafermine*
Cafertabs*
Cafertrate*
Caffedrine
Caffeine And Sodium Benzoate*
Capron*
Carisopodol*
Cenaid*
Children's 217*
Citra*
Codalan*
Codophen-R*
Cortiforte*
CP2 Tablets*
C3*
C4*
Darvon Compound-65*
Darvon-N Compound*
DasiKon*
Dasin*

Dewitt's Pills for Backache & Joint Pain*
Dietac*
Dilone*
Doan's Pills*
Dolene Compound-65*
Dolor*
Double-E Alertness
Drinophen*
Duradyne*
Dynosal*
Efed II*
Emagrin*
Empirin Compound*
Emprazil*
Emprazil-C*
Ercaf*
Ercatab*
Ergocaf*
Esgic*
Excedrin*
Ex-Apap*
Femcaps*
Fiorinal*
Fiorinal-C1/2*
Fiorinal-C1/4*
Fiorinal With Codeine*
Goody's Headache Powder*
Histosal*
Hungrex Plus*
Kolephrin*
Korigesic*
Makoz
Meadache*
Medache*
Medigesic Plus*
Midol*
Migral*
Migralam*
Migrastat*
Monacet with Codeine*
Neopirine Co. with Codeine*
Neopirine Co. No.35*
Nilain*
Nodoz
Norgeis Forte*
Norgesic*
Norgesic Forte*
Novopropoxyn Compound*
PAC*
P-A-C Compound*
PAC Compound with Codeine*
Panodynes Analgesic*
Percobarb*
Percodan*
Percodan-Demi*
Permathene H2Off*
Permathene-12*
Phenacodein 002*
Phenacodein 003*
Phrenilin*
Pre-Mens Forte*
Quick-Pep
Repan*
Rid-A-Pain*
S-A-C*
Salatin with Codeine*
Saleto-D*
Sal-Fayne*
Sedacane*
Sinexin*
SK-65 Compound*
Slim One*
Soma Compound with Codeine*
Soprodol*
S.P.C.*
Stanback*
Stim-Tabs
Summit*
Supac*
Super Odrinex*
Synalgos*
Synalgos-DC*
S45 Anti-Pain Compound*
Tabloid Brand A.P.C. with Codeine*
Talwin Compound*
Tirend
Tisma*
Trigesic*
Two-Dyne*
Vanquish Caplet*

Verb T.D.
Vivarin
Wigraine*
217*
217 MEP*
217 Strong*
222*
282*
282 MEP*
292*
293*
294*
692*
812*

CAJEPUT OIL
Dewitt's Oil for Ear Use*

CALAMINE
Caladryl*
Caladryl Hydrocortisone*
Calamatum*
Calamine*
Calamox
Cal-ZO Dressing*
Dome-Paste Bandage*
Ivarest*
Rhulihist*
Rhulispray*

CALCIFEDIOL
Calderol

CALCITONIN
Calcimar

CALCITRIOL
Rocaltrol
Rolcaltrol

CALCIUM
Calcivitam
Calora
Cal-M*
Ca-Plus
Dicalgin
Fosfree*
Gramacal
Iromin-G*
Mission Prenatal*
Neo-Calglucon Syrup
Surbex 750 with Iron*
Surbex 750 with Zinc*

CALCIUM BROMIDOLACTOBIONATE
Calcibronat

CALCIUM CARBIMIDE
Dipsan
Temposil

CALCIUM CARBONATE
Albicon*
Alka-Mints
Alka-2 Chewable Antacid
Alkets*
Amitone
Anti-Acid No.1*
BiSoDol*
Calcet*
Calcilac*
Calglycine*
Caltrate 600 + D*
Camalox*
Chooz*
Co-Gel Liquitabs*
Dicarbosil
Dimacid*
Equilet
Glycate*
Glycogel*
Krem*
Lo-sal*
Mallamint
Marblen*
Os-Cal*
Os-Cal-Gesic*
Os-Cal 500
Pepto-Bismol*
Ratio*
Spastosed*
Titralac
Trialka
Tums

CALCIUM CASEINATE
Casec
Casilan

CALCIUM CYCLOBARBITAL
Hexodorm

CALCIUM GLUCONATE
Akes-N-Pain*
Calcet*
Sedacane*
Supac*

CALCIUM GLYCEROPHOSPHATE
Calphosan B-12*

CALCIUM HYDROXIDE
Percy Medicine*
CALCIUM IODIDE
Calcidrine*
CALCIUM LACTATE
Calcet*
Calphosan
Calphosan B-12*
CALCIUM LEVULINATE
Levucal
CALCIUM PANTOTHENATE
Alba-Lybe*
Cal-Pan
Vergo*
Wart-Aid*
CALCIUM PENTASULFIDE
Vleminckx*
CALCIUM PHOSPHATE
Perio Cal-D*
CALCIUM POLYSTYRENE SULFONATE
Resonium Calcium
CALCIUM POLYSULFIDE
Vlemasque*
Vlem-Dome*
CALCIUM SUCCINATE
Dolcin*
CALCIUM THIOSULFATE
Vlemasque*
Vleminckx*
Vlem-Dome*
CALCIUM UNDECYLENATE
Caldesene
Caldesene Medicated Powder
Cruex
Cruex Medicated Powder
Jockex
CALCIUM-IODINE COMPLEX
Synthaloids*
CALUSTERONE
Methosarb
CAMPHOR
Analbalm*
Banalg Liniment*
Betuline*
Blistex*
Blistr Klear
Boil-Ease*
Calamatum*
Cal-ZO Dressing*
Campho-Phenique*
Dalidyne*
Dasin*
Dermaphill*
Dewitt's Oil for Ear Use*
Emul-O-Balm*
Heet Analgesic Liniment*
Heet Spray Analgesic*
Minut-Rub*
Panalgesic*
Pazo Hemorrhoid*
Rhulicream*
Rhuligel*
Rhulispray*
Soltice Quick Rub*
Sting-Eze*
Vatronol Nose Drops*
Vicks Inhaler*
Vicks Sinex Decongestant Nasal Spray*
Vicks Throat Lozenges*
Vicks Vaporub*
Vicks Vaposteam*
Vicks Vatronol Nose Drops*
CANDICIDIN
Candeptin
Candimon
Vanobid
CANTHARIDIN
Canthacur
Cantharone
CANTHAXANTHINE
Orobronze
CAPREOMYCIN
Capastat
Caprocin
CAPRYLIC ACID
Deso-Creme*
CAPSICUM
Throat Discs Throat Lozenges
CAPTODIAME
Covatin
Suvren
CAPTOPRIL

Capoten
Capozide*
CARAMIPHEN
Aid-Tuss*
Bay-Ornade*
Caramiphen Edisylate*
Panparnit
Parpanit
Toryn
Tuss-Ade*
Tuss Allergine*
Tuss-Ornade*
CARBACHOL
Carbacel Oph
Carcholin
Doryl
Isopto Carbachol
Isopto Carbachol Ophthalmic
Lentin
Miostat
Mistura C
P.V. Carbachol
CARBAMAZEPINE
Tegretol
CARBAMIDE PEROXIDE
Amosan
Auro Ear Drops
Benadyne Ear Drops
Cank-Aid
Debrox
Ear Drop By Murine*
Gly-Oxide
Murine Ear Wax Removal System/ Murine Ear Drops*
Periolav
Proxigel
CARBASPIRIN CALCIUM
Calurin
Fiogesic*
Ursinus*
CARBAZOCHROME SALICYLATE
Adrenosem Salicylate
Adrenoxyl
Adrestat F
Salicylate
Statimo
CARBENICILLIN
Anabactyl
Geocillin
Geopen
Geopen Oral
Gripelin
Pyopen
CARBENOXOLONE
Biogastrone
Biorex
Carbenoline
Duogastrone
CARBETAPENTANE
Rynatuss*
Toclase
Toclonol with Codeine*
Toclonol Expectorant*
Tussar-SF*
Tussar-2*
CARBIDOPA
Sinemet*
CARBIMAZOLE
Neo-Mercazole
CARBINOXAMINE
Allergefon
Baydec*
Brexin*
Carbodec*
Clistin
Clistin-D*
Rondec*
Rondec-DM*
Rondec-TR*
CARBOMYCIN
Magnamycin
CARBON DIOXIDE
Evac-Q-Kit*
CARBOPROST
Prostin
CARBOXYMETHYLCELLULOSE
Anorexin*
Appedrine*
Bacid*
Carmethose
Dialose*
Dialose Plus*
Diet-Trim*
Dioctalose*
Diocto*

Disolan Forte*
Disoplex*
Kaodene*
Kaolin Pectin
Suspension*
Scrip-Lax*
Spantrol*
Tri-Sof*
CARBROMAL
Adalin
Carbrital*
Fydalin
Nyctal
Panelex*
CARBUTEROL
Bronsecur
CARISOPRODOL
Carisoma
Rela
Sanoma
Soma
Soma Compound with
Codeine*
Soprodol
Soprodol*
CARMUSTINE
BiCNU
CARPHENAZINE
Proketazine
CASANTHRANOL
Afko-Lube Lax*
Alko-Lube Lax*
Bu-Lax Plus*
Cassa-Laud*
Comfolax Plus*
Constiban*
Dialose Plus*
Dioctalose*
Diocto*
Diolax*
Diothron*
Disanthrol*
Disolan Forte*
Doctase*
D-S-S Plus*
Hydrocil Fortified*
Lane's Pills
Molatoc-CST*
Peri-Colace*
Peri-Conate*
Peri-Doss*
Peristim Forte
Scrip-Lax*
Tri-Sof*
CASCARA SAGRADA
Amlax*
Biolax
Biolax SP
Bio-Tab
Caroid Laxative*
Cas-Evac
Casyllium*
Kondremul with
Cascara Sagrada*
Milk of Magnesia-
Cascara
Suspension*
Nature's Remedy
Candy Coated
Nature's Remedy
Juniors
Nature's Remedy
Regular
Oxothalein*
Petrogalar*
Stimulax*
CASTILE SOAP
Fleet Bagenema
CASTOR OIL
Alphamul
Covicone*
Decubitex*
Fleet Prep Kit 4*
Fleet Prep Kit 5*
Fleet Prep Kit 6*
Granulex*
G-W Emulsoil
Neoloid
Purge
Ricifruit
Unisoil
CEDAR LEAF OIL
Vicks Vaporub*
CEFACLOR
Ceclor
CEFADROXIL
Duricef
Ultracef
CEFAMANDOLE
Mandol

CEFAZOLIN
  Ancef
  Kefzol
CEFONICID
  Monocid
CEFOPERAZONE
  Cefobid
CEFOTAXIME
  Claforan
CEFOXITIN
  Mefoxin
CEFTAZIDIME
  Fortaz
CEFTIZOXIME
  Cefizox
CEFTRIAXONE
  Rocephin
CEFUROXIME
  Zinacef
CELLULASE
  Converzyme*
  Kutrase*
  Ku-Zyme*
CELLULOSE
  Pentazyme*
CEPHALEXIN
  Cephorex
  Cepor
  Ceporex
  Ceporexine
  Keflex
  Keforal
CEPHALOGLYCIN
  Kafocin
  Kefglycin
CEPHALORIDINE
  Cephalomycin
  Ceporan
  Ceporin
  Keflodin
  Kefloridin
  Kefspor
  Loridine
CEPHALOTHIN
  Ceporacin
  Keflin
  Keflin Neutral
  Seffin
  Sefflin
CEPHAPIRIN
  Cefadyl
CEPHRADINE
  Anspor
  Sefril
  Velosef
CERULETIDE
  Tymtran
CETALKONIUM
  Isodettes Super*
  Trokettes*
  Zettyn
CETRIMIDE
  Cetavlon
  Cetril
  Drapolex
  Savlon
  Savlon-Hospital
    Concentrate
CETYL ALCOHOL
  Absorbine Arthritic
    Pain*
  Cetaphil*
  Derm-Aid
CETYLPYRIDINIUM
  Axon*
  Bactalin*
  Ceepryn
  Cepacol
  Cepacol Troches*
  Conex Lozenge*
  Kank-A*
  Lanazets*
  Laryngine
  Merocet
  Mycinettes*
  Mycinettes Sugar
    Free*
  Oradex-C*
  Semets*
  Sinex Decongestant
    Nasal Spray*
  Trokettes*
  Vicks Medi-Trating*
  Vicks Sinex
    Decongestant Nasal
    Spray*
  Vicks Throat
    Lozenges*
  Watkins Antiseptic
CHARCOAL
  Charcocaps
  Medicoal

CHARCOAL, ACTIVATED
Digestalin*
Liquid-Antidose
CHENODIOL
Chendol
Chenix
Cheno
CHINIOFON
Quinoxyl
Yatren
CHLOPHEDIANOL
Detigon
Ulo
CHLORAL BETAINE
Beta-Chlor
CHLORAL HYDRATE
Aquachloral
Chloralex
Chloralvan
Cohidrate
Felsules
Lorinal
Lycoral
Nigracap
Noctec
Novochlorhydrate
Oradrate
Rectules
Somni Sed
Somnos
SK-Chloral Hydrate
CHLORAMBUCIL
Chloraminophene
Leukeran
CHLORAMINE-T
Chloralone
Nuklorene
CHLORAMPHENICOL
Alficetyn
Amphichlor
Amphicol
Antibiopto
Ophthalmic*
Chlomin
Chloromycetin
Chloromycetin
Hydrocortisone*
Chloromyxin*
Chloroptic
Chloroptic S.O.P.
Cylphenicol
Econochlor
Ophthalmic
Elase-Chloromycetin
Ointment*
Enicol
Fenicol
Isopto Fenicol
Kemicetine
Leukomycin
Mychel
Mycin
Nova-Phenicol
Ophthalmic
Novochlorocap
Ophthochlor
Pantofenicol
Pentamycetin
Sopamycetin
CHLORAZANIL
Daquin
CHLORCYCLIZINE
Di-Paralene
Fedrazil*
Mantadil*
Perazil
CHLORDANTOIN
Sporostacin*
CHLORDIAZEPOXIDE
A-Poxide
Chlordinium Sealets*
Clindex*
Clioxide*
Clipoxide*
Corax
C-Tran
Librax*
Librelease
Libritabs
Librium
Lidinium*
Limbitrol*
Medilium
Menrium
Nack
Novopoxide
Pentrium*
Relaxil
SK-Lygen
Solium
Trilium
Via-Quil

CHLORHEXIDINE
  Bactigras
  Hibicare
  Hibiclens
  Hibistat
  Hibitane
  Hibitane Tincture*
CHLORHYDROXYQUINOLINE
  Loroxide Acne Lotion*
  Loroxide-HC Lotion*
  Vanoxide*
CHLORIODIZED OIL
  Iodochlorol
CHLORISONDAMINE
  Ecolid
CHLORMERODRIN
  Mercloran
  Mercuroxyl
  Neohydrin
CHLORMEZANONE
  Clorilax
  Trancopal
CHLOROBUTANOL
  Akwa Tears*
  Baciguent Ophthalmic*
  Chloretone
  Fluress*
  Glukor Injection*
  Myciguent*
  Neo-Delta-Cortef*
  Neo-Medrol*
  Neosone*
  Ows Blue*
  Tears Plus*
CHLOROGUANIDE
  Paludrine
CHLOROPHYLLIN
  Chloresium
  Derifil
  Sudroma
  Voids
CHLOROPROCAINE
  Nesacaine
  Versacaine
CHLOROQUINE
  Aralen*
  Avlochlor
  Quinachlor
CHLOROTHEN
  Tagathen
CHLOROTHIAZIDE
  Aldoclor*
  Chloroserpine*
  Chlotride
  Diupres*
  Diupres-250*
  Diuril
  Ro-Chlorozide
  Ro-Chloro-Serp*
  Saluric
  SK-Chlorothiazide
  Supres*
CHLOROTHYMOL
  Dalidyne*
  Medicated Foot Powder*
  NP-27 Liquid*
  Rid-Itch Liquid*
  Solvex Athlete's Foot Spray*
  Solvex Powder*
CHLOROTRIANISENE
  PMB 200
  Tace
CHLOROXINE
  Capitrol Cream Shampoo
CHLOROXYLENOL
  Benzodyne Drops*
  Ice-O-Derm
  Ice-O-Derm Lotion
  Ice-O-Derm Skin Cleanser
  O.B. Liquid
  Orlex H.C. Otic*
  Orlex Otic
  Otall Ear Drops*
  Otic-HC Ear Drops*
  Podiaspray*
  Zetar Shampoo*
CHLORPHEDIANOL
  Ulone
CHLORPHENESIN
  Maolate
  Mycil
CHLORPHENIRAMINE
  Advanced Formula Dristan*
  Aid-Tuss*
  Alamine*

Alamine-C*
Alamine Expectorant*
Al-Ay*
Alermine
Alersule*
Alka-Seltzer Plus*
Allerbid
Allerest Regular and Children's*
Allerest Sinus Pain Formula*
Allerform*
Allergesic*
Allergin*
Allergy Relief Medicine*
Allerid
Allerid-D.C.*
Allerprop*
Aller-Chlor
AL-R
Alumadrine*
Amaril D*
Anafed*
Anamine*
Anamine T.D. Caps*
Anatuss*
Anodynos Forte*
Aspirin Free Dristan*
Atlachlor
Atussin D.M. Expectorant*
Atussin Expectorant*
Bayaminic Syrup*
Bayer Decongestant*
Bayhistine*
Breacol*
Cenaid*
Cheracol Plus*
Childrens Co Tylenol*
Chlorafed Timecelles*
Chlorated Adult Timecells*
Chlorofed Injection*
Chloro-Pro
Chloro-100
Chlorphen
Chlortab
Chlor-Rest*
Chlor-Trimeton
Chlor-Trimeton Decongestant*
Chlor-Trimeton Expectorant*
Chlor-Trimeton Expectorant with Codeine*
Chlor-Tripolon
Citra*
Codimal*
Codimal-L.A. Cenules*
Codrin L.A*
Colrex*
Colrex Antitussive*
Colrex Cough Syrup*
Coltab*
Comhist*
Comtrex*
Conex*
Conex with Codeine*
Contac*
Contac Severe Cold Formula*
Cophene*
Coricidin*
Coricidin "D"*
Coricidin Antitussive*
Coricidin Demilets*
Coricidin Medilets*
Corlin Infant Drops*
Corsym*
Cortiforte*
Coryban-D*
Cotrol-D*
Covanamine*
Covangesic*
Co-Pyronil*
Co Tylenol*
Co Tylenol Cold Formula for Children*
CoTylenol Liquid Cold Formula*
Dallergy*
Dasikon*
Decohist*
Deconade*
Deconamine*
Decongestabs*

Deconsmine*
Dehist*
Demazin*
Deproist*
Donatussin Drops*
Donatussin Syrup*
Dristan*
Dristan Advanced Formula*
Dristan Antitussive*
Dristan Ultra*
Dristan Ultra Coughs Formula*
Drize*
Duadacin*
Duphrene*
Duradyne-Forte*
Duralex*
Efricon*
Extendac*
Extendryl*
Fedahist*
Fedahist Expectorant*
Fedahist Syrup*
Fernhist*
Ginsopan*
Hal-Chlor
Headway*
Histabid Duracap*
Histaject*
Histalet*
Histalet DM*
Histalet Forte*
Histalon
Histaspan
Histaspan-D*
Histaspan-P*
Histaspan-Plus*
Histatab*
Hista-Compound No.5*
Hista-Phen-S.A.*
Hista-Vadrin*
Histex
Historal*
Histor-D Syrup*
Histor-D Timecelles*
Hot Lemon*
Hournaze*
H-Stadur
Ibioton
Imotep*
Intensin*
Isoclor*
Kiddisan*
Kleer Chewable*
Kolephrin*
Kophane Cough & Cold Formula*
Korigesic*
Kronofed-A Kronocaps*
Kronohist Kronocaps*
Lanatuss*
Lanatuss Expectorant*
Midran Decongestant*
Naldecon*
Naldelate*
Napril Plateau Caps*
Narspan*
Nasahist*
Nasahist II*
Nasalspan*
Nazac Timed-Disintegration Decongestant*
N.D. Clear T.D.*
ND-Gesic*
N.D.-Stat*
Neotep*
Nilcol*
N-N Cough*
Nogest*
Nolamine*
Noraminic Syrup*
Norel Plus*
Norel Plus Injection*
Nor-Lief*
Noscosed
Novafed A*
Novahistine*
Novahistine DH*
Novahistine Elixir*
Novahistine Expectorant*
Novahistine Fortis*
Novahistine LP*
Novahistine Sinus*
Novamor*
Novopheniram
Omnicol*

Orahist*
Oraminic*
Ornade*
Ornade 2 Liquid for Children*
Pediacof*
Pentuss*
Phenate*
Phenetron
Phenetron Lanacaps
Phenhist Elixir*
Piriton
Polaronil
Probacon*
Probacon II*
Pseudo-Hist*
Pseudo-Hist Expectorant*
Pyrralan Expectorant*
Pyrroxate*
Quadra-Hist*
Quelidrine*
Quiet-Nite*
Relemine*
Reletuss*
Resaid T.D.*
Rhinafed-Ex*
Rhinex*
Rhinex D-Lay*
Rhinex DM*
Rhinocyn-DM*
Rhinocyn-PD*
Rhinogesic*
Rhinolar*
Rhinolar-Ex*
Rhinosyn*
Romex*
Romilar*
Ru-Tuss*
Ru-Tuss II*
Rynatan*
Rynatuss*
Ryna-C Liquid*
Ryna Liquid*
Ryna-Tussadine Expectorant*
Salphenyl*
Sinapils*
Sinarest*
Sinarest Nasal Spray*
Sinexin*
Sine-Off*
Sine-Off-Aspirin Formula*
Sine-Off Aspirin-Free Extra Strength*
Singlet*
Sinocon*
Sinovan Timed*
Sino-Comp*
Sinulin*
Sinurex*
Sinusol-D*
Sinutab Extra Strength*
Spantac*
Spantuss*
Sudafed Plus*
Supercitin*
T.D. Alermine
Teldrin
Telodron
Timed Cold*
Tonecol*
T.P.I.*
Triaminicin*
Triaminicin Allergy*
Triaminicin Chewables*
Triaminic Allergy*
Tricodene Forte*
Tricodene NN*
Trihista-Phen*
Trind*
Trind DM*
Tri-Nefrin*
Tri-Phen-Chlor*
Trymegen
Tudecon*
Tussanil Syrup*
Tussar DM*
Tussar-SF*
Tussar-2*
Tussi-Organidin*
Tussi-Organidin DM*
Tuss-Ade*
Tuss Allergine*
Tus-Oraminic*
Tymcaps
Valihist*

Vernate*
Viromed*
Wesmatic Forte*
CHLORPHENIRAMINE MALEATE
Chloramate Unicelles
CHLORPHENOXAMINE
Clorevan
Phenoxene
Systral
CHLORPHENTERMINE
Chlorophen
Lucofen
Pre-Sate
CHLORPROCAINE
Nesacaine-CE
CHLORPROMAZINE
Chloramead
Chlorprom
Chlor-Promanyl
Chlor-PZ
Cromedazine
Elmarine
Hibanil
Largactil
Megaphen
Ormazine
Promachel
Promapar
Promaz
Promosol
Psychozine
Sonazine
Thorazine
Thorazine Spansules
Tranzine
CHLORPROPAMIDE
Chloromide
Chloronase
Diabetoral
Diabinese
Glucamide
Insulase
Mellinese
Novopropamide
Stabinol
CHLORPROTHIXENE
Taractan
Tarasan
Truxal
CHLORQUINALDOL
Gynoterax
Sterosan
CHLORTETRACYCLINE
Aureomycin
Chrysomysin
CHLORTHALIDONE
Combipres*
Demi-Regroton*
Hygroton
Hygroton-Reserpine*
Igroton
Novothalidone
Regroton*
Tenoretic*
Thalitone
Uridon
CHLORZOXAZONE
Chlorofon-F*
Chlorzoxazone w/APAP*
Flexaphen*
Lobac*
Miflex*
Myoforte*
Paraflex
Parafon Forte*
Saroflex*
Spasgesic*
Tuzon*
Zoxaphen*
CHOLECALCIFEROL
Alphamettes*
Andoin*
Aquasol A & D*
Cal-M*
Deltalin
Desitin Ointment*
Jay Leith
Jayleth
Ostoforte
Ostogen
Proctodon*
Radiostol
Scott's Emulsion*
Tri-Vi-Flor*
Tri-Vi-Flor w/Iron Drops*
Tri-Vi-Sol*
Tri-Vi-Sol with Iron*

Vi-Daylin ADC Drops*
Vi-Daylin/F ADC + Iron Drops*
Vi-Daylin/F ADC Drops*
Vi-Daylin Plus Iron ADC Drops*

CHOLESTYRAMINE RESIN
Cuemid
Questran

CHOLINE BITARTRATE
Co-Salt*

CHOLINE MAGNESIUM TRISALICYLATE
Trilisate

CHOLINE SALICYLATE
Arthropan
Teejel

CHONDRUS
Kondremul*
Kondremul with Cascara Sagrada*
Kondremul with Phenolphthalein*

CHORAMPHENICOL
Ophthocort*

CHROMIC PHOSPHATE
Chromphosphotope
Phosphocol P32

CHYMOPAPAIN
Chymodiactin

CHYMOTRYPSIN
Alpha Chymar
Alpha Chymolean
Avazyme
Biozyme*
Catarase
Chymar
Chymase
Chymetin
Chymolase
Chymoral
Chymotest
Enzeon
Orenzyme*
Quimotrase
Zolyse
Zonulyn

CICLOPIROX
Loprox

CIMETIDINE
Novo-Cimetine
Peptol
Tagamet

CINCHOPHEN
Atophan

CINNAMEDRINE
Midol*

CINNARIZINE
Apomiteral
Corathiem
Glanil
Mitronal
Roin
Sturgeon
Stutgeron

CINOXACIN
Cinobac

CISPLATIN
Neoplatin
Platinol

CITRIC ACID
Albatussin*
Alka-Seltzer Effervescent Antacid*
Alka-Seltzer Effervescent Pain Reliever and Antacid*
Bicitra-Sugar Free*
Bromo-Seltzer*
Instant Mix Metamucil*
Polycitra*
Polycitra-K*
Polycitra-LC--Sugar-Free*
Renacidin*
Sal Hepatica*

CLAVULANIC ACID
Augmentin*

CLEMASTINE
Tavegil
Tavist
Tavist-D*

CLEMIZOLE
Allercur

CLIDINIUM
Chlordinium Sealets*

Clindex*
Clioxide*
Clipoxide*
Librax*
Lidinium*
Quarzan

CLINDAMYCIN
Cleocin
Dalacin C
Sobelin

CLIOQUINOL
Aristform*
Aristform D*
Aristform R*
Caquin Cream*
Domeform-HC*
Dreniform*
Formtone-HC*
Hexaderm I.Q. Modified Cream*
Hydroquin*
Hysone Ointment*
Iodocort Cream*
Mity-Quin Cream*
Propaderm C*
Racet Cream*
Racet LCD Cream*

CLOBETASOL
Dermovate

CLOBETASONE
Eumovate

CLOCORTOLONE
Cloderm

CLOFAZIMINE
Lamprene

CLOFIBRATE
Amotril
Atromidin
Atromid-S
Azionyl
Claripex
Liposid
Liprinal
Novofibrate
Skleromexe

CLOMIPHENE
Clomid
Dyneric

CLOMIPRAMINE
Anafranil

CLONAZEPAM
Clonopin
Iktorivil
Rivotril

CLONIDINE
Catapres
Catapres-TTS
Combipres*

CLOPENTHIXOL
Sordinol

CLORAZEPATE
Azene
Tranxene
Tranxilene Azene

CLOREXOLONE
Flonatril
Nefrolan

CLORTERMINE
Voranil

CLOTRIMAZOLE
Canesten
Canesten-1
Gyne-Lotrimin
Lotrimin
Mycelex
Mycelex-G
Mycelex Troche
Trimysten

CLOXACILLIN
Bactopen
Cloxapen
Cloxilean
Novocloxin
Orbenin
Staphobristol-250
Tegopen

CO-TRIMOXAZOLE
Bactrim DS
Bactrim IV
Eusaprim
Novo-Trimel
Septan
Septra
Septra DS
Septra IV
Sulfatrin
Trimethoprim-Sulfa

COAL TAR
A.T.S.*
Balnetar*

Denorex*
Doak Oil
Doak Oil Forte
Estar
Lavatar
Locon*
L.C.D.
Mazon*
Neutratar
Oxipor VHC Lotion for Psoriasis*
Pentrax Tar Shampoo
Polytar*
Pragmatar*
Psorex Medicated
Psorigel
Racet LCD Cream*
Sebutone*
Supertah*
Tarbonis
Targel
Targel S.A.
Tarlene*
Tarsum*
Tar Distillate "Doak"
Tar-Doak Lotion*
Tersa-Tar
Ul-tar
Ultra Clear Medicated Shampoo
Unguentum Bossi*
Vanseb-T*
Xseb-T Shampoo*
Zetar
Zetar Emulsion
Zetar Shampoo*

COBALAMIN
Trinsicon*
Trinsicon M*

COCCIDIOIDIN
Spherulin

CODEINE
Acetaco*
Acetaminophen With Codeine Elixir*
Actifed-C*
Actifed with Codeine Cough Syrup*
Acutuss Expectorant With Codeine*
Alamine-C*
Alamine Expectorant*
Ambenyl Expectorant*
Ancasal Compound No.1*
Ancasal Compound No.2*
Ancasal Compound No.3*
Anexsia with Codeine*
Apa-Deine*
APC with Codeine*
A.S.A. and Codeine Compound*
Ascodeen-30*
Ascriptin*
Atasol-15*
Atasol-30*
Atasol-8*
Bancap With Codeine*
Broncho-Tussin*
Bufferin with Codeine No. 3*
Calcidrine*
Capital With Codeine*
Cerose*
Cetro-Cirose*
Cheracol*
Chlor-Trimeton Expectorant with Codeine*
Coastaldyne*
Codalan*
Codasa*
Codimal PH*
Codophen-R*
Conex with Codeine*
Copavin*
Coryphen-Codeine*
Cosanyl Cough*
Cotussis*
Co-Xan*
C3*
C4*
Dimetapp with Codeine*
Efricon*
Empirin With Codeine*
Empracet with Codeine Phosphate No. 3*

Empracet with
  Codeine Phosphate
  No. 4*
Empracet-30*
Emprazil-C*
Entrophen with
  Codeine*
Fiorinal-C1/2*
Fiorinal-C1/4*
G-3*
Hasacode*
Histadyl EC*
Liquix-C*
Lo-Tussin*
Maxigesic*
Mercodol with
  Decapryn*
Mersyndol with
  Codeine*
Monacet with
  Codeine*
Naldecon-CX*
Neopirine Co. with
  Codeine*
Noratuss*
Novahistine DH*
Novahistine
  Expectorant*
Nucofed*
Nucofed Pediatric
  Expectorant*
Panadol with
  Codeine*
Paveral
Pediacof*
Pentuss*
Phenacodein 002*
Phenacodein 003*
Phenaphen with
  Codeine*
Phenaphen-650 with
  Codeine*
Poly-Histine
  Expectorant with
  Codeine*
Prunicodeine*
PAC Compound with
  Codeine*
Robaxisal C-1/4*
Robaxisal C-1/8*
Robitussin A-C*
Robitussin DAC*
Rounox + Codeine*
Ryna-Cx Liquid*
Ryna-C Liquid*
Salatin with
  Codeine*
SK-APAP with
  Codeine*
Soma Compound with
  Codeine*
Tabloid Brand A.P.C.
  with Codeine*
Tolu-Sed*
Triaminic
  Expectorant with
  Codeine*
Tricodene C-V*
Tussar-SF*
Tussar-2*
Tussi-Organidin*
Tylenol #1*
Tylenol #2*
Tylenol #3*
Tylenol #4*
Tylenol with
  Codeine*
Tylenol No.1 Forte*
222*
282*
282 MEP*
292*
293*
294*

COLCHICINE
  ColBenemid*
  Colsalide
  Novocolchine

COLESTIPOL
  Colestid Granules

COLISTIMETHATE
  Coly-Mycin M
    Parenteral

COLISTIN
  Coly-Mycin
  Coly-Mycin S Otic*

COLLAGENASE
  Biozyme-C
  Santyl

COLLODIAL OATMEAL
  Sebaveen*

CONJUGATED ESTROGENS
- C.E.S.
- Estrocon
- Evestrone
- Kestrin
- Menotab
- Oestrilin
- Oestrilin with Methyltestosterone*
- Ovest
- Premarin with M.T.*
- Sodestrin
- Sodestrin H

COPPER
- Dequasine*

COPPER OLEATE
- Cuprex*

COPPER UNDECYLENATE
- Verdefam Cream*
- Verdefam Solution*

CORN STARCH
- Lobana*

CORTICOTROPIN
- Actest
- ACTH
- Acthar
- Cortrophin
- Cortrophin-Zinc
- Depo-ACTH
- Duracton
- H.P. Acthar Gel
- Tubex

CORTISOL
- Orabase HCA
- Racet Cream*
- Racet LCD Cream*

CORTISONE
- Cortelan
- Cortistab
- Cortogen
- Cortone
- Neosone*

COSYNTROPIN
- Corthrosyn
- Cortrosyn
- Synacthen Depot

CREOSOTE
- Creo-Terpin*

CRESOL
- Emer-Cide

CROMOLYN
- Aarane

CROMOLYN SODIUM
- Aarane
- Fivent
- Intal
- Lomudal
- Nasalcrom
- Nasmil
- Opticrom
- Rynacrom

CROTAMITON
- Eurax

CRUDE COAL TAR
- Polytar*

CRUDE COAL TAR EXTRACT
- Alphosyl-HC Lotion & Cream*
- Alphosyl Lotion & Cream*
- Tegrin For Psoriasis*

CRYPTENAMINE
- Diutensen*
- Unitensen

CYANOCOBALAMIN
- Alba-Lybe*
- Anacobin
- Bedoz
- Berubigen
- Betalin 12 Crystalline
- Bevidox
- Bio-12
- Brevatine-12
- B-Twelv-Ora
- Cabadon M
- Calphosan B-12*
- Cenalene*
- Chromagen*
- Cobadoce Forte
- Cobione
- Crystwel
- Cyanabin
- Cyredin
- Depinar
- Docibin
- Dodecamin
- Dodecavite
- Dodex
- Ducobee
- Geravite Elixir*

Hemocyte Injection*
Hepcovite
Hepp-Iron Drops*
Laud-Iron Plus
Chewing*
Neo-Rubex
Neuro B-12 Forte
Injectable*
Neuro B-12
Injectable*
Niferex-150 Forte*
Normocytin
Nova-Rubi
Perihemin*
Pinkamin
Poyamin
Pronemia*
Redisol
Rhodavite
Rubion
Rubramin
Rubramin PC
Sytobex
Thera-Combex H-P*
Tia-Doce Injectable
Univial*
TriHemic 600*
Tri-Tinic*
Trophite*
Troph-Iron*
Troph-Iron Liquid*
Vibalt
Vitron-C-Plus*
Vi-Twel
Willcotrin
CYCLACILLIN
Cyclapen
Cyclapen-W
CYCLANDELATE
Cyclanfour
Cyclospasmol
Cydel
Cyvaso
CYCLIZINE
Marezine
Marzine
Migral*
Valoid
CYCLOBARBITAL
Phanodorn
CYCLOBENZAPRINE
Flexeril
CYCLOCUMAROL
Cumopyran
CYCLOFENIL
Sexovid
CYCLOMETHYCAINE
Surfacaine
CYCLOPENTAMINE
Aerolone*
Hista-Clopane*
CYCLOPENTOLATE
Ak-Pentolate
Cyclogyl
Cyclomydril*
Mydplegic
Mydrilate
Novo-Cyclo
Optopentolate
CYCLOPHOSPHAMIDE
Cytoxan
Endoxan
Neosar
Procytox
CYCLOSERINE
Closina
Oxamycin
Serociclina
Seromycin
Tisomycin
CYCLOSPORINE
Sandimmune
CYCLOTHIAZIDE
Anhydron
Fluidil
CYCRIMINE
Pagitane
CYPROHEPTADINE
Nuran
Periactin
Vimicon
CYSTEINE
Dequasine*
CYTARABINE
Cytosar

D

DACARBAZINE
DTIC-Dome
DACTINOMYCIN

Cosmegen
Meractinomycin
DANAZOL
Cyclomen
Danocrine
DANTHRON
Danivac
Danthross*
Doctate-P*
Dorbane
Dorbantyl*
Dorbantyl Forte*
Doxan*
Doxidan*
DOSS* (Canada)
Istizin
Laxatyl*
Magcyl*
Modane*
Modane Mild
Modane Plus*
Regulex-D*
Roydan
Ruc-Dane*
Tonelax
Unilax*
Valax*
DANTROLENE
Dantrium
Relaxant
DAPSONE
Disulone
Udolac
DAUNORUBICIN
Cerubidine
Daunoblastin
Ondena
DEANOL ACETAMIDOBENZOATE
Cervoxan
Deaner
Deaner-100
DEBRISOQUINE
Declinax
DECAMETHONIUM
Eulissin
Syncurine
DEFEROXAMINE
Desferal
DEHYDROCHOLIC ACID
Bilax*
Bilezyme*
Bilostat
Bio-Cholin
Cholan DH
Cholypyl
Dehydrocholin
Dilabil
Dycholium
Hepahydrin
Hykolex
Idrocrine
Ketochol
Neocholan
Neolax*
Procholon
Sarolax*
Transibyl
Triketol
Trilax*
DEMECARIUM
Humorsol
Tosmilen
DEMECLOCYCLINE
Declomycin
Declostatin*
Demeclor
Ledermycin
Novociclina
Tollerclin
DENATONIUM BENZOATE
Thumz
DEQUALINIUM
Dequadin
Quoticidine
DESERPIDINE
Enduronyl*
Enduronyl Forte*
Harmonyl
Oreticyl*
Raunormine
DESIPRAMINE
Norpramin
Pertofrane
DESLANOSIDE
Cedilanid-D
Cedilanid Injection
DESMOPRESSIN
DDAVP
Minirin
Stimate
DESONIDE

Tridesilon
DESOXIMETASONE
Aubason
Esperson
Ibaril
Topicort
Topisolon
DESOXYCHOLIC ACID
Bilezyme*
Bilogen*
Oxycholine
DESOXYCORTICOSTERONE
Cortate
Decostrate
Descotone
Doca Acetate
Dorcostrin
Doxatone
Percorten
Percorten Acetate
Syncortin
DESOXYEPHEDRINE
Vicks Inhaler*
DESOXYRIBONUCLEASE
Elase*
Elase-Chloromycetin Ointment*
DEXAMETHASONE
Aeroseb-Dex
Ak-Dex
Dalone
Decaderm
Decadrol
Decadron
Decadron Eye-Ear Solution
Decadron Phosphate Respihaler
Decajet-L.A.
Decameth L.A.
Decaspray
Delladec
Demasone L.A.
Deronil
Dexameth
Dexasone
Dexo-LA
Dexon
Dexone
Gammacorten
Hexadrol
L.A.Dezone
Maxidex
Maxidex Ophthalmic
NeoDecadron*
Novadex
Optomethasone
Savacort-D
SK-Dexamethasone
Solurex-L.A.
Turbinaire Decadron Phosphate
Wexaphos
DEXBROMPHENIRAMINE
Disomer
Disophrol*
Drixoral*
Duo-hist*
Efedra P.A.*
Histarall*
Pseudo-Mal*
DEXCHLORPHENIRAMINE
Polaramine
Polaramime Expectorant*
DEXPANTHENOL
Ilopan
Panol
DEXTRAN 150
Dextraven
DEXTRAN 40
Gentran 40
LMD 10%
Rheomacrodex
Rheotran
DEXTRAN 70
Macrodex
DEXTRAN 75
Gentran 75
DEXTRANOMER
Debrisan
DEXTRIFERRON
Astrafer
DEXTROAMPHETAMINE
Biphetamine*
Dexampex
Dexamyl*
Dexedrine
Eskatrol*
Ferndex

Obetrol*
Obotan
Oxydess II
Spancap No.1
Synatan

DEXTROMETHORPHAN
Albatussin*
Ambenyl-D Decongestant Cough Formula*
Anatuss*
Anti-Tuss DM*
Atussin D.M. Expectorant*
Balminil DM
Bayaminicol*
Baydec*
Bayer Cough for Children*
Baytussin DM*
Benylin DM*
Breacol*
Broncho-Grippol-DM
Carbodec*
Cerose DM*
Cheracol D*
Cheracol Plus*
Chexit*
Children's Hold 4 Hour Cough Suppressant*
Chloraseptic DM Cough Control Lozenges*
Codimal DM*
Codistan*
Colrex Antitussive*
Colrex Cough Syrup*
Comtrex*
Congespirin
Consotuss*
Contac Cough*
Contac Jr. Childrens' Cold Medicine*
Contac Severe Cold Formula*
Contac Severe Cold Formula Night Strength*
Coryban-D Antitussive*
Cosanyl DM Improved Formula*
CoTylenol Liquid Cold Formula*
Cremacoat 1
Cremacoat 3*
Cremacoat 4*
Delsym
Demo-Cineol Antitussive
Dextrotussin*
Dextro-Tuss GG*
Dimacol*
DM
DM-4 Children's Cough Control*
DM-8*
Donatussin Syrup*
Dorcol Pediatric*
Dormethan
Dristan Antitussive*
Dristan Ultra*
Dristan Ultra Coughs Formula*
Endotussin-NN*
Endotussin-NN Pediatric*
Formula 44*
Formula 44 Cough Discs
Formula 44-D*
Glydm*
G-Tussin DM*
Guaimid*
Halls*
Histalet DM*
Histivite-D*
Hold*
Hold Liquid Cough Suppressant*
Hold 4 Hour Cough Suppressant
Kleer Chewable*
Kolephrin GG*
Kophane Cough & Cold Formula*
Liquitussin DM*
Mediquell
Methorate
Multi-Symptom*
Naldetuss*

Nasalspan
  Expectorant*
Nilcol*
N-N Cough*
Novahistine DMX*
Nyquil Nighttime
  Colds Medicine*
Omnicol*
Ornacol*
Orthoxicol*
Pertussin
Pertussin Cough for
  Children*
Pertussin 8-Hour
  Cough Formula
Promatussin DM*
Pyrralan Expectorant*
Quelidrine*
Queltuss*
Quiet-Nite*
Reletuss*
Rem*
Rhinex DM*
Rhinocyn-DM*
Rhinosyn DM*
Rhinosyn-X*
Robidex
Robitussin-CF*
Robitussin-DM*
Robitussin-DM Cough
  Calmers
Robitussin Night
  Relief*
Romex*
Romilar*
Romilar
Romilar Children's
Romilar CF*
Romilar III*
Rondec-DM*
Sedatuss
Sediodal-DM
Silence Is Golden
Silexin*
Soltice*
Sorbutuss*
Spantuss*
Spec-T Sore Throat/
  Cough Suppressant*
St. Joseph Cough for
  Children
Sucrets Cough
  Control Formula
Sudafed Cough*
Supercitin*
Symptom I
Syracol*
Tolu-Sed DM*
Tonecol*
Triaminicol*
Triaminicol
  Decongestant Cough*
Triaminic-DM Cough
  Formula*
Tricodene DM
Tricodene Forte*
Tricodene NN*
Tricodene Pediatric*
Triminicol Cough
  Syrup*
Trind DM*
Troutman's
Tussagesic*
Tussaminic*
Tussar DM*
Tussi-Organidin DM*
Tussorphan
Tus-Oraminic*
Unproco*
Vicks Cough*
Vicks Cough Silencer
Vicks Formula 44
  Cough Control
  Discs*
Vicks Formula 44
  Cough Mixture*
Vicks Formula 44D
  Decongestant Cough
  Mixture*
Vicks Nyquil
  Nighttime Colds
  Medicine*
2/G-DM*

DEXTROSE
Cartose
Glucodex
L. A. Formula*
Plova*
Syllact*
Syllamalt
  Effervescent*

DEXTROTHYROXINE

Choloxin
Hypaque
DIATRIZOATE MEGLUMINE
Anglovist 370
Cardiografin
Cystografin
Gastrografin*
Gastrovist
MD-76
Renografin
Reno-M-DIP
Reno-M-30
Renovist*
Renovist II*
Sinografin*
Urovist
DIATRIZOATE SODIUM
Gastrografin*
Hypaque M*
Hypaque Oral
Hypaque Sodium
Renovist*
Renovist II*
Urovist Sodium 300
DIAZEPAM
Apaurin
Apo-Diazepam
Atensine
D-Tran
E-Pam
Lembrol
Meval
Neo-Calme
Noan
Novodiazepam
Novodipam
Paxel
Rival
Serenack
Setonil
Stress-Pam
Tensium
Tranimul
Valium
Valrelease
Vatran
Vivol
DIAZOXIDE
Hyperstat
Proglycem
DIBUCAINE
Corticaine Cream*
D-Caine
Dibucaine Ointment
Neo-Hydro*
Nupercainal
Nupercainal Suppositories
Nupercaine
Nuperlone
Otocort Ear Drops*
Otoreid-HC*
DICALCIUM PHOSPHATE
D.C.P.
D.C.P. 340
DICHLORALPHENAZONE
Chloralol
Midrin*
DICHLOROACETIC ACID
Bichloracetic Acid
DICHLOROPHEN
Anthiphen
DICHLOROPHENARSINE
Dichlor-Mapharsen
DICHLORPHENAMIDE
Daranide
Oratrol
DICLOFENAC
Voltaren
DICLOXACILLIN
Diclocil
Dycill
Dynapen
Pathocil
Veracillin
DICUMAROL
Dicuman
Dufalone
DICYCLOMINE
Antispas
Bentyl
Bentylol
Bentylol with Phenobarbital*
Bentyl with Phenobarb*
Cyclobec
Dibent
Dibent-PB*
Dicen
Dilomine
Di-Spaz

Dyspas
Formulex
Menospasm
Merbentyl
Neoquess Injectable
Niospaz
Or-Tyl
Pasmin
Rocycle-20
Rocyclo-10
Spasmoban
Spasmoban-PH*
Spasmoject
Spastyl with Phenobarbital*
Viscephen*
Viscerol
Wyovin

DIENESTROL
AVC with Dienestrol*
DV Cream/ Suppositories
Estraguard
Ortho Dienestrol Cream
Synestrol
Willnestrol

DIETHAZINE
Diparcol

DIETHYLAMINE SALICYLATE
Algesal Cream

DIETHYLAMINOBARBITAL
Upnos

DIETHYLCARBAMAZINE
Banocide
Franocide
Hetrazan

DIETHYLPROPION
Depletite
Derfon
Dietec
D.I.P.
Nobesine
Regenon
Regibon
Tenuate
Tenuate Dospan
Tepanil
Tepanil Ten-Tab

DIETHYLSTILBESTROL
A.T.V.
DV
Estrosyn
Honvol
Makarol
Micrest
Prin V/S
Stibilium
Stilbestrol
Stilbetin
Stilphostrol
Tylosterone*
Vagestrol

DIFLORASONE DIACETATE
Florone
Maxiflor

DIFLUNISAL
Dolobid

DIGALLOYL TRIOLEATE
Sunstick
Sunswept

DIGITALIS
Digifortis
Digiglusin
Pil-Digis

DIGITOXIN
Cardidigin
Crystodigin
De-Tone-2
Digisidin
Digitaline Nativelle
Purodigin
Unidigin

DIGOXIN
Lanoxicaps
Lanoxin
Natigoxine Nativelle
Novodigoxin
SK-Digoxin
Winoxin

DIHEXYVERINE
Metaspas
Spasmalex

DIHYDROERGOTAMINE
D.H.E. 45
Plexonal*

DIHYDROQUINIDINE
Hydroquine

DIHYDROTACHYSTEROL

A.T.10
DHT
Hytakerol
Tachystin
DIHYDROXYALUMINUM ACETATE
Aluscop*
DIHYDROXYALUMINUM AMINOACETATE
Alamino
Alglyn
Alminate
Alzinox
Arthritis Strength Bufferin*
Aspogen
Bufferin*
Bufferin with Codeine No. 3*
Dimothyn
Doraximin
Prodexin
Robalate
Tralmag*
DIHYDROXYALUMINUM SODIUM CARBONATE
Rolaids
DIHYPRYLONE
Sedulon
DILOXANIDE FUROATE
Furamide
DILTIAZEM
Cardizem
DIMENHYDRINATE
Dimenest
Dimentabs
Dinate
Dommanate
Dramaban
Dramamine
Dramilin
Dramocen
Dramoject
Dymenate
Dymenol
Eldodram
Faston
Gravol
Hydrate
Marmine
Motion-Aid
Nauseal
Nauseatol
Nico-Vert*
Novodimenate
Prevenause
Ram
Reidamine
Solbrine
Tega-Vert*
Travamine
Trav-Arex
Vertiban
Wehamine
DIMERCAPROL
BAL in Oil
Sulfactin
DIMETHICONE
Covicone*
DIMETHINDENE
Fenistil
Forhistal
Triten
DIMETHISOQUIN
Quotane
DIMETHISTERONE
Secrosteron
DIMETHYL SULFOXIDE
Demasorb
Demeso
Dromisol
Kemsol
Rimso-50
DINOPROSTONE
Prostin E2
DIOXYBENZONE
Solbar*
DIOXYLINE
Paveril
Paverone
DIPERODON
Allersone*
Diothane
Dodds Hemoraids
Emeroid*
Epimycin "A"*
Mity-Mycin*
Proctodon*
DIPHEMANIL
Prantal

DIPHENADIONE
  Dipaxin
DIPHENHYDRAMINE
  Allerdryl
  Ambenyl Expectorant*
  Belix
  Benadryl
  Benadryl with Ephedrine*
  Bena-D
  Benahist
  Bendylate
  Benoject
  Benylin
  Benylin Decongestant*
  Benylin DM*
  Benylin Pediatric Cough
  Caladryl*
  Caladryl Hydrocortisone*
  Calmex
  Diahist
  Dihydrex
  Diphen
  Diphenadril
  Di-Delamine*
  Eldadryl
  Fenylhist
  Hydril Cough
  Hyrexin
  Insomnal
  Nautamine
  Noradryl
  Nordryl
  Nytol(Canada)
  Phen-Amin
  Robalyn
  Rodryl
  Sedicin
  SK-Diphenhydramine
  Sominex (Canada)
  Sominex Formula 2
  Somnium
  Standryl
  Sting-Eze*
  Tusstat
  T-Dryl
  Valdrene
  Wehdryl
  Ziradryl Lotion*
DIPHENIDOL
  Vontrol
DIPHENOXYLATE
  Diaction*
  Diarsed
  Di-Atro*
  Diphenatol*
  Elmotil*
  Enoxa*
  Lofene*
  Loflo*
  Lomotil*
  Lonox*
  Lo-Trol*
  Low Quel*
  Nor-Mil*
  Retardin
  SK-Diphenoxylate*
DIPHENYLPYRALINE
  Diafen
  Hispril
  Hista-Nil
  Novahistex*
DIPHTHERIA TOXOID
  Tri-Immunol*
  Triogen*
  Wyeth*
DIPIPANONE
  Pipadone
DIPIVEFRIN
  Propine
DIPYRIDAMOLE
  Persantine
DISOPYRAMIDE
  Norpace
  Norpace CR
  Rythmodan
DISULFIRAM
  Abstinyl
  Antabuse
  Refusal
  Ro-Sulfiram
DITHIAZANINE
  Abminthic
  Delvex
  Telmid
DOBUTAMINE
  Dobutrex

DOCUSATE CALCIUM
- Doxical
- Doxidan*
- Pro-cal-sof
- Surfak

DOCUSATE POTASSIUM
- Dialose
- Dialose*
- Dialose Plus*
- Kasof
- Rectalad*

DOCUSATE SODIUM
- Aerosol OT
- Afko-Lube
- Afko-Lube Lax*
- Alko-Lube Lax*
- Bilax*
- Bu-Lax
- Bu-Lax Plus*
- Cassa-Laud*
- Colace
- Coloctyl
- Comfolax
- Comfolax Plus*
- Constiban*
- Coprola
- Correctol*
- Danthross*
- Definate
- Dilax
- Dilax-250
- Dioctalose*
- Diocto*
- Dioctyl
- Dioeze
- Diolax*
- Diosuccin
- Diothron*
- DioMedicone
- Dio-Sul
- Disanthrol*
- Disolan*
- Disolan Forte*
- Disonate
- Disoplex*
- Di-Sosul
- Doctase*
- Doctate
- Doctate-P*
- Dorbantyl*
- Dorbantyl Forte*
- DOSS* (Canada)
- DOSS (USA)
- Doxan*
- Doxinate
- D-S-S
- D-S-S Plus*
- Dual Formula Feen-A-Mint*
- Dulcodos*
- Duosol
- Dynoctol
- Ex-Lax Extra Gentle*
- Extra Gentle Ex-Lax*
- Feen-A-Mint Pills*
- Ferro-Sequels*
- Gentlax S*
- Ilosoft
- Konlax
- Laxatyl*
- Laxinate
- Laxinex 100
- Liqui-Doss*
- Magcyl*
- Milkinol*
- Modane Plus*
- Modane Soft
- Molatoc-CST*
- Molofac
- Neolax*
- Peri-Colace*
- Peri-Conate*
- Peri-Doss*
- Regulex
- Regulex-D*
- Regul-Aid
- Regutol
- Ruc-Dane*
- Sarolax*
- Schoenfeld
- Scrip-Lax*
- SenoKap DSS*
- Senokot-S*
- Sof-Lax Wafers*
- Stimulax*
- Stulax
- Super Doss*
- Trilax*
- TriHemic 600*
- Tri-Sof*

Unilax*
Valax*
DOMIPHEN
Bradosol
DOMPERIDONE
Motilium
DOPAMINE
Dopastat
Intropin
Revimine
DOXAPRAM
Dopram
Doxapril
Stimulexin
DOXEPIN
Adapin
Aponal
Curatin
Sinequan
DOXORUBICIN
Adriamycin
Adriblastina
DOXYCYCLINE
Doxychel
Doxy-II
Doxy-Lemmon
Doxy-Tabs
Doxy 100
Doxy 200
Vibramycin
Vibra-Tabs
DOXYLAMINE
Bay-Ornade*
Bendectin*
Consotuss*
Contac Severe Cold Formula Night Strength*
Cremacoat 4*
Decapyryn
Doxine*
Formula 44*
Mercodol with Decapryn*
Mersyndol with Codeine*
Nyquil Nighttime Colds Medicine*
NyQuil*
Unisom
Vicks Formula 44 Cough Mixture*
Vicks Nyquil Nighttime Colds Medicine*
DROCODE
Paracodin
Ru-Lor-N
Synalgos-DC*
DROMOSTANOLONE
Drolban
Masterid
Masteril
Masterone
DRONABINOL
Marinol
DROPERIDOL
Droleptan
Inapsine
Innovar*
DYCLONINE
Dyclone
Resolve
DYDROGESTERONE
Duphaston
Gynorest
DYPHYLLINE
Aerophylline
Airet
Dilin
Dilor
Dilor G Tabs*
Droxine L.A.
Droxine S.F.
Dyflex
Dyflex G Tabs*
Iphyllin
Lufyline-EPG TABS*
Lufyllin
Lufylline G Tabs*
Neophyl
Neothylline
Neothylline-GG*
Neutraphylline
Oxystat
Protophylline

E

ECHOTHIOPHATE IODIDE
Echodide

Ecodide
Phospholine Iodide
ECONAZOLE
Ecostatin
Gyno-Pevaryl 150
Pevaryl
Prevaryl
Spectazole
EDETATE CALCIUM DISODIUM
Calcium Disodium Versenate
Chealamide
E.D.T.A.
Endrate Disodium
Mosatil
Sodium Versenate
Sormetal
Versenate
EDETIC ACID
Adapettes*
Aqua-Flow*
Boil n Soak*
Cleaning & Soaking*
Comfort Drops*
Contique Dual Wet*
Lensine Extra Strength*
Lensrins*
Lens-Mate*
Lens-Wet*
Sequestrene A
Versene Acid
EDROPHONIUM
Tensilon
ELECTROLYTES, MULTIPLE
Pedialyte
EMYLCAMATE
Striatran
ENFLURANE
Ethrane
ENOXOLONE
Biosone
ENTSUFON
PhisoCare
PhisoDerm
PhisoLan
EPHEDRINE
Amesec*
Amodrine*
Asma-Lief*
Asminorl Improved*
Asminyl*
Asthmacon*
Asthmagyl*
Azma Aid*
Benadryl with Ephedrine*
Bronitin*
BronKaid*
BronKolixir*
BronKotabs*
Chemfedral*
Chemphyl*
Collyrium Drops*
Co-Xan*
Derma Medicone-HC Ointment*
Efedron Nasal Jelly
Efed II*
Ephedsol
Eunuretrol
Femcaps*
Flavedrin Mild*
Guiaphed Elixir*
Histadyl EC*
Histivite-D*
HTO Stainless Manzan Hemorrhoidal Tissue Ointment*
Hydromax Syrup*
Hydrophed Tabs*
I-Sedrin Plain
Isogen Compound*
Isogen Compound Elixir*
Isuprel Compound Elixir*
KIE*
Lardet Expectorant Tabs*
Lardet Tabs*
Lufyline-EPG TABS*
Marax*
Mudrane*
Mudrane GG*
Mudrane GG Elixir*
Nasdro No.3
Nyquil Nighttime Colds Medicine*
NyQuil*
Pazo Hemorrhoid*

PBZ with ephedrine*
PBZ Expectorant w/Ephedrine*
Phedral*
Primatene M*
Primatene P*
Pyrralan Expectorant*
Quadrinal*
Quelidrine*
Quibron Plus*
Quiet-Nite*
Relasma*
Respirol*
Roamphed*
Rynatuss*
Tedral*
Tedral Elixir*
Tedral Expectorant*
Tedral SA*
Tedral-25*
T.E.P.*
Thalfed*
Thecord*
Theodrin Pediatric Suspension*
Theofedral*
Theophedrizine*
Theophenyllin*
Theoral*
Theotabs*
Theozine*
Tossecol*
Va-Tro-Nol
Vatronol Nose Drops*
Verequad*
Verquad*
Vicks Nyquil Nighttime Colds Medicine*
Vicks Vatronol Nose Drops*
Wesmatic Forte*
Wyanoids Hemorrhoidal Suppositories*
Wyanoids HC Rectal Suppositories*
1-Sedrin Plain

EPINEPHRINE
Adrenalin
Adrenaline Chloride Solution, Injectable
Adrenalin in Oil
Adrenatrate
Asmatane Mist
Asmolin
AsthmaHaler
AsthmaNefrin
Breatheasy
Bronitin Mist
BronKaid Mist
BronKaid Mistometer
Dysne-Inhal
E-Carpine*
Epifrin
E-Pilo*
E-Pilo-1
E-Pilo-2
Epinal
EpiPen Jr.
Epitrate
E1
E1/2
E2
Glaucon
IOP
Lyophrin
Medihaler-Epi
Micronefrin
Mistura E
Murocoll
Mytrate
Primatene Mist
P1E1*
P2E1*
P3E1*
P4E1*
P6E1*
Simplene
Suprarenin
Sus-Phrine
Vaponefrin

EPINEPHRYL BORATE
Eppy
Eppy/N

ERGOCALCIFEROL
Calcet*
Calciferol
Dical-D with Iron*
Drisdol
Dristol Deltalin
Geltabs
Os-Cal*

Os-Cal-Gesic*
Perio Cal-D*
Sterogyl-15
ERGOLOID MESYLATES
Circanol
Deapril-sT
Gerimal
H.E.A.
Hydergine
Trigot
ERGONOVINE
Ergobasine
Ergotrate
ERGOTAMINE
Bellergal*
Bellergal-S*
Bellermine-O.D.*
Cafergot*
Cafermine*
Cafertabs*
Cafertrate*
Ercaf*
Ercatab*
Ergobel*
Ergocaf*
Ergoklinine
Ergomar
Ergostat
Femergin
Gynergen
Lingraine
Medihaler-Ergotamine
Migrastat*
Wigraine*
ERYTHRITYL TETRANITRATE
Cardilate
Cardilate-P*
Cordilate
ERYTHROMYCIN
Benzamycin*
Dowmycin E
E-Mycin
Eryc
ERYC
Eryderm
Erymycin
Eryped
Ery-Tab
Erythrocin
Erythrogran
Erythroguent
Erythromid
Ilosone
Ilotycin
Novorythro
Pediamycin
Pfizer-E Film Coated
Revrocin
Robimycin
RP-Mycin
SK-Erythromycin
Staticin*
T-Stat
Wyamycin
ERYTHROMYCIN ETHYLSUCCINATE
E.E.S.
E-Mycin E Liquid
Pediazole*
ERYTHROMYCIN STEARATE
Bristamycin
Eramycin
Erypar
Erythrocin Stearate Filmtab
Ethril
Ethril 250
Pfizer-E
ESTERIFIED ESTROGENS
Menotrol
Neo-Estrone
ESTRADIOL
Aquadiol
Delestrogen
Depanate
Depestro
Dep-Gynogen
Depogen
Depo-Testadiol*
Dimenformon
Diogyn
Diogynets
Dioval
Di-Ovocylin
Dura-Estrin
Duragen
E-Cypionate
E. Ionate P.A.
E-Lonate P.A.
Estate
Estrace
Estraldine

Estraval P.A.
Estraval 2X
Estra-Cyp
Estra-D
Estroject-L.A.
Femogen CYP
Femogex
Ferminate-10
Hormogen Depot
Hormonin*
L.A.E. 20
Mal-O-Fem CYP
Menaval-10
Ovocylin
Progynon
Progynon B
Progynova
Testaval 90/4*
Test-Estrin*
Valergen-10
ESTRAMUSTINE
Emcyt
ESTRIOL
Hormonin*
Theelol
ESTROGENS, CONJUGATED
Premarin
Premarin w/
Methyltestosterone*
ESTROGENS, ESTERFIED
Evex
Formatrix*
ESTROGENS, ESTERIFIED
Amnestrogen
Climestrone
Estabs
Estertest H.S.*
Estratab
Estratest*
Estromed
Menest
ESTRONE
Bestrone
Di-Genik*
Duogen*
Estequa
Estroject-2
Estronol
Estrusol
Femogen
Foygen
Gravigen
Gynogen
Hormestrin
Hormogen-A
Hormonin*
Kestrone
Menformon A
Spanestrin P
Theelin
Theogen
Unigen
Wehgen
ESTROPIPATE
Ogen
Sulestrex
ETAFEDRINE
Nethamine
ETHACRYNATE
Sodium Edecrin
ETHACRYNIC ACID
Edecrin
Hydromedin
Reomax
Taladren
ETHAMBUTOL
Etibi
Myambutol
ETHAMIVAN
Emivan
Vandid
ETHAVERINE
Cebral
Circubid
Eta-Lent
Ethaquin
Ethatab
Isovex-100
Rothav-150
ETHCHLORVYNOL
Arvynol
Placidyl
Serensil
ETHER
Compound W*
Freezone*
ETHINAMATE
Valmid
Valmidate
ETHINYL ESTRADIOL

Brevicon*
Brevicon-28*
Demulen*
Demulen 1/35*
Demulen-28*
Diogyn E
Estinyl
Ethinoral
Eticylol
Feminone
Gynetone*
Halodrin*
Inestra
Loestrin*
Lo/Ovral*
Lynoral
Mepilin*
Modicon*
Nordette*
Norinyl 1+35*
Norlestrin*
Nylestin
Ortho-Novum 10/11*
Ortho-Novum 7/7/7*
Ovcon*
Ovral*
Tri-Norinyl*
Triphasil*
Zorane*

ETHIODIZED OIL
Ethiodol

ETHIONAMIDE
Trecator
Trecator-SC
Trescatyl

ETHISTERONE
Lutocylol
Ora-Lutin
Pranone
Prodoxan
Progestab
Progestoral
Syngestrotabs
Trosinone

ETHOHEPTAZINE
Equagesic*
Meprogesic*
Zactane
Zactirin*

ETHOPROPAZINE
Lysivane
Parsidol
Parsitan

ETHOSUXIMIDE
Capitus
Petinimid
Suxinutin
Thilopemal
Zarontin

ETHOTOIN
Peganone

ETHOXAZENE
Serenium

ETHOXZOLAMIDE
Cardrase
Ethamide

ETHYL BISCOUMACETATE
Stabilene
Tromexan

ETHYL DIBUNATE
Neodyne
Tussets

ETHYLESTRENOL
Maxibolin

ETHYLNOREPINEPHRINE
Bronkephrine

ETHYNODIOL
Demulen*
Demulen 1/35*
Demulen-28*
Ovulen*

ETIDOCAINE
Duranest

ETIDRONATE DISODIUM
Didronel

ETOFYLLINE
Bio-Phylline

ETOMIDATE
Amidate
Hypnomidate

ETOPOSIDE
VePesid

ETRETINATE
Tegison

ETYMEMAZINE
Nuital
Sergetyl

EUCALYPTOL
Saratoga*
Soltice Quick Rub*

Sting-Eze*
Vatronol Nose Drops*
Vicks Sinex Decongestant Nasal Spray*
Vicks Vatronol Nose Drops*

EUCALYPTUS OIL
Banalg Liniment*
Jen-Balm*
Vicks Throat Lozenges*
Vicks Vaporub*
Vicks Vaposteam*

EUCATROPINE
Euphthalmine

EUGENOL
Benzodent*
Counter Pain Rub*
Emerdent
Mentholatum Toothache Remedy

F

FACTOR IV COMPLEX
Konyne
Profilinine
Proplex

FENCLOFENAC
Flenac

FENFLURAMINE
Ganal
Ponderal
Ponderax
Pondimin

FENOPROFEN
Fenopron
Nalfon
Nalgesic

FENOTEROL
Berotec
Berotec Inhaler
Partusisten

FENTANYL
Innovar*
Sublimaze

FERRIC PYROPHOSPHATE
Dical-D with Iron*
Troph-Iron*

FERROCHOLINATE
Chel-Iron
Chel-Iron Liquid
Chel-Iron Pediatric Drops
Ferrolip

FERROGLYCINE SULFATE
Ferronord

FERROUS ASCORBATE
Ascofer

FERROUS FUMARATE
Cefera*
Chromagen*
C-Ron*
C-Ron Forte*
C-Ron Freckles*
Femiron
Femiron with Vitamins*
Fe-O.D.*
Feostat
Ferancee*
Ferancee-HP*
Ferosorb-C*
Feroton
Ferrobid*
Ferro-Sequels*
Fersamal
Fumaral Elixir and Spancaps*
Fumasorb
Fuma Drops
Fumerin
Hematon
Hemocyte
Hemocyte-F*
Hemocyte Injection*
Hemocyte Plus Tabules*
Hemo-Vite*
Ircon
Irolong*
Iron with C*
Laud-Iron Plus Chewing*
Laun-Iron
Monster Vitamins & Iron*
Moro Pills

Novofumar
Palafer
Palmiron
Palmiron-C*
Perihemin*
Pronemia*
Recoup*
Red Pills
Span-FF
Tabron Filmseal*
Toleron
Tolifer
TriHemic 600*
Trinsicon*
Trinsicon M*
Tri-Tinic*
Vitron-C*
Vitron-C-Plus*
Zentinic*
Zentrol Chewable*
Zintinic*

FERROUS GLUCONATE
Fergon
Fergon with C Caplets*
Ferralet
Ferroid
Fertinic
I.L.X. B12*
Iromin-G*
Ironate
Novoferrogluc
Simron
Sym-Fer*

FERROUS SUCCINATE
Cerevon

FERROUS SULFATE
Arne Timesules
Cytoferin*
Feosol
Feosol Spansules
Fer-In-Sol
Fer-In-Sol Drops,
Fermalox
Fero-Grad
Fero-Gradumet
Fero-Grad-500*
Ferrosulph
Fesofor
Folvron*
Fumaral Elixir and Spancaps*
Heptuna Plus*
Ironized Yeast*
Mol-Iron
Mol-Iron with Vitamin C*
Novoferrosulfa
Slow-Fe
Vi-Daylin/F + Iron*
Vi-Daylin/F ADC + Iron Drops*
Vi-Daylin Plus Iron ADC Drops*
Zentron Liquid*

FIBRINOGEN
Fibrogen
Parenogen

FIBRINOLYSIN
Elase*
Elase-Chloromycetin Ointment*

FIBRINOLYSIN, HUMAN
Actase
Thrombolysin

FLAVOXATE
Urispas

FLECAINIDE
Tambocor

FLORANTYRONE
Zanchol

FLOXACILLIN
Fluclox

FLOXURIDINE
Fudr
FUDR

FLUCYTOSINE
Ancobon
Ancotil

FLUDROCORTISONE
Alflorone
Cortef-F
Florinef Acetate
Fludrocortone

FLUMETHASONE
Flucort
Locacorten
Locacorten-Vioform*
Locorten

FLUMETHIAZIDE

Ademil
Ademol
FLUNISOLIDE
Aerobid
Nasalide
Rhinalar
Syntaris
FLUNITRAZEPAM
Narcozep
Rohypnol
FLUOCINOLONE
Dermalar
Fluocin Cream
Fluocinolone Acetonide
Fluoderm
Fluonid
Flurosyn
Jellin
Neo-Synalar*
Synadone
Synalar
Synalar-HP
Synamol
Synemol
Viaderm-F.A.
FLUOCINONIDE
Lidemol
Lidex
Metosyn
Topsyn Gel
FLUORESCEIN
AK-Fluor
Fluorescite
Fluor-L-Strip A.T.
Fluress*
Ful-Glo
Funduscein-10
FLUORIDE
Acidflud
Cari-Tab Softab*
Poly-Vi-Flor*
Poly-Vi-Flor with Iron*
Tri-Vi-Flor*
Tri-Vi-Flor w/Iron Drops*
FLUOROMETHOLONE
FML Liquifilm
Neo-Oxylone*
Oxylone
Trilcin
FLUOROURACIL
Adrucil
Efudex
Fluoroplex
FLUOXYMESTERONE
Halodrin*
Halotestin
Oratestin
Ora-Testryl
Ultandren
FLUPENTIXOL
Fluanxol
FLUPHENAZINE
Dapotom
Modecate
Moditen
Permitil
Prolixin
Trancin
FLUPREDNISOLONE
Alphadrol
FLURANDRENOLIDE
Alondra-F
Cordran
Dreniform*
Drenison
Drocort
Haldrone-F
Sermaka
FLURAZEPAM
Dalmane
Novo-Flupam
FLURBIPROFEN
Ansaid
FLUROTHYL
Indoklon
FLUROXENE
Fluoromar
FLUSPIRILENE
Imap
Redeptin
FOLIC ACID
Berocca*
En-Cebrin F*
Fero-Folic-500*
Folbal
Foldine
Folvite

Folvron*
Hemocyte-F*
Hemocyte Injection*
Mission Prenatal*
Niferex-150 Forte*
Novofolacid
Perihemin*
Pronemia*
Trinsicon*
TriHemic 600*
Tri-Tinic*
Vitron-C-Plus*
Zentinic*
Zintinic*
FONAZINE
Banistyl
Migristene
Promaquid
FRAMYCETIN
Soframycin
Sofra-Tulle
FURALTADONE
Altafur
Darifur
Valsyn
FURAZOLIDONE
Furoxone
FUROSEMIDE
Furoside
Fursemide
Lasilix
Lasix
Laxur
Neo-Renal
Novosemide
Seguril
Uritol
FUSIDIC ACID
Fucidin

G

GELSEMINIUM
Cafacetin*
GEMFIBROZIL
Lopid
GENTAMICIN
Apogen
Bristagen
Cidomycin
Garamycin
Garamycin Ophthalmic
Garamycin Otic
Genoptic*
Gentalline
Gentalyn
Genticin
Jenamicin
Refobacin
Sulmycin
GENTIAN VIOLET
Genapex
GVS Vaginal
Hyva
Hyva Vaginal
GITALIN
Gitaligin
GLIPIZIDE
Glucotrol
GLOBULIN, IMMUNE
Gamimune
GLUCONIC ACID
Renacidin*
GLUCOSE
Glucosol
GLUCOSE OXIDASE REAGENT
Clinistix
Diastix
GLUCOSULFONE
Promin
GLUCUROLACTONE
Glucurone
GLUTAMIC ACID
Acidogen
Acidoride
Acidulin
Antalka
Cerebro-Nicin*
Dizyme*
Glukor Injection*
Glutan Hydrochloride
Hydrionic
Kanulase*
Magacin*
Miclo-Zyme
Muriamic
Muripsin*
GLUTARAL

Cidex
GLUTETHIMIDE
Doriden
Elrodorm
Rolathimide
Somide
GLYBURIDE
Daonil
Diabeta
Dia Beta
Euglucon
Micronase
GLYCERIN
Agoral*
Agoral Plain*
Americaine-Otic*
Benzodyne Drops*
Blistex*
Buf Foot-Care Soap*
Calamine*
Calglycine*
Concentrated Milk of Magnesia*
Dewitt's Baby Cough*
Ear Drop By Murine*
Fleet Babylax
Glyrol
Kerid Ear Drop*
Lubriderm*
Murine Ear Drops*
Murine Ear Wax Removal System/ Murine Ear Drops*
Neo-Hydro*
Ophthalgan
Ortega Otic M*
Osmoglyn
Otoreid-HC*
Procolin*
Rectalad*
Rhinocyn-DM*
Rhinocyn-PD*
Rhinosyn*
Tucks Pads*
Ultra derm*
GLYCINE
Glytinic*
GLYCOBIARSOL
Broxolin
Milibis
Wintodon
GLYCOPYRROLATE
Glycopyrrolate*
Nodapton
Robinul
Robinul Forte
Robinul-PH*
Robinul-PH Forte*
Tarodyl
GOBULIN, IMMUNE
Gamastan
Gammar
Immuglobin
Immune Globulin
Immune Serum Globulin Gammar
Immu-G
GOLD SODIUM THIOMALATE
Myochrysine
GONADORELIN
Factrel
GONADOTROPIN
Anteron
Choranid
Gestasol Dry
Libigen
GONADOTROPIN, CHORIONIC
Antuitrin-S
A.P.L.
Entromone
Follutein
Fullutein
Glukor Injection*
Pranturon
Pregnesin
Pregnyl
Profasi
GONADOTROPIN, SERUM
Gonadin
Gonadogen
GRAMICIDIN
Cortisporin Cream*
Gramoderm
Kenacomb*
Mycolog*
Myco Triacet Cream & Ointment*
Mytrex*
Neosporin-G Cream*
Nysolone*
Polysporin*
Spectrocin*

Tricilone NNG*
Tri-Statin*
GRISEOFULVIN
Cortussin
Dilyn
Fulvicin P/G
Fulvicin-U/F
Grifulvin-V
Grisactin
Grisactin Ultra
Grisovin-FP
Grisowen
Gris-Peg
Likuden
GUAIFENESIN
Acet-Am Expectorant*
Actifed-C*
Actifed Expectorant*
Actol Expectorant*
Acutuss Expectorant With Codeine*
Adatuss D.C. Expectorant*
Alamine Expectorant*
Albatussin*
Ambenyl-D Decongestant Cough Formula*
Ambenyl Expectorant*
Amonidrin*
Anatuss*
Anti-Tuss
Anti-Tuss DM*
Asbron G Inlay*
Atussin D.M. Expectorant*
Atussin Expectorant*
Balminil Expectorant
Bayaminic Extract*
Baytussin
Baytussin DM*
Biotussin
Breonesin
Brexin*
Bronchial Capsules*
Bronchicide
Broncholate*
Broncho-Grippex
Brondecon*
Bronitin*
BronKaid*
BronKolixir*
BronKotabs*
Cheracol*
Cheracol D*
Chlor-Trimeton Expectorant*
Chlor-Trimeton Expectorant with Codeine*
Choledyl Expectorant*
Codistan*
Colrex Expectorant*
Conar Expectorant*
Conex*
Conex with Codeine*
Congestac*
Congress Jr.*
Congress Sr.*
Coricidin Antitussive*
Corutol Expectorant
Coryban-D Antitussive*
Co-Xan*
Cremacoat 2
Cremacoat 3*
Demo-Cineol
Demo-Cineol Expectorant
Dextro-Tuss GG*
Dilor G Tabs*
Dimacol*
Dimetane Expectorant*
Dimetane Expectorant-DC*
Donatussin Drops*
Donatussin Syrup*
Dorcol Pediatric*
Dyflex G Tabs*
Elixophyllin-GG Oral Liquid
Entair*
Entex*
Entex LA*
Entuss Expectorant & Liquid*
Fedahist Expectorant*
Formula 44-D*

Gaiapect
Gee Gee
GG-Cen
G G Tussin
Glyate
Glycerol-T*
Glycotuss
Glydm*
Glytuss
G-Tussin DM*
Guaiahist TT Tempotrol*
Guaianesin
Guaifed*
Guaimid*
Guiaphed Elixir*
G-200
Head & Chest Cold Medicine*
Hycotuss*
Hylate-tabs*
Hytuss
Hytuss 2X
Kleer Comp*
Kolephrin GG*
Lanatuss*
Lanatuss Expectorant*
Lanophylline-GG Capsules*
Lardet Expectorant Tabs*
Liquitussin
Liquitussin DM*
Lo-Tussin*
Lufyline-EPG TABS*
Lufylline G Tabs*
Malotuss
Midatane Expectorant*
Mor-Tussin P.E.*
Motussin
Mudrane GG*
Mudrane GG Elixir*
Mudrane GG-2*
Naldecon-CX*
Naldecon-Ex Pediatric*
Nasalspan Expectorant*
Neophiban*
Neothylline-GG*
Nilcol*
Normatane Expectorant*
Nortussin
Novahistine DMX*
Novahistine Expectorant*
Nucofed Pediatric Expectorant*
Pediaquill*
Pertussin Cough for Children*
Polaramime Expectorant*
Pseudo-Bid*
Pseudo-Hist Expectorant*
P-V Tussin*
Queltuss*
Quibron*
Quibron Plus*
Reletuss*
Respair-S.R.*
Respinol L.A.*
Resyl
Rhinosyn DM*
Rhinosyn-X*
Rhinspec*
Robitussin
Robitussin A-C*
Robitussin-CF*
Robitussin DAC*
Robitussin-DM*
Robitussin-PE*
Romex*
Rotane Expectorant*
Rymed-TR*
Ryna-Cx Liquid*
Ryna-Tussadine Expectorant*
Sedatuss Expectorant
Silexin*
Slo-Phyllin GG*
Soltice*
Sorbutuss*
S.T. Expectorant
S-T Forte*
Sudafed Cough*

Synophylate-GG*
Tedral Expectorant*
Theolair-Plus 250*
Theo-Guaia*
Tolu-Sed*
Tolu-Sed DM*
Tonecol*
Triaminic
Expectorant*
Triaminic
Expectorant with
Codeine*
Tri-Medex*
Triphenyl
Expectorant*
Tussanca
Tussar-SF*
Tussar-2*
Tussciden Expectorant
Tussend Expectorant*
Unproco*
Verequad*
Verquad*
Vicks Cough*
Vicks Formula 44D
Decongestant Cough
Mixture*
Voxin-PG*
Wesmatic Forte*
Zephrex*
Zephrex-La*
2/G
2/G-DM*

GUANABENZ
Wytensin

GUANADREL
Hylorel

GUANETHIDINE
Esimil*
Ismelin
Ismelin-Esidrix*
Visutensil

H

HALAZEPAM
Paxipam

HALCINONIDE
Halciderm
Halog

HALOPERIDOL
Haldol
Serenace

HALOPROGIN
Halotex

HALOTHANE
Fluothane
Somnothane

HEMICELLULASE
Festal*

HEMIN
Panhematin

HEPARIN
Calciparine
Depo-Heparin Sodium
Hepalean
Heparinar
Hepathrom
Hep-lock
Lipo-Hepin
Liquaemin
Panheprin

HEPATITIS B IMMUNE GLOBULIN
H-BIG

HEPATITIS B IMMUNE GLOBULIN, HUMAN
Hep-B-Gammagee
Hyper Hep

HEPATITIS B VACCINE
Heptavax-B

HEPTABARBITAL
Medomin

HETACILLIN
Natacilline
Penplenum
Verapen-K
Versapen
Versapen-K

HETASTARCH
Hespan

HEXACHLOROPHENE
Burdeo*
Dermohex
Fomac
Fung-O-Spray*
Gamophen

Germa-Medica
G-11
Hexamead-PH
PhisoHex
Phiso Scrub
Septisol
Septi-Soft
Soy Dome Cleanser
Surgi-Cen
WescoHex

HEXACYCLONATE
Gevilon

HEXADIMETHRINE
Polybrene

HEXAFLUORENIUM
Mylaxen

HEXAMETHONIUM
Bistrium
Hexathide
Methium
Vegolysen
Vegolysen-T

HEXAMIDINE
Desomedine
Esomedina
Hexomedine

HEXETIDINE
Hexoral
Sterisil
Sterisol

HEXOBARBITAL
Evipal
Percobarb*
Sombucaps
Sombulex
Somnalert

HEXOCYCLIUM
Tral

HEXYLCAINE
Cyclaine

HEXYLRESORCINOL
Caprokol
Crystoids
Listerine
S.T. 37
Sucrets

HOMATROPINE
Bilamide*
Dia-Quel Liquid*
DIA-quel*
Homapin
Homatrisol
Homatrocel
Hycodan*
Isopto Homatropine
Malcotran
Matropinal*
Matropinal Forte Inserts*
Matropinal Inserts*
Mesopin
Murocal
Novatrin
Novatropine
Panzyme*
Probilagol
Ru-Spas No.2
Sed.Tens.Se

HOMOSALATE
Suntan

HUMAN DIPLOID CELL RABIES VACCINE
Imovac
Wyvac

HYALURONIDASE
Alidase
Diffusin
Enzodase
Hyazyme
Infiltrase
Wydase

HYCANTHONE
Etrenol

HYDRALAZINE
Apresazide*
Apresoline
Dralserp*
Dralzine
Hydrap-ES*
Hyser Plus*
Lopress
Nor-Pres
R-HCTZ-H*
Rolazine
Ser-Ap-Es*
Serpasil-Apresoline*
Unipres*

HYDROCHLOROTHIAZIDE
Aldactazide*
Aldoril*

Apo-Triazide*
Apresazide*
Aquarius
Butiserpazide*
Capozide*
Chlorzide
Decaserpyl Plus*
Diaqua
Direma
Diuchlor H
Diu-Scrip
Dyazide*
Esidrix
Esimil*
Fluvin
Hydrap-ES*
Hydrochlor 50
Hydromal
Hydropres*
Hydroserp*
Hydroserpine*
Hydrotensin*
Hydrozide
Hydro-Aquil
HydroDiuril
Hydro-Saluric
Hydro-Z
Hyperetic
Hyser Plus*
Inderide*
Ismelin-Esidrix*
Lexxor
Liquapres*
Manuril
Maxzide*
Moduret*
Moduretic*
Natrimax
Neo-Codema
Novohydrazide
Novotriamzide*
Novo-Doparil*
Novo-Triamzide*
Oretic
Oreticyl*
R-HCTZ-H*
Serpasil-Esidrix*
Ser-Ap-Es*
SK-Hydrochlorothiazide
Thianal
Thiaserp*
Thiuretic
Timolide*
Unipres*
Urozide
Zide

HYDROCODONE
Adatuss D.C. Expectorant*
Bancap HC*
Codone
Corutol DH
Dicodid
Entuss Expectorant & Liquid*
Hycodan*
Hycomine*
Hycotuss*
Mercodinone
Norcet*
Pseudo-Hist Expectorant*
P-V Tussin*
Robidone
S-T Forte*
Tussend*
Tussend Expectorant*
Tussionex*
Vicodin
Vicoprin*

HYDROCORTAMATE
Magnacort

HYDROCORTISONE
Acetate-AS
Acticort-100
Aeroseb-HC
Allersone*
Alphaderm
Alphosyl-HC Lotion & Cream*
Anugard-HC*
Anusol-HC*
A-Hydrocort
Bactine Hydrocortisone
Barbseb*
Barseb HC
Barsed Thera-Spray*

Caladryl
  Hydrocortisone*
Caldecort
Caquin Cream*
Carmol HC Cream
Cetacort
Chloromycetin
  Hydrocortisone*
Clinicort
Coly-Mycin S Otic*
Corque*
Cortaid
Cortamed
Cortef
Cortenema
Corticaine Cream*
Corticreme
Cortifoam
Cortiment
Cortisporin Cream*
Cortisporin Ointment*
Cortisporin Ointment
  Ophthalmic*
Cortisporin
  Ophthalmic
  Suspension*
Cortisporin Otic
  Solution*
Cortisporin Otic
  Suspension*
Cortispray
Cortizone-5
Cortril
Cort-Dome
Cort-Quin*
Delacort
Dermacort
Dermarex*
Derma Medicone-HC
  Ointment*
Dermicort
Dermolate
Dermtex
Domeform-HC*
Dureze Otic Drops*
Eldecort
Emo-Cort
Epicort
Epifoam
EpiForm-HC*
F-E-P Creme*
Formtone-HC*
Fungotic*
Gynecort
HC-Form*
Hc-Jel
HCV Creme*
Heb-Cort
Hexaderm Cream
  Modified
Hexaderm I.Q.
  Modified Cream*
Hill Cortac Lotion*
Hyderm
Hydrocortone
Hydrocortone Acetate
Hydroquin*
Hydro-Cortilean
Hydro-Cortone
  Acetate Ophthalmic
Hysone Ointment*
Hytone
H2 Cort
Indocort*
Iodocort Cream*
Iodosone*
Komed HC*
Lanacort
Lanvisone*
Lidaform-HC*
Locoid
Loroxide-HC Lotion*
Mantadil*
Manticor
Microcort
Mity-Quin Cream*
Mycort
Mysone
Neo-Cortef*
Neo-Cort-Dome*
Neo-Hydro*
Novohydrocort
Nutracort
Nystaform-HC*
Ophthocort*
Optef
Orlex H.C. Otic*
Ortega Otic M*
Otall Ear Drops*
Otic-HC Ear Drops*

Otic Neo-Cort-Dome*
Otocort Ear Drops*
Otoreid-HC*
Pedi-cort V*
Pharma-Cort
Pramosone
Pro-cort M
Proctocort
Proctofoam-HC
Pyocidin-Otic*
Racet Resicort
Rectacort*
Rectal Medicone-HC Suppositories*
Rectoid
Relecort
Rhulicort
S-Cortilean
Sensacort
Solu-Cortef
Stera-Form*
Steramine Otic*
Synacort
Terra-Cortril*
Terra-Cortril Spray with Polymyxin B*
Texacort
Theracort*
Ulcort
Unicort
Uremol HC*
Vioform-Hydrocortisone*
Viopramosone*
Vio Hydrosone*
VoSol HC Otic Solution*
Vytone*
Wellcortin
Westcort
Wyanoids HC Rectal Suppositories*

HYDROFLUMETHIAZIDE
Di-Ademil
Diucardin
Hydrenox
Saluron
Salutensin*
Salutensin-Demi*

HYDROGEN IODIDE
Hydriodic Acid Cough

HYDROGEN PEROXIDE
PerOxyl

HYDROMORPHONE
Dilaudid
Dilaudid-HP
Hymorphan

HYDROQUINOLONE
Meltex*

HYDROQUINONE
Artra
Black and White Bleaching Cream
Eldopaque
Eldoquin
Esoterica
HQC
Melanex
Porcelane
Quinnone
Solaquin

HYDROXOCOBALAMIN
AlphaRedisol
Alpha-Ruvite
Codroxomin
Droxomin
Ducobee-Hy
Hydroxo B12
HY-12
Neo-Betalin 12
Rubranova
Sytobex-H

HYDROXYAMPHETAMINE
Paredrine

HYDROXYCHLOROQUINE
Plaquenil

HYDROXYDIONE SODIUM SUCCINATE
Viadril

HYDROXYETHYLCELLULOSE
Aqua-Flow*
Hy-flow*

HYDROXYPHENAMATE
Listica

HYDROXYPROGESTERONE
Delalutin
Deprolutin-250
Duralutin
Hydrosterone
Hylutin

Hyproval P.A.
Pro-Depo
HYDROXYPROPYL
METHYLCELLULOSE
Lens-Mate*
Liquifilm Wetting*
HYDROXYQUINOLINE
Benzodent*
Medicone Dressing
Cream*
NP-27 Cream*
Solvex Powder*
HYDROXYUREA
Hydrea
Litalir
HYDROXYZINE
Asminorl Improved*
Atarax
Ataraxoid*
Cartrax*
Durrax
Enarax*
Equipoise
E-Vista
Hydromax Syrup*
Hydrophed Tabs*
Hyzine-50
Hy-Pam
Marax*
Orgatrax
Pas Depress
Quiess
Sedaril
Theophedrizine*
Theozine*
Vistacon
Vistaject
Vistaril
Vistrax*
HYMENOPTER VENOM
EXTRACT
Pharmalgen
Venomil
HYOSCINE
Donnatal*
Donnatal Extentabs*
HYOSCINE BUTYLBROMIDE
Buscopan
HYOSCYAMINE
Anaspaz
Anaspaz PB*
Arco-Lase Plus*
Barbidonna*
Bellaphen*
Bellastal*
Butabell HMB*
Comhist*
Cystospaz
Digestamic*
Dolonil*
Dolsed*
Donnagel*
Donnagel-PG*
Donnamor Elixir*
Donnatal*
Donnatal Extentabs*
Donnazyme*
Donphen*
Ergobel*
Hasp*
Hybephen*
Hyosophen*
Kinesed*
Kutrase*
Levamine
Levsin
Levsinex with
Phenobarbital
Timecaps*
Levsinex Timecaps
Levsin with
Phenobarbital*
Malatal*
Neoquess Tablets*
Omnibel*
Palbar No. 2*
Panzyme*
Prosed*
Pylora*
Pyridium Plus*
Quiagel*
Quiagel PG*
Relaxadon*
Ru-Tuss*
Seds*
Sidonna*
Spalix*
Spasaid*
Spaslin*
Spasmolin*

Spasmophen*
Spasmorel*
Spasquid*
Susano*
Trac*
Tri-Cone Plus*
UAA*
Uralgic*
Uramine*
Urised*
Urisedamine*
Urisep*
Uritab*
Uritabs W.O.*
Urithol*
Uroblue*
Urostat-Forte*
Vanatal*
Vanodonnal*

I

IBUPROFEN
Advil
Amersol
Brufen
Inabrin
Motrin
Nuprin
Rufen
ICHTHAMMOL
Boil-Ease*
Boyol*
Derma Medicone-HC Ointment*
Derma Medicone Ointment*
Ichthyol
IDOXURIDINE
Dandrid
Dendrid
Herplex
Herplex-D Liquifilm
Kerecid
S.O.P.
Stoxil
IMIPRAMINE
Antipress
Apo-Imipramine
Berkomine
Dynaprin
Imavate
Impril
Janimine
Melipramin
Novopramine
Praminil
Presamine
Ropramine
SK-Pramine
Tofranil
Tofranil-PM
INDAPAMIDE
Lozol
INDOCYANINE GREEN
Cardio-Green
INDOMETHACIN
Amuno
Apo-Indomethacin
Indocid
Indocin
Indocin SR
Indomed
Indomee
Indo-Lemmon
Infrocin
Metacen
Novo-Methacin
INDORAMIN
Baratol
INFLUENZA VIRUS VACCINE
Fluogen
Fluzone
INOSIPLEX
Isoprinosine
INOSITOL NIACINATE
Linodil
Palohex
INSULIN [SUSPENSION] ISOPHANE
Insulatard
Mixtard*
NPH Iletin
NPH Insulin
Protaphane NPH Insulin
INSULIN [SUSPENSION] PROTAMINE ZINC

PZI
INSULIN HUMAN
Human N
Human R
Humulin
Humulin N
SHI
INSULIN ISOPHANE
Protaphane MC
INSULIN ISOPHANE, HUMAN
Protaphane, Human
INSULIN PROTAMINE ZINC
Protamine, Zinc & Iletin
INSULIN REGULAR
Actrapid MC
Iletin Regular
Toronto Insulin
INSULIN REGULAR, HUMAN
Actrapid, Human
INSULIN ZINC
Monotard MC
INSULIN ZINC [SUSPENSION] EXTENDED
Iletin Ultralente
Insulin Ultralente
Mixtard*
Ultralente
Ultralente Iletin
Ultralente Insulin
Ultratard
INSULIN ZINC [SUSPENSION] PROMPT
Iletin Semilente
Insulin Semilente
Semilente Iletin
Semilente Insulin
Semitard
INSULIN ZINC SUSPENSION
Iletin Lente
Insulin Lente
Lentard
Lente Iletin
Lente Insulin
Monotard
INSULIN ZINC, HUMAN
Monotard, Human
INSULIN,HUMAN
BHI
INTRINSIC FACTOR
Al-Vite*
Hemo-Vite*
Perihemin*
Pronemia*
Trinsicon*
Trinsicon M*
TriHemic 600*
INVERT SUGAR
Emetrol
IOCETAMIC ACID
Choledbrine
IODAMIDE MEGLUMINE
Renovue-DIP
Renovue-65
IODINATED GLYCEROL
Ipsatol
Organidin
Theo-Organidin*
Tussi-Organidin*
Tussi-Organidin DM*
IODINE
Dequasine*
Diodine
Gastrografin*
Iodex
Lugol's Solution*
Nova-Kelp
Pliacide
Roma-Nol
IODIPAMIDE MEGLUMINE
Cholografin
Cholografin Meglumine
Sinografin*
IODIZED OIL
Lipiodol
IODOALPHIONIC ACID
Bilombrine
Priodax
IODOCHLORHYDROXYQUIN
Corque*
Dermarex*
Domeform
EpiForm-HC*
F-E-P Creme*
HC-Form*
HCV Creme*
Indocort*

Iodosone*
Lanvisone*
Lidaform-HC*
Locacorten-Vioform*
Mycoquin
Nystaform-HC*
Nystaform Ointment*
Pedi-cort V*
Quinambicide
Quin III
Quin-O-Creme
Stera-Form*
Tar-Doak Lotion*
Vioform
Vioform-Hydrocortisone*
Viopramosone*
Vio Hydrosone*

IODOHIPPURATE
Nephroflow

IODOPYRACET
Diodrast
Pyelosil

IODOQUINOL
Cort-Quin*
Diodoquin
Floraquin
Gynovules
Ioquin Suspension
Moebiqine
Quinadome
Sebaquin
Vytone*
Yodoxin

IODOXAMATE MEGLUMINE
Cholovue

IOPANOIC ACID
Telepaque

IOPHENDYLATE
Ethiodan
Myelodil
Myodil

IOPHENOXIC ACID
Teridax

IOTHALAMATE SODIUM
Angio-Conray
Conray-325
Conray-400

IPECAC FLUIDEXTRACT
Cerose*
Cerose DM*
Cetro-Cirose*
Dr. Drake's
Quelidrine*
Sorbutuss*

IPODATE
Bilivist
Oragrafin

IPRATROPIUM
Atrovent

IPRONIAZID
Marsilid

IRON
Abdec Teens with Iron*
Albafort Injectable*
AVP Natal*
Bilron*
Calcicaps with Iron*
Chocks-Bugs Bunny Plus Iron*
Chocks Plus Iron*
Dayalets Plus Iron*
Dequasine*
Enzymacol*
Feraplex Liquid*
Fero-Folic-500*
Fe-Plus
Flintstones Plus Iron*
Fosfree*
Glytinic*
Golden Bounty B Complex with Vitamin C
Hepp-Iron Drops*
I.L.X. B12 Elixir*
Incremin with Iron*
L-Glutavite*
Maltlevol*
Maltlevol 12*
Mission Prenatal*
Niferex-150
Niferex-150 Forte*
Nu-Iron
Nu-Iron-V*
One-A-Day Plus Iron*
Pals with Iron
Poly-Vi-Flor with Iron*

Poly-Vi-Sol with Iron*
Stresstabs 600 with Iron*
Stresstabs 600 with Zinc*
Surbex 750 with Iron*
Tri-Vi-Flor w/Iron Drops*
Tri-Vi-Sol with Iron*
Tri-Vi-Sol with Iron Drops*
Troph-Iron Liquid*
Unicap Plus Iron*
Vigran Plus Iron*
Vi-Daylin Plus Iron*

IRON DEXTRAN
Ferrospan
Imferon
Proferdex

IRON SORBITEX
Jectofer

ISOBORNYL THIOCYANOACETATE
Bornate
Cidalon

ISOCARBOXAZID
Marplan

ISOETHARINE
Beta-2
Bronkometer
Bronkosol
Dey-Dose
Dispos-a-Med

ISOFLURANE
Forane

ISOFLUROPHATE
D.F.P.
Floropryl

ISOMETHEPTENE
Isometh
Octin
Spazoc

ISOMETHEPTENE MUCATE
Midrin*
Migralam*

ISONIAZID
Armazide
Cotinazin
Di-Isopacin*
Dinacrin
Ditubin
Double Isopacin*
Hyzyd
Inapasade-SQ*
Isolyn
Isotamine
INH
Laniazid
Niconyl
Nidaton
Nydrazid
Panazid
P-HV Forte
Pycazide
Pyrizidin
Rifamate*
Rimactane/INH Dual Pack*
Rimifon
Rolazid
Teebaconin
Tisin
Tyvid

ISOPROPAMIDE
Combid*
Combid Spansule*
Darbid
Iso-Perazine TR*
Isopro T.D.*
Ornade*
Priamide
Probacon II*
Prochlor-Iso*
Pro-Iso*
Tyrimide

ISOPROPYL ALCOHOL
Absorbine Arthritic Pain*
Acnederm Lotion*
Akne Drying*
Alcojel
Alcorub
Alkoisol
Aurocaine*
Auro-Dri*
Barbseb*
Barsed Thera-Spray*
Dawson Rubbing Compound

Hibitane Tincture*
Hill Cortac Lotion*
Komed*
Komed HC*
Mercurochrome II*
Neutrogena
Acne-Drying Gel*
Rhulicaine*
Rhulispray*
Sal-Dex*
Thru Penetrating
Liquid*
Tinver*

ISOPROPYL MYRISTATE
Barsed Thera-Spray*

ISOPROTERENOL
Aerolone*
Aludrin
Duohaler*
Duo-Medihaler*
Iprenol
Isonorin
Isuprel
Isuprel-Neo
Mistometer*
Luf-Iso
Medihaler-Iso
Neo-Epinine
Norisodrine
Prenomiser Forte
Proternol
Saventrine
Vapo-Iso
Vapo-N-Iso

ISOSORBIDE
Ismotic

ISOSORBIDE DINITRATE
Carvasin
Coronex
Dilatrate-SR
Isogard
Isoket
Isordil
Isordil Tembids
Isordil Titradose
Isotrate
Isotrate Timecelles
Iso-Bid
Laserdil
Onset
Risordan
Sorate
Sorbide
Sorbitat
Sorbitrate
Sorbitrate SA
Sorquad

ISOTRETINOIN
Accutane
Accutane

ISOXSUPRINE
Dilavase
Duvadilin
Nasodilan
Vasodilan
Vasoprine

ITRAMIN TOSYLATE
Nilatil
Tostram

J

JUNIPER TAR
Boil-Ease*
Polytar*

K

KANAMYCIN
Kamycine
Kanabristol
Kanecidin
Kantrex

KAOLIN
Amogel*
Amogel PG*
BellKatal*
Bisilad*
Diabismul*
Dia-Eze*
Donnagel*
Donnagel-MB*
Donnagel-PG*
Kaodene*
Kaodonna*
Kaodonna-PG*
Kaolin Pectin
Suspension*

Kaomead*
Kaomead with Belladonna*
Kaopectate*
Kaopectate Concentrate*
Kao-Con*
K-P*
K-Pek*
Parepectolin*
Pargel*
Pecto-Kalin*
Pektamalt*
Quiagel*
Quiagel PG*
Ru-K-N*
Woodward's K.P.*

KERATIN
Jeri-Bath Oil*
Jeri-Lotion*

KETAMINE
Ketaject
Ketalar
Ketaset

KETOCONAZOLE
Nizoral

KETOPROFEN
Airheumat
Orudis

KETOTIFEN
Zaditen

KHELLIN
Ammivin
Khelisem
Khelloyd
Visammin

L

LABETALOL
Normodyne
Trandate

LACTASE
Lactaid
Lactrase
Lact-Iron

LACTIC ACID
Duofilm*
Gordofilm*
Panscol*
P&S Shampoo*
Viranol*

LACTOBACILLUS ACIDOPHILUS
Bacid*
Lactinex*

LACTOBACILLUS BULGARICUS
Lactinex*

LACTULOSE
Cephulac
Chronulac
Duphalac

LANOLIN
Alpha Keri*
Alpha Keri Soap*
Balmex*
Balneol*
Balnetar*
Boyol*
Cutemol*
Ice Mint
Jeri-Lotion*
Kerasol Bath Oil*
Lubriderm*
Mediconet*
Nivea Skin Oil*
Perifoam*
Surgi-Kleen*
Ultra derm*
Ultra-Derm Bath Oil*

LAUDEXIUM METHYLSULFATE
Laudolissin

LEUCOVORIN
Wellcovorin

LEVALLORPHAN
Lorfan

LEVAMFETAMINE
Cydril

LEVARTERENOL
Levophed

LEVODOPA
Bendopa
Dopaidan
Dopar
Lardopa
Larodopa
Levopa

L-Dopa
Prolopa*
Sinemet*
LEVONORDEFRIN
Carbocaine Hydrochloride 2% With Neo-Cobefrin Injection*
LEVONORGESTREL
Microval
Nordette*
LEVOPROPOXYPHENE
Novrad
Regretos
LEVORPHANOL
Levo-Dromoran
LEVOTHYROXINE
Eltroxin
Letter
Levoid
Levothroid
LTS
Noroxine
Roxstan
Synthroid
LIDOCAINE
Anestacon
Bactine Antiseptic Anesthetic*
Clinicaine
Dilocaine
Dolicaine
Duo-Trach Kit
L-Caine
Lidaform-HC*
Lida-Mantle
Lidoject
Lidosporin Otic Solution*
LidoPen Auto-Injector
Medi-Quik*
Mercurochrome II*
Nervocaine
Nulicaine
Octocaine
Topilidon
Ultracaine
Unguentine Plus*
Xylocaine
Xylocaine Endotracheal Aerosol
Xylocaine Jelly
Xylocaine Ointment
Xylocaine Topical Spray
Xylocaine Viscous
Xylocard
LINCOMYCIN
Cillimycin
Lincocin
Mycivin
LINDANE
Gamene
Gbh
Gexane
Kwell
Kwellada
Scabane
LIOTHYRONINE
Armour Thyroid*
Cynomel
Cytomel
Cytomine
Tertroxin
Thyroid Strong*
Tyjodin
LIOTRIX
Euthroid
Thyrolar
LIPASE
Arco-Lase*
Arco-Lase Plus*
Converzyme*
Enzymacol*
Festal*
Festalan*
Kutrase*
Ku-Zyme*
Phazyme*
Phazyme-PB*
Phazyme-95*
Tri-Cone*
Tri-Cone Plus*
LITHIUM CARBONATE
Camcolit
Carbolith
Cibalith-S
Eskalith

Eskalith CR
Hypnorex
Lithane
Lithizine
Lithobid
Lithonate
Lithotabs
Priadel
PFI-Lithium
LITHIUM CITRATE
Lithonate-S
LOBELINE
Nikoban
LOMUSTINE
Ceenu
CeeNU
LOPERAMIDE
Imodium
LORAZEPAM
Ativan
Emotival
Larpose
Lorax
Psicopax
Tavor
Temesta
LORMETAZEPAM
Noctamid
LOXAPINE
Daxolin
Daxolin C
Loxapac
Loxitane
LUTUTRIN
Lutrexin
LYPRESSIN
Diapid Nasal Spray
LYSERGIDE
Delysid
LYSINE
Alba-Lybe*
Dequasine*
Enisyl
Geravite Elixir*

M

MAFENIDE
Marfanil
Sulfamylon Cream

MAGALDRATE
Riopan
Riopan Plus*
Rioplus*
MAGESIUM SALICYLATE
Analate
MAGNESIUM
Buffergel*
Cal-M*
Chemdrox*
Chemgastric*
Chemlox*
Dequasine*
Magacin*
Mg-Plus
Neosorb Plus*
Neutralca-S*
Neutralox*
Niarb Super*
Univol*
MAGNESIUM CARBONATE
Albicon*
Alkets*
Antacid Powder*
Anti-Acid No.1*
Arthritis Strength Bufferin*
BiSoDol*
Bufferin*
Bufferin with Codeine No. 3*
Dewitt's Antacid Powder*
Dimacid*
Di-Gel*
Escot*
Estomul-M*
Flacid*
Formula Magsic*
Glycogel*
Krem*
Kudrox*
Marblen*
Noraiac*
Noralac*
Ratio*
Silain-Gel*
Spastosed*
Syntrogel*
MAGNESIUM CHLORIDE
Magnelium

MAGNESIUM CITRATE
- Citro-Mag
- Evac-Q-Kit*
- Evac-Q-Kwik*
- National Laxative
- Tridate Bowel Kit*

MAGNESIUM GLUCOHEPTONATE
- Magnesium Rougier

MAGNESIUM GLUCONATE
- Erimag

MAGNESIUM GLUTAMATE HYDROBROMIDE
- Bromalate

MAGNESIUM HYDROXIDE
- Algemol*
- Algenic Alka Improved Tablets*
- Alumid Suspension*
- Alurex*
- Alurex No.2
- Aluscop*
- Arthritis Pain Formula*
- Ascriptin*
- Ascriptin A/D*
- Banacid*
- B-A*
- Cama*
- Concentrated Milk of Magnesia*
- Cope*
- Diovol*
- Diovol Ex*
- Flacid*
- Gelusil Extra Strength Liquid*
- Haley's M-O*
- Kessadrox*
- Kolantyl*
- Laxsil*
- Liquid Antacid*
- Lo-sal*
- Maalox*
- Maalox #1*
- Maalox #2*
- Maalox Plus*
- Magenion
- Magmalin*
- Magna Gel*
- Milk of Magnesia
- Milk of Magnesia-Cascara Suspension*
- Mygel*
- Mylanta*
- Mylanta II*
- Mylanta-2 Extra Strength*
- Nutramag*
- Phillip's Milk of Magnesia*
- Rolox*
- Rulox*
- Simaal Gel*
- Simeco*
- Syntrogel*
- Tralmag*
- WinGel*

MAGNESIUM NICOTINATE
- Athemol-N*

MAGNESIUM OXIDE
- Albicon*
- Alkets*
- Aludrox*
- Aluscop*
- Beelith*
- BiSoDol*
- Buffaprin*
- Buffinol*
- Camalox*
- Creamalin*
- Delcid*
- Di-Gel*
- Estomul-M*
- Gelusil*
- Gelusil II*
- Gelusil M*
- Kolantyl*
- Kudrox*
- Magnatril*
- Magnesia and Alumina Oral Suspension*
- Mag-Ox 400
- Maox
- Maxamag Suspension*
- Par-Mag
- Phillip's Milk of Magnesia*
- Silain-Gel*
- Uro-Mag

MAGNESIUM SALICYLATE
- Argesic*

Arthrin
Arthrogesic*
Dalca*
Doan's Pills*
Durasal
Efficin
Lorisal
Magan
Mobigesic*
MSG-600
MAGNESIUM SULFATE
Adlerika
Bilagog*
English Style Health Salts
Epsom Salt
Mag-5
MAGNESIUM TRISILICATE
Almacone*
Antacid Powder*
Azolid-A*
A.M.T.*
Banacid*
Bronkaid*
Chooz*
Dewitt's Antacid Powder*
Escot*
Gaviscon Antacid*
Gaviscon-2 Antacid*
Gelumina*
Magnatril*
Neutracomp*
Neutrasil
Noraiac*
Noralac*
Pama*
Trimagel*
Trimax
Trisogel*
Trisomin
Tri-Sil
MALATHION
Prioderm
MALT SOUP EXTRACT
Maltsupex
Syllamalt*
Syllamalt Effervescent*
MANGANESE
Dequasine*
MANNITOL
Isotol
Osmitrol
Resectisol
MANNITOL HEXANITRATE
Manexin
Manite
Mannex
Maxitate
Nitranitol
Ruhexatal with Reserpine*
MAPROTILINE
Ludiomil
MAZINDOL
Mazanor
Sanorex
MEASLES AND RUBELLA VIRUS VACCINE
M-R-VaxII
MEASLES VIRUS VACCINE
Attenuvax
MEASLES, MUMPS AND RUBELLA VIRUS VACCINE
M-M-RII
MEBENDAZOLE
Telmin
Vermox
MEBUTAMATE
Capla
MECAMYLAMINE
Inversine
MECHLORETHAMINE
Dichloren
Mustargen
Sinalost
MECLIZINE
Ancolan
Antivert
Antivert/25
Bonamine
Bonine
Dizmiss
Motion Cure
Vertrol
Wehvert
MECLOCYCLINE SULFOSALICYLATE

Meclan
MECLOFENAMATE
Meclomen
MEDAZEPAM
Nobrium
MEDROGESTONE
Colpro
Colprone
MEDROXYPROGESTERONE
Amen
Curretab
Depo-Provera
Gesinal
Oragest
Provera
MEDRYSONE
HMS Liquifilm
Medrocort
Visudrisone
MEFENAMIC ACID
Coslan
Parkemed
Ponstan
Ponstel
MEGESTROL
Megace
Ovaban
Pallace
MEGLUMINE
Angiografin
Biligrafin
Conray
Cysto-Conray
Endografin
Fortombrine 'M'
Hypaque M*
Reno-M-60
Transbilix
MELARSONYL
Trimelarsan
MELARSOPROL
Arsobal
MEL-B
MELPHALAN
Alkeran
MENADIOL
Kapilon
Kappadione
Synkavite
Synkayvite
Thylokay
MENADIONE
Hykinone
Kanone
Kappaxin
Kayquinone
Thyloquinone
MENINGOCOCCAL POLYSACCHARIDE VACCINE
Menomune A
Menomune-A/C
MENOTROPINS
Pergonal
MENTHOL
Absorbine Arthritic Pain*
Ambenyl Expectorant*
Analbalm*
Analgesic Balm*
Banalg Liniment*
Baumodyne*
Ben-Gay External Analgesic*
Ben-Gay Ointment*
Betuline*
Counter Pain Rub*
Dalidyne*
Denorex*
Dermaphill*
Derma Medicone-HC Ointment*
Derma Medicone Ointment*
Dermoplast Aerosol Spray*
Dewitt's Oil for Ear Use*
Di-Delamine*
Doans Rub*
Emul-O-Balm*
Heet Spray Analgesic*
Icy Hot*
Jen-Balm*
Mercurochrome II*
Minut-Rub*
Num-zit jel*
Panalgesic*
Rhulicaine*
Rhulicream*

Rhuligel*
Rhulispray*
Soltice Quick Rub*
Vatronol Nose Drops*
Vicks Cough Drops
Vicks Formula 44 Cough Control Discs*
Vicks Sinex Decongestant Nasal Spray*
Vicks Throat Lozenges*
Vicks Vaporub*
Vicks Vaposteam*
Vicks Vatronol Nose Drops*
Zemo*

MENTHYL ANTHRANILATE
A-FIl*

MEPARFYNOL
Atempol
Dormison
Somnesin

MEPARTRICIN
Tricandil

MEPAZINE
Pacatal

MEPENZOLATE
Cantil

MEPERIDINE
Atropine with Demerol*
Demer-Idine
Demerol
Dolantal
Dolantin
Mefedina
Mepergan*
Phytadon

MEPHENESIN
Dioloxol
Mephson
Oranixon
Sinan
Tolseram
Tolserol
Tolyspaz

MEPHENOXALONE
Lenetran
Transpoise
Trepidone

MEPHENTERMINE
Biocidin
Wyamine

MEPHENYTOIN
Mesantoin
Phenantoin

MEPHOBARBITAL
Mebaral
Mebroin*
Menta-Bal
Mephoral
Phemitone
Prominal

MEPIVACAINE
Carbocaine
Carbocaine Hydrochloride 2% With Neo-Cobefrin Injection*
Isocaine

MEPREDNISONE
Betapar
Betapred

MEPROBAMATE
Aneural
Deprol*
Equagesic*
Equanil
Equanitrate*
Lan-Dol
Meditran
Mepavlon
Meprogesic*
Meprospan
Meprospan-400
Meprotabs
Mepro-Hex*
Mep-E
Micrainin*
Milpath*
Milprem
Milspan
Miltown
Miltrate*
Neo-Tran
Novomepro
Pathibamate*
Pensive

PMB-400
Probal
Quietal
Robamate
Saronil
SK-Bamate
Tamate
Tranmep
Tranquiline
Trelmar
VioBamate
217 MEP*
282 MEP*
MEPRYLCAINE
Oracaine
MERALEIN
Merodicein
Thantis
MERALLURIDE
Mercardon
Mercuhydrin
MERBROMIN
Mercurochrome*
MERCAPTOMERIN
Thiomerin
MERCAPTOPURINE
Purinethol
MERCUFENOL
Myringacaine
Salicresin
MERCUMATILIN
Cumertilin
MERCURIC IODIDE
Neko
MERETHOXYLLINE PROCAINE
Dicurin Procaine*
MERSALYL
Salyrgan
Theo-Sly-R*
MESORIDAZINE
Lidanar
Serentil
MESTANOLONE
Androstalone
MESTRANOL
Enovid*
Enovid-E*
Norinyl 1+50*
Norinyl 1+80*
Norinyl 2*
Ortho-Novum*
Ovulen*
METABUTETHAMINE
Unacaine
METABUTOXYCAINE
Primacaine
METAPROTERENOL
Alupent
Dosalupent
Metaprel
METARAMINOL
Aramine
Pressonex
Pressoral
METAXALONE
Skelaxin
METFORMIN
Diabexyl
Glucophage
METHACHOLINE
Mecholyl
METHACYCLINE
Molciclina
Rondomycin
METHADONE
Adanon
Althose
Amidone
Dolophine
Physeptone
Westadone
METHALLENESTRIL
Vallestril
METHAMPHETAMINE
Desoxedrine
Desoxyn
Desyphed
Methampex
Methedrine
Neodrine
Norodin
Obedrin-LA
Semoxydrine
Syndrox
METHANDRIOL
Methostan
Stenediol
METHANDROSTENOLONE
Danabol
Dianabol

METHANTHELINE
  Banthine
METHAPHENILENE
  Diatrin
METHAPYRILENE
  Allerest*
  Apcohist Allergy*
  Compoz*
  Cope*
  Dormin
  Dozar
  Histadyl
  Hista-Clopane*
  Histadyl EC*
  Histivite-D*
  Lullamin
  M-P
  Nervine
  Nervine Effervescent
  Nite Rest*
  Nytol(U.S.A.)
  Pyrathyn
  Relax-U-Caps
  Sedacaps
  Semikon
  Sinurex*
  Sleepinal
  Sominex (USA)*
  Somnicaps
  Super-Decon*
  Thenylene
  Tranqium
  Tranquil*
  Tri-Nefrin*
  Twilight*
METHAQUALONE
  Hyptor
  Mequelon
  Mequin
  Optinoxan
  Parest
  Quaalude
  Quaalude-300
  Rouqualone "300"
  Sedalone
  Somnafac
  Sopor
  Triador
  Tualone-300
  Tuazole
  Vitalone
METHARBITAL
  Gemonil
METHAZOLAMINE
  Neptazane
METHDILAZINE
  Dilosyn
  Disyncran
  Tacaryl
METHENAMINE
  Cystex*
  Dolsed*
  Formin
  Methandine
  Prosed*
  Trac*
  UAA*
  Uralgic*
  Uramine*
  Urised*
  Urisep*
  Uritab*
  Uritabs W.O.*
  Urithol*
  Uritone
  Uroblue*
  Urostat-Forte*
  Urotropin
  Uro-Phosphate*
METHENAMINE HIPPURATE
  Hiprex
  Urex
METHENAMINE MANDELATE
  Azo-Mandelamine*
  Maldex*
  Mandalay
  Mandelamine
  Mandelets
  Prov-U-Sep
  Renelate
  Sterine
  Thiacide*
  Urisedamine*
  Uroqid-Acid*
  Uroqid-Acid No.2*
METHENAMINE SULFOSALICYLATE
  Hexalet
  Unguentum Bossi*
METHICILLIN
  Azapen
  Celbenin

Dimocillin-RT
Penistaph
Staphcillin
Synticillin
METHIMAZOLE
Mercazole
Tapazole
METHIODAL
SKiodan
METHIONINE
Odor-Scrip
METHISAZONE
Marboran
METHIXENE
Tremaril
Tremonil
Trest
METHOCARBAMOL
Delaxin
Forbaxin
Marbaxin-750
Methocarbamol w/ASA*
Metho-500
Robaxin
Robaxisal*
Robaxisal C-1/4*
Robaxisal C-1/8*
Spenaxin
Tresortil
METHOHEXITAL
Brevimytal Natrium
Brevital
Brietal
METHOSERPIDINE
Decaserpyl
Decaserpyl Plus*
METHOTREXATE
Mexate
METHOTRIMEPRAZINE
Levoprome
Nozinan
Veractil
METHOXAMINE
Vasoxyl
METHOXSALEN
Meloxine
Methoxa-Dome
Oxsoralen
Soloxsalen
METHOXYFLURANE
Methofane
Penthrane
METHOXYPHENAMINE
Orthoxicol*
Orthoxine
Pyrroxate*
METHSCOPOLAMINE
Alersule*
Dallergy*
Extendryl*
Hista-Phen-S.A.*
Histaspan-D*
Historal*
Histor-D Timecelles*
MSC Triaminic*
Narspan*
Pamine
Rhinolar*
Sinovan Timed*
SKopyl
METHSUXIMIDE
Celontin
Petinutin
METHYCLOTHIAZIDE
Aquatensen
Diutensen*
Diutensen-R*
Duretic
Enduron
Enduronyl*
Enduronyl Forte*
Eutron*
METHYL SALICYLATE
Absorbine Arthritic Pain*
Analbalm*
Analgesic Balm*
Banalg Liniment*
Baumodyne*
Ben-Gay External Analgesic*
Ben-Gay Ointment*
Betuline*
Counter Pain Rub*
Doans Rub*
Emul-O-Balm*
Ger-o-Foam*
Gordogesic Cream
Heet Analgesic Liniment*
Heet Spray Analgesic*

Icy Hot*
Jen-Balm*
Minut-Rub*
Panalgesic*
Sloan's Liniment*
Soltice Quick Rub*
Vicks Inhaler*
Zemo*

METHYLBENZETHONIUM
Bactine*
Dalidyne*
Delavan
Diaparene
Fordustin
Hyseptine
Lobana*
Surgi-Kleen*

METHYLCELLULOSE
Adsorbotear
Bro-Lac
BFL
Cellogran
Cellothyl
Cellumeth
Cologel
Contactisol
Hydrolose
Isopto Alkaline
Isopto Plain
Isopto Tears
Lacril
Lyteers
Methocel
Methopto*
Methulose
Methylose
Murine Ear Drops*
Nicel
Odrinex*
Ows Blue*
Prolens*
Tearisol
Tears Naturale
Ultratears
Visalens Wetting*
Visculose

METHYLDOPA
Aldoclor*
Aldomet
Aldoril*
Dopamet
Medimet-250
Novomedopa
Novo-Doparil*
Presinol
Sembrina
Supres*

METHYLDOPATE
Aldomet Ester

METHYLENE BLUE
Dolsed*
M-B Tabs
MG-Blue
Prosed*
Trac*
UAA*
Uralgic*
Uramine*
Urised*
Urisep*
Uritab*
Urithol*
Uroblue*
Urolene Blue
Urostat-Forte*

METHYLNICOTINATE
Absorbine Arthritic Pain*

METHYLPHENIDATE
Centedrin
Methidate
Ritalin
Ritalin-SR

METHYLPREDNISOLONE
A-MethaPred
Depo-Medrol
Depo-Predate 80
Dep Medalone
D-Med-80
Duralone-40
Duralone-80
Dura-Meth
Medralone-40
Medralone-80
Medrate
Medrol
Medrol Acetate
Medrol Acne Lotion*
Medrol Topical
Medrone

Med-Depo
Mepred
Metastab
Methylone
M-Prednisol
Neo-Medrol*
Neomedrol Acne Lotion*
Nisolone
Pre-Dep-40
Pre-Dep-80
Rep-Pred 40
Rep-Pred 80
Solu-Medrol
Urbason
Wyacort

METHYLTESTOSTERONE
Android
Estertest H.S.*
Estratest*
Formatrix*
Gynetone*
Mepilin*
Metandren
Neo-Hombreol
Oestrilin with Methyltestosterone*
Oraviron
Orchisterone-M
Oreton Methyl
Premarin w/ Methyltestosterone*
Synandrets
Synandrotabs
Testaform
Testora
Testred
Tylosterone*
Virilon

METHYLTHIOURACIL
Muracin
Thyreostat

METHYPRYLON
Noludar

METHYSERGIDE
Deseril
Desernil
Sansert

METOCLOPRAMIDE
Cerucal
Maxeran
Maxolon
Primperan
Reglan

METOCURINE IODIDE
Metubine Iodide

METOLAZONE
Diulo
Zaroxolyn

METOPROLOL
Betaloc
Lopressor
Seloken

METRIZAMIDE
Amipaque

METRONIDAZOLE
Clont
Flagyl
Flagylstatin*
Metryl
Neo-Tric
Novonidazol
Protostat
Satric
Trichazol
Trikacide
Trikamon

METYRAPONE
Metopirone

METYROSINE
Demser

MEXILETINE
Mexitil

MEZLOCILLIN
Mezlin

MIANSERIN
Bolvidon

MICONAZOLE
Daktarin
Micatin
Monistat
Monistat 3
Monistat 7 Vaginal Cream

MINERAL OIL
Agoral*
Agoral Plain*
Alpha Keri*
Alpha Keri Soap*
Balneol*

Balnetar*
Blandlube
Dewitt's Oil for Ear Use*
Fleet Enema Mineral Oil
Fleet Enema Oil Retention
Formula Magsic*
Haley's M-O*
Hydrol
Jeri-Bath Oil*
Jeri-Lotion*
Kerasol Bath Oil*
Kondremul*
Kondremul Plain
Kondremul with Cascara Sagrada*
Kondremul with Phenolphthalein*
Liqui-Doss*
Lowila Cake*
Lubriderm*
Milkinol*
Neo-Cultol
Nephrox Suspension*
Nivea Skin Oil*
Nujol
Petrogalar*
Petro-Syllium No. 1 Plain*
Petro-Syllium No. 2 with Phenolphthalein*
Ultra derm*
Ultra-Derm Bath Oil*
Zymenol

MINERALS, MULTIPLE
Abdol with Minerals*
Adabee with Minerals*
Aprisac*
Chenatal*
Citrotein*
Eldec Kapseals*
Eldercaps*
Eldertonic*
En-Cebrin*
En-Cebrin F*
Filibon*
Glutofac*
Hemocyte Plus Tabules*
Heptuna Plus*
Lonalac*
Maltlevol-M*
Materna*
Megadose*
Mevanin-C*
Mi-Cebrin*
Mi-Cebrin T*
Natacomp-FA*
Natafort Filmseal*
NaturSlim II*
Niferex-PN*
One-A-Day Vitamins Plus Minerals*
Optilets-M-500
Os-Cal Forte*
Os-Cal Plus*
Paladac with Minerals*
Pramet FA*
Pramilet FA*
Ragus*
Rovite*
Sclerex*
Stuartnatal*
Stuart Prenatal*
Theragran-M*
Therapeutic Vitamins and Minerals*
Vicon-C*
Viopan-T*
VG*

MINOCYCLINE
Minocin
Ultramycin
Vectrin

MINOXIDIL
Loniten

MITHRAMYCIN
Mithracin

MITOMYCIN
Ametycin
Mitocin-C
Mutamycin

MITOTANE
Lysodren

MITOXANTRONE
Novantrone*

MOLINDONE
  Lidone
  Moban
MONOBENZONE
  Alba-Dome
  Benoquin
  Pigmex
MONOETHANOLAMINE
  Monolate
MONOSODIUM PHOSPHATE
  Sal Hepatica*
MORPHINE
  Duramorph PF
  Epimorph
  M.O.S.
  Roxanol
  RMS
MOXALACTAM
  Moxam
MUMPS VIRUS VACCINE
  Mumpsvax

N

NABILONE
  Cesamet
NADOLOL
  Corgard
  Corzide*
NAFCILLIN
  Nafcil
  Nallpen
  Unipen
NALBUPHINE
  Nubain
NALIDIXIC ACID
  Cybis
  NegGram
  Nogram
  Wintomylon
NALORPHINE
  Lethidrone
  Nalline
  Norfin
NALOXONE
  Narcan
  Talwin Nx*
NALTREXONE
  Trexan
NANDROLONE
  Deca-Durabolin
  Dekabolin
  Durabolin
NAPHAZOLINE
  Ak-Con Ophthalmic
  Albalon
  Albalon-A*
  Albalon Liquifilm
  Allerest Eye Drops
  Antistine-Privine*
  Clear Eyes
  Degest-2
  Naphcon
  Naphcon Forte
  Optozoline
  Privine
  Rhino-Mex
  Rhino-Mex-N
  Vasocon
  Vasocon A*
  Vasocon Regular
  Vaso Clear
  Zincfrin-A*
  20/20 Eye Drops
  4-Way*
  4-Way Nasal Spray*
NAPROXEN
  Anaprox
  Naprosyn
  Naxen
  Novonaprox
NATAMYCIN
  Natacyn
NEFOPAM
  Acupan
NEOMYCIN
  Alba-3 Ointment*
  Bacimycin*
  Biozyme*
  BPN Ointment*
  Clinicydin*
  Coly-Mycin S Otic*
  Cortisporin Cream*
  Cortisporin
    Ointment*
  Cortisporin Ointment
    Ophthalmic*
  Cortisporin
    Ophthalmic
    Suspension*

Cortisporin Otic Solution*
Cortisporin Otic Suspension*
Epimycin "A"*
Herisan Antibiotic
Kenacomb*
Mity-Mycin*
Mycifradin
Mycifradin Sulfate
Myciguent*
Mycitracin*
Mycolog*
Myco Triacet Cream & Ointment*
N.B.P.*
Neobiotic
Neocin
Neomedrol Acne Lotion*
Neomixin*
Neosone*
Neosporin*
Neosporin-G Cream*
Neosporin G.U. Irrigant*
Neotal*
Neo-Cortef*
Neo-Cort-Dome*
NeoDecadron*
Neo-Delta-Cortef*
Neo-Hydeltrasol*
Neo-Hydro*
Neo-Medrol*
Neo-Oxylone*
Neo-Polycin*
Neo-Synalar*
Neo-Thrycex*
Nysolone*
Ortega Otic M*
Otic Neo-Cort-Dome*
Otobiotic
Otocort Ear Drops*
Otoreid-HC*
Polyspectrin Ophthalmic*
Poly-Pred Drops*
Pyocidin*
Relespor*
Septal*
Spectrocin*
Statrol Ophthalmic*
Tricilone NNG*
Triple Antibiotic*
Tri-Statin*

NEOSTIGMINE
Prostigmin
Prostigmin Bromide

NETILMICIN
Netromycin

NIACIN
A.C.N.*
Cal-M*
Cerebro-Nicin*
Geriliquid
Lipo-Nicin*
Magacin*
Menic*
Nicamin
Nicobid
Nicocap
Nicolar
Niconacid
Nicotinex Elixir
Nicozol*
Nico-Metrazol*
Nico-Span
Nico-Vert*
Nico-400
Novoniacin
Ru-Vert*
SK-Niacin
Tega-Span
Tega-Vert*
Verstat*
Vertex*
Wampocap

NIACINAMIDE
Alba-Lybe*
Cenalene*
Cerebro-Nicin*
Geravite Elixir*
Magacin*
Niarb Super*
Thera-Combex H-P*
Vita-Metrazol*

NIACINAMIDE HYDROIODIDE
Iodo-Niacin*

NIALAMIDE

Niamid
NICLOSAMIDE
Niclocide
Yomesan
NICOTINE
Nicorette
NICOTINYL ALCOHOL
Niacol
Radecol
Roniacol
NICOTINYL ALCOHOL TARTRATE
Speniacol
NIFEDIPINE
Adalat
Procardia
NIFURTIMOX
Lampit
NIKETHAMIDE
Anacardone
Coramine
Corvotone
Nikethyl
Nikorin
NIRIDAZOLE
Ambilhar
NITHIAMIDE
Pleocide
Tritheon
NITRAZEPAM
Megadon
Mogadon
NITROCELLULOSE
Covicone*
NITROFURANTOIN
Chemiofuran
Cyantin
Dantafur
Fua-Med
Furadantin
Furalan
Furan
Furanex
Furatine
Furatoin
Ituran
Ivadantin
J-Dantin
Macrodantin
Nephronex
Nifuran
Nitrex
Nitrodan
Novofuran
N-Toin
Parfuran
Sarodant
Urotoin
NITROFURAZONE
Eldezol
Furacin
Furacin Soluble Dressing
NITROGLYCERIN
Angised
Ang-O-Span
Cardabid
Klavi Cordal
Myocon
Niong
Nitrobon
Nitrocap T.D.
Nitrodisc
Nitroglyn
Nitrolin
Nitrol Ointment
Nitronet
Nitrong
Nitrospan
Nitrostabilin
Nitrostat
Nitrostat IV
Nitrotest
Nitro-Bid Ointment
Nitro-Bid Plateau Caps
Nitro-Dur
Nitro-T.D.
Ro-Nitro
Susadrin
Transderm-Nitro
Trates
Tridil
NITROMERSOL
Metaphen
NOMIFENSINE
Merital
NONOXYNOL
Because
Gynol

Intercept
Koronoex
Semicid

NONOXYNOL 9
Conceptrol
Delfen
Emko Contraceptive Foam
Encare
Ortho-Creme

NORETHANDROLONE
Nilevar

NORETHINDRONE
Agestin
Aygestin
Brevicon*
Brevicon-28*
Loestrin*
Micronor
Modicon*
Noriday
Norinyl 1+35*
Norinyl 1+50*
Norinyl 1+80*
Norinyl 2*
Norlestrin*
Norlutate
Norlutin
Nor-Q.D.
Ortho-Novum*
Ortho-Novum 10/11*
Ortho-Novum 7/7/7*
Ovcon*
Tri-Norinyl*
Zorane*

NORETHYNODREL
Enovid*
Enovid-E*

NORGESTREL
Lo/Ovral*
Microlut
Ovral*
Ovrette
Triphasil*

NORTRIPTYLINE
Acetexa
Allegron
Altilev
Avantyl
Aventyl
Noritren
Pamelor
Vividyl

NOSCAPINE
Actol Expectorant*
Conar*
Conar Expectorant*
Conar Suspension*
Coscopin
Coscotabs
Isotil Tabs*
Nectadon
Noscatuss
Tusscapine

NOVOBIOCIN
Albamycin
Cardelmycin
Cathomycin
Inamycin

NUTMEG OIL
Vicks Vaporub*

NYLIDRIN
Arlidin
Circlidrin
Dilatyl
Perdilatal
Pervadil
Rolidrin

NYSTATIN
Achrostatin V*
Candex
Comycin*
Declostatin*
Flagylstatin*
Kenacomb*
Korostatin Vaginal
Moronal
Mycolog*
Mycostatin
Myco Triacet Cream & Ointment*
Mytrex*
Nadostine
Nilstat
Nyaderm
Nysolone*
Nystaform-HC*
Nystaform Ointment*
O-V Statin
Terrastatin*

Tetrastatin*
Tricilone NNG*
Tri-Statin*
Viaderm-N

O

OAK EXTRACT
Rhus-All Antigen*
OATMEAL COMPOUND
Aveeno Preparations
OIL OF CAMPHOR
Sloan's Liniment*
OIL OF CLOVES
Numzident*
OIL OF EUCALYPTUS
Baumodyne*
OIL OF PINE
Sloan's Liniment*
OLEANDOMYCIN
Metromycin
Romicil
OLEORESIN CAPSICUM
Heet Analgesic Liniment*
OPIPRAMOL
Ensidon
Insidon
OPIUM
Amogel*
Diabismul*
Donnagel-PG*
Infantol Pink*
Pantopon
Parelixir*
Quiagel PG*
ORPHENADRINE
Banflex
Brocasipal
Disipal
Flexoject
Flexon
K-Flex
Marflex
Mephenamine
Myolin
Myotrol
Norflex
Norgeis Forte*
Norgesic*
Norgesic Forte*
O'Flex
X-Otag
OX BILE
Bilagog*
Bilamide*
OX BILE EXTRACT
Bilogen*
Pentazyme*
OXACILLIN
Bactocill
Bristopen
Penstapho
Prostaphlin
Resistopen
OXAMNIQUINE
Vansil
OXANAMIDE
Quiactin
OXANDROLONE
Anavar
Lonavar
Protivar
Vasorome Kowa
OXAZEPAM
Adumbran
Limbial
Praxiten
Serax
Serenid-D
Serepax
Seresta
OXELADIN
Pectamol
Silopentol
Tussimol
OXETHAZAINE
Oxaine
OXOLINIC ACID
Oxobid
Utibid
OXOPHENARSINE
Mapharsen
Mapharside
OXPRENOLOL
ISET
Slow-Trasicor
Traisicor
Trasicor

OXTRIPHYLLINE
Brondecon*
Choledyl
Choledyl Expectorant*
OXYBENZONE
Block-Aid*
Block Out*
Chapstick Sunblock*
PreSun 15*
Solbar*
Sundown Sunblock*
Sun Dare 15*
SunGer Sunblock*
Super Shade*
Total Eclipse Sunscreen*
OXYBUTYNIN
Ditropan
OXYCHLOROSENE
Chlorpactin XCB
OXYCODONE
Eudol
Mictoben
Percobarb*
Percocet*
Percocet-Demi*
Percocet-5*
Percodan*
Percodan-Demi*
Proladone
Supeudol
Tylox*
OXYMETAZOLINE
Afrin
Afrin Pediatric
Dristan Long Lasting Nasal Mist
Dristan Long Lasting Vapor Spray
Drixine
Duration
Duration Mentholated Vapor Spray
Hazol
Nafrine
Neo-Synephrine 12-Hour
St. Joseph Decongestant for Children
St. Joseph Nasal Spray/Drops
OXYMETHOLONE
Adroyd
Anadrol
Anapolon 50
Androyd
Synasternol
OXYMORPHONE
Numorphan
OXYPHENBUTAZONE
Alka-Tandearil
Iridil
Oxalid
Oxybutazone
Reducin
Tandearil
Tanderil
OXYPHENCYCLIMINE
Daricon
Enarax*
Gastrix
Naridan
Setrol
Vio-Thene
Vistrax*
W-T Anticholinergic
Zamanil
OXYPHENONIUM
Antrenyl
OXYQUINOLINE
Aci-Jel*
Derma Medicone-HC Ointment*
Derma Medicone Ointment*
Oxyzal West*
Rectal Medicone-HC Suppositories*
Rectal Medicone Suppositories*
Rectal Medicone Unguent*
OXYTETRACYCLINE
Abbocin
E.P. Mycin
Imperacin
Otetryn
Oxlopar
Oxymycin
Oxy-Tetrachel

Terramycin
Terramycin with Polymyxin B*
Terramycin Ointment*
Terramycin Ophthalmic*
Terramycin Ophthalmic Ointment*
Terramycin Otic Ointment*
Terramycin Topical Ointment*
Terramycin Vaginal*
Terrastatin*
Terra-Cortril*
Terra-Cortril Spray with Polymyxin B*
Tetramine
Uri-Tet
Urobiotic-250*

OXYTOCIN
Pitocin
Syntocinon
Uteracon

P

PADIMATE
Chapstick Sunblock*
Original Eclipse Sunscreen*
Partial Eclipse Suntan*
PreSun 15*
Sundown Sunblock*
Sun Dare 15*
SunGer Sunblock*
Super Shade*
Total Eclipse Sunscreen*

PADIMATE O
Block Out*

PAMABROM
Cardui*
Maximum Cramp Relief*
Pamprin*
Premesyn PMS*
Sunril*
Trendar*

PANCREATIN
Bilogen*
Digestalin*
Digolase*
Dizyme*
Donnazyme*
Elzyme 303
Entozyme*
Enzypan*
Gasticans*
Kanulase*
Panteric
Panzyme*
Pentazyme*
Viokase
Zypan*

PANCRELIPASE
Accelerase
Cotazym
Cotazyme
Digestive Enzymes-PXP*
Ilozyme
Ku-Zyme HP
Pancrease

PANCURONIUM
Pavulon

PANGAMATE CALCIUM
Nyamik 15*

PANGAMIC ACID
Nyamik 15*

PANTHENOL
Cozyme
Ilopan
Motilyn
Panthoderm
Thera-Combex H-P*

PAPAIN
Caroid
Digestalin*
Digestamic*
Gasticans*
Hydrocare
Panafil Ointment*
Panafil-White Ointment*

PAPAVERINE
Cerebid
Cerespan
Copavin*
Delapav

Dilart
Dipav
Durapar
Kavrin
Lapav Graduals
Myobid
Orapav Timecelles
Papacon
Parasule
Pavabid HP
Pavabid Plateau Caps
Pavacap Unicelles
Pavacen
Pavadur
Pavadyl
Pavagen
PavaKey
Pavatran TD
Pavatym
Pava-Mead T.D.
Pava Par
Pava Rx
Paverine Spancaps
Paverolan Lanacaps
P.T.-300
P-200
Therapav
Tri-Pavasule
Vasal Granucaps
Vasocap
Vasospan

PARACHLOROMETAXYLENOL
Dureze Otic Drops*
Fungotic*
Metasep
Metasep Medicated Shampoo
Nu-Flow
Sween Karaya Powder
Unguentine Plus*

PARAMETHADIONE
Paradione

PARAMETHASONE
Alondra
Dilar
Haldrate
Haldrona
Haldrone
Monocortin
Stemex

PARATHYROID
Para-Thor-Mone
Paroidin

PAREGORIC
Amogel PG*
Corrective Mixture with Paregoric*
DIA-quel*
Kaodonna-PG*
Pabizol with Paregoric*
Parepectolin*
Pecto-Kalin*
Ru-K-N*

PARGYLINE
Eudatine
Eutonyl
Eutron*

PAROMOMYCIN
Humagel
Humatin

PAROXYPROPIONE
Frenantol
Possipione

PASINIAZID
InPas

PECTIN
Amogel*
Amogel PG*
Diabismul*
Diarkote*
Diar-Aid*
Diatrol*
DIA-quel*
Dia-Quel Liquid*
Donnagel*
Donnagel-MB*
Donnagel-PG*
Infantol Pink*
Kaodene*
Kaodonna*
Kaodonna-PG*
Kaolin Pectin Suspension*
Kaomead*
Kaomead with Belladonna*
Kaopectate*
Kaopectate Concentrate*

Kao-Con*
K-P*
K-Pek*
Parelixir*
Parepectolin*
Pargel*
Pecto-Kalin*
Pektamalt*
Polymagma Plain*
Quiagel*
Quiagel PG*
Ru-K-N*
Woodward's K.P.*

PEMOLINE
Cylert
Deltamine
Kethamed
Pioxol
Stimul
Volital

PENICILLAMINE
Cuprimine
Depen Titratabs
Distamine

PENICILLIN G
Ben-P
Crystapen
Duracillin
Estencilline
Falapen
Forpen
Forticillin
Genecillin-400
G-Recillin
G-Recillin-T
Ka-Pen
K-Cillin 250
K-Cillin 500
K-Pen
Liquapen
Megacillin
Megapen
M-Cillin D 400
Neolin
Novopen
Novopen-G
Palocillin
Penalev
Pencitabs
Penidural
Penioral-500
Penisem
Pentids
Pfizerpen G
P.G.A.
Pronapen
P-50
Quidpen G
SK-Penicillin G
Sugracillin
Tardocillin
TuCillin
Wycillin
Wycillin and Probenecid*

PENICILLIN G BENZATHINE
Bicillin
Bicillin L-A
Duapen
Megacillin Suspension
Permapen

PENICILLIN G PROCAINE
Ayercillin
Crysticillin 300 A.S.
Crysticillin 600 A.S.
Duracillin A.S.
Pfizerpen-AS

PENICILLIN V
Pen-Vee
Redpen-VK
V-Cillin

PENICILLIN V POTASSIUM
Beepen-VK
Betapen-VK
Cocillin V-K
Compocillin V
Compocillin-VK
Deltapen-VK
Genecillin-VK-500
Hi-Pen
Ledercillin VK
LV Penicillin
Nadopen-V
Novopen-V
Novopen-V-500
Penapar
Penapar VK
Penbec-V

Pen-Vee K
Pen VK
Pfizerpen VK
PVF
PVF K
Repen-VK
Robicillin VK
Suspen
SK-Penicillin VK
Uticillin-K
Uticillin-VK
Veetids '125'
Veetids '250'
Veetids '500'
V-Cillin-K
V-Cil-K
VC-K 500
Wincillin-VK
Win-V-K
PENICILLINASE
Neutrapen
PENTAERYTHRITOL TETRANITRATE
Angitrate
Antora
Blaintrate
Cartrax*
Covap*
Dilanca
Duotrate Plateau Caps
El Petn
Equanitrate*
Kaytrate
Miltrate*
Myocardol
Naptrate
Neo-Corovas
Penetra
Pennpheno*
Pentafin
Pentestan
Pentritol
Pentrium*
Pentryate
Pentylan with Phenobarbital*
Peritrate
Peritrate with Phenobarbital*
Quintrate PB*
Rate-20
SDM No.22
SDM No.23
SDM No.35
Tranite
Vasitol
Vasodiatol
Vaso-80 Unicelles
PENTAGASTRIN
Gastrodiagnost
Peptavlon
PENTAMIDINE
Lomidine
PENTAPIPERIDE
Lyspafen
PENTAPIPERIDE METHYLSULFATE
Quilene
PENTAZOCINE
Fortalgesic
Fortral
Pentazin
Sosegon
Talwin
Talwin Compound*
Talwin Nx*
Talwin 50
PENTHIENATE
Monodral
PENTOBARBITAL
Butylone
Carbrital*
Dorsital
Hypnotal
Ibatal
Nebralin
Nembutal
Nova-Rectal
Pentanca
Pentogen
Triaprin*
WANS*
PENTOLINIUM
Ansolysen
Tensilest
PENTOXIFYLLINE
Trental
PENTYLENETETRAZOL
Cardiazol
Cenalene*

Cerebro-Nicin*
Geravite Elixir*
Leptazol
Menic*
Metalex-P
Metrazol
Nelex-100
Nicozol*
Nico-Metrazol*
Nioric
Pentrazol
Ru-Vert*
Verstat*
Vita-Metrazol*

PEPPERMINT
Numzident*

PEPPERMINT OIL
Betuline*
Blistex*

PEPSIN
Corrective Mixture*
Corrective Mixture with Paregoric*
Digestalin*
Digestive Enzymes-PXP*
Dizyme*
Donnazyme*
Entozyme*
Enzypan*
Fermentol
Kanulase*
Muripsin*
Normacid*
Panazyme Digestant
Panzyme*
Pentazyme*
Zypan*

PERICIAZINE
Aolept
Neulactil
Neuleptil

PERPHENAZINE
Etrafon*
Etrafon-A*
Etrafon Forte*
Fentazin
Phenazine
Triavil*
Trilafon

PERTUSSIS IMMUNE GLOBULIN, HUMAN
Hypertussis

PERTUSSIS VACCINE
Triogen*
Tri-Immunol*

PERUVIAN BALSAM
Anugard-HC*
Anusol*
Anusol-HC*
Anusol Ointment*
Anusol Suppositories*
Balmex*
Decubitex*
Granulex*

PETROLATUM
Buf Foot-Care Soap*
Cutemol*
Lip Therapy
Nivea Skin Oil*
RVPaba Lip Stick*
Saratoga*
Ultra derm*

PHENACAINE
Holocaine

PHENACEMIDE
Epiclase
Phenurone

PHENACETIN
Apac*
Asphac-G*
Buffets*
Cafacetin*
Carisopodol*
Cortiforte*
CP2 Tablets*
Soprodol*

PHENAGLYCODOL
Acalo
Remin
Ultran

PHENAZOCINE
Narphen
Prinadol
Xenagol

PHENAZOPYRIDINE
Azodine
Azomine
Azo-standard
Azosul*

Azotrex*
Azo Gantanol*
Azo Gantrisin*
Azo-Mandelamine*
Azo-Soxazole*
Azo-Sulfisoxazole*
Azo-Sulfstat*
Baridium
Di-Azo
Dolonil*
Mallophene
Microsul-A*
Phenazo
Pyridiate
Pyridium
Pyridium Plus*
Sedural
Signa Sul-A*
Suladyne
Suldiazo*
Thiosulfil-A*
Thiosulfil-A Forte*
Thiosulfil Duo-Pak*
Uremide*
Uri-pak*
Urobiotic-250*
Urodine
Uro-Gantanol*

PHENDIMETRAZINE
Adphen
Anorex
Aptrol
Bacarate
Bontril PDM
Dietrol
Ex-Obese
Limit
Melfiat
Melfiat-105 Unicelles
Metra
Obalan
Obepar
Obestrol
Obeval
Obezine
Omnibesel
PDM
Phendimead
Phenzine
Plegine
Prelu-2
Ropledge
Sprx
Statobex
Trimstat
Trimtabs
Weightrol

PHENELZINE
Monoten
Nardelzine
Nardil
Stinerval

PHENETHICILLIN
Broxil
Chemipen
Darcil
Maxipen
Syncillin

PHENFORMIN
DBI
Dibotin
Insoral
Meltrol
Meltrol-50

PHENINDAMINE
Cerose*
Cerose DM*
Comhist*
Nolamine*
Omnicol*
P-V Tussin*
Thephorin

PHENINDIONE
Danilone
Hedulin
Indon

PHENIPRAZINE
Catron
Cavodil

PHENIRAMINE
Bayaminicol*
Chexit*
Citra*
Dextrotussin*
Dristan Nasal Spray*
Extendac*
Fiogesic*
Inhiston
MSC Triaminic*

Nazac Timed-
Disintegration
Decongestant*
Panadyl*
Poly-Histine-D*
Poly-Histine-D
Elixir*
Ru-Vert*
S-T Forte*
Timed Cold*
Tossecol*
Triaminic*
Triaminicol*
Triaminicol
Decongestant
Cough*
Triaminic
Expectorant*
Triaminic
Expectorant with
Codeine*
Trihista-Phen*
Trimeton
Triminicol Cough
Syrup*
Tussagesic*
Tussaminic*
Ursinus*
Vasominic TD*
Vernacel Ophthalmic*
Verstat*
Vertex*

PHENMETRAZINE
Preludin

PHENOBARBITAL
Alised*
Amobell*
Amodrine*
Anaspaz PB*
Antrocol*
Arco-Lase Plus*
Asma-Lief*
Asminyl*
Asthmagyl*
Atrobarb*
Atrobarbital*
Atrosed*
Azma Aid*
Barbenyl
Barbidonna*
Barbita
Barbivis
Belladenal*
Belladenal-S*
Bellaphen*
Bellastal*
Bellergal*
Bellergal-S*
Bellermine-O.D.*
Bellkatal*
Bellophen*
Bentylol with
Phenobarbital*
Bentyl with
Phenobarb*
Bilamide*
Bronkolixir*
Bronkotabs*
Cardilate-P*
Chardonna-2*
Chemfedral*
Dibent-PB*
Donnamor Elixir*
Donnatal*
Donnatal Extentabs*
Donnazyme*
Donphen*
Ergobel*
Eskabarb
Gardenal
Gaysal*
Glycopyrrolate*
Guiaphed Elixir*
Hasp*
Henotal
Hybephen*
Hyosophen*
Hypnolone
Isogen Compound*
Isogen Compound
Elixir*
Isuprel Compound
Elixir*
Kinesed*
Lardet Expectorant
Tabs*
Lardet Tabs*
Levsinex with
Phenobarbital
Timecaps*

Levsin with
Phenobarbital*
Levsin-PB
Liquital
Lufyline-EPG TABS*
Luminal
Malatal*
Matropinal*
Matropinal Forte
Inserts*
Matropinal Inserts*
Mediphen
Mudrane*
Mudrane GG*
Mudrane GG Elixir*
Neoquess Tablets*
Nova-Phase with
Pheno*
Nova-Pheno
Panzyme*
Pennpheno*
Pentylan with
Phenobarbital*
Peritrate with
Phenobarbital*
Phazyme-PB*
Phedral*
Phenonyl
Pheno-Bella*
Pheno-Squar
Plexonal*
Primatene P*
Pro-Banthine with
Phenobarbital*
Pylora*
Quadrinal*
Quintrate PB*
Relaxadon*
Respirol*
Robinul-PH*
Robinul-PH Forte*
Salibar Jr.*
Seds*
SK-Phenobarbital
Solfoton
Solu-Barb
Spalix*
Spasaid*
Spaslin*
Spasmoban-PH*
Spasmolin*
Spasmophen*
Spasmorel*
Spasquid*
Spastyl with
Phenobarbital*
Stental
Susano*
Talpheno
Tedral*
Tedral Elixir*
Tedral Expectorant*
Tedral SA*
T.E.P.*
Thalfed*
Thecord*
Theodrin Pediatric
Suspension*
Theofedral*
Theophenyllin*
Theoral*
Theotabs*
Valpin 50-PB*
Vanatal*
Vanodonnal*
Verequad*
Verquad*
Viscephen*
Wesmatic Forte*

PHENOBUTIODIL
Biliodyl
Vesipaque

PHENOL
Anbesol Antiseptic
Anesthetic*
Boil-Ease*
Calamatum*
Cal-ZO Dressing*
Campho-Phenique*
Castellanis Paint*
Cepastat
Cherry Chloraseptic*
Chloraseptic DM
Cough Control
Lozenges*
Chloraseptic Gel*
Chloraseptic
Lozenges*
Chloraseptic Spray*
Dermaphill*

Hemocyte Injection*
HTO Stainless Manzan
Hemorrhoidal
Tissue Ointment*
Menthol
Chloraseptic*
Neo-Castaderm*
Panscol*
Procolin*
Rhus Tox Lotion*
Sting-Eze*
Unguentine Plus*

PHENOLATE SODIUM
Menthol
Chloraseptic*

PHENOLPHTHALEIN
Agoral*
Alophen
Amlax*
Caroid Laxative*
Correctol*
Correctol Liquid
Disolan*
Dual Formula
Feen-A-Mint*
Espotabs
Evac-Q-Kit*
Evac-Q-Kwik*
Evac-U-Gen
Extra Gentle Ex-Lax*
Ex-Lax
Ex-Lax Extra Gentle*
Ex-Lax Pills
Feen-A-Lax
Feen-A-Mint
Feen-A-Mint Gum
Feen-A-Mint Pills*
Fructines-Vichy
Kondremul with
Phenolphthalein*
Oxothalein*
Petrogalar*
Petro-Syllium No. 2
with
Phenolphthalein*
Phenolax
Prulet
Prulet Liquitab
Sarolax*
Trilax*

PHENOLSULFONPHTHALEIN
Test P.S.P.

PHENOPERIDINE
Operidine

PHENOXYBENZAMINE
Dibenzyline

PHENPROCOUMON
Liquamar
Marcumar

PHENSUXIMIDE
Lifene
Milontin

PHENTERMINE
Adipex
Adipex-P
Duromin
Fastin
Ionamin
Mirapront
Obephen
Obermine
Obesamead
Obestin
Parmine
Phentermyl
Phentrol
Phermine
Pronidin
Rolaphent
Teramine
Tora
Wilpowr

PHENTOLAMINE
Regitine
Rogitine

PHENYL AMINOSALICYLATE
Pheny-PAS-Tebamin

PHENYL SALICYLATE
Corrective Mixture*
Corrective Mixture
with Paregoric*
Pabizol with
Paregoric*
Trac*
Uralgic*
Uramine*
Urisep*
Uritab*
Uritabs W.O.*
Urithol*

Uroblue*
Urostat-Forte*

PHENYLBUTAZONE

Algoverine
Alkabutazone
Alka Butazolidin
Anevral
Azolid
Azolid-A*
Buffazone
Busone
Butagesic
Butagesic-B
Butalgan
Butazolidin
Butazolidin Alka
Butone
Ecobutazone
Intrabutazone
Malgesic
Malgesic-Alk
Nadozone
Neo-Zoline
Novobutazone
Phenbutazone
Tazone

PHENYLEPHRINE

Acutuss Expectorant With Codeine*
Advanced Formula Dristan*
AK-Dilate Ophthalmic
AK-Nefrin Ophthalmic
Alamine*
Alamine-C*
Alamine Expectorant*
Al-Ay*
Albatussin*
Alconefrin
Alersule*
Allerest Nasal
Amaril D*
Anatuss*
Anodynos Forte*
Aspirin Free Dristan*
Atussin D.M. Expectorant*
Atussin Expectorant*
Biomydrin
Blephamide Liquifilm*
Brocon Chewable*
Brocon C.R.*
Bromophen*
Cenagesic*
Cenaid*
Cerose*
Cerose DM*
Chlor-Trimeton Expectorant*
Chlor-Trimeton Expectorant with Codeine*
Citra*
Clistin-D*
Codimal DM*
Codimal PH*
Colrex*
Colrex Antitussive*
Colrex Cough Syrup*
Coltab*
Comhist*
Conar*
Conar Expectorant*
Conar Suspension*
Congespirin Chewable Cold Tablets for Children*
Contac Nasal Mist
Cophene*
Cordamine*
Coricidin Demilets*
Coricidin Nasal Spray
Coryban-D Antitussive*
Covanamine*
Covangesic*
Cyclomydril*
Dallergy*
Decohist*
Decongestabs*
Degest
Demazin*
Dimetane Decongestant*
Dimetane Expectorant*
Dimetane Expectorant-DC*

Dimetapp with
  Codeine*
Dimetapp Elixir*
Dimetapp Extentabs*
Donatussin Drops*
Donatussin Syrup*
Dristan*
Dristan Antitussive*
Dristan Nasal Spray*
Duadacin*
Duohaler*
Duo-Medihaler*
Duphrene*
Duradyne-Forte*
Efricel
Efricon*
Emagrin Forte*
Emeroid*
Entex*
Epicel
Extendryl*
Eyephrine*
Eye Cool
Fendol*
Ginsopan*
Guaiahist TT
  Tempotrol*
Histalet Forte*
Histaspan-D*
Histaspan-P*
Histaspan-Plus*
Histatab*
Histatapp Elixir*
Histatapp T.D.*
Hista-Compound No.5*
Hista-Phen-S.A.*
Hista-Vadrin*
Histor-D Syrup*
Histor-D Timecelles*
Hot Lemon*
Hydra
Imotep*
Isophrin
Isopto-Frin
Isuprel-Neo
  Mistometer*
Kiddisan*
Kleer Chewable*
Kolephrin*
Korigesic*
Mercodol with
  Decapryn*
Midatap*
Midran Decongestant*
Mistura D
Mydfrin
Naldecon*
Naldelate*
Napril Plateau Caps*
Narspan*
Nasahist*
Nase-X
Naso Mist
Neotep*
Neozin*
Neo-Synephrine
Neo-Synephrine
  Compound*
Neo-Synephrine Eye
  Drops
Newphrine
Normatane*
Nor-Lief*
Nostril
Nostrilla
Novahistex*
Novahistine Fortis*
Novahistine LP*
ND-Gesic*
NTZ
Omnicol*
Optigene II
Optised Ophthalmic*
Optocrymal
Pediacof*
Pediaquill*
Phenatapp Extend*
Phenoptic
Phenylzin*
Prefrin
Prefrin-A*
Prefrin Liquifilm
Prefrin Z
Purebrom*
Puretapp Elixir*
Puretapp PA*
Pyracort-D
Quadra-Hist*
Quelidrine*
Rectagene Balm*

Relemine*
Respinol L.A.*
Rhinex*
Rhinex DM*
Rhinogesic*
Rhinspec*
Robitussin Night Relief*
Romex*
Romilar*
Rotapp*
Ru-Tuss*
Rymed-TR*
Rynatan*
Rynatuss*
Ryna-Tussadine Expectorant*
Salphenyl*
Sinaphen-Nasal
Sinarest Nasal Spray*
Sinex
Sinexin*
Sinex Decongestant Nasal Spray*
Singlet*
Sino-Comp*
Sinocon*
Sinovan Timed*
Soltice Nasal Spray
Soothe(Canada)
Spantuss*
Spec-T Sore Throat/ Decongestant*
S.T. Decongest*
S-T Forte*
Sucraphen
Sulfadrin Nasal Suspension*
Super Anahist Nasal Spray
Super-Decon*
Synasal
Tagatap*
Tamine*
Tear-Efrin
Tonecol*
T.P.I.*
Triaminicin Nasal Spray*
Tri-Phen*
Tri-Phen-Chlor*
Tudecon*
Tussanil Syrup*
Tussar DM*
Tympagesic*
Tyrohist
Vacon
Valihist*
Vasosulf*
Veltap*
Vernacel Ophthalmic*
Vicks Sinex Decongestant Nasal Spray*
Visadron
Westapp*
Zincfrin
4-Way*
4-Way Cold*
4-Way Nasal Spray*

PHENYLMERCURIC ACETATE
Blinx*
Trimo-San

PHENYLMERCURIC NITRATE
Clean-N-Soak
Merlenate*

PHENYLPROPANOLAMINE
Acutrim
Aid-Tuss*
Alka-Seltzer Plus*
Allerest*
Allerest Regular and Children's*
Allerest Sinus Pain Formula*
Allerform*
Allergesic*
Allergin*
Allergy Relief Medicine*
Allerprop*
Alumadrine*
Amaril D*
Anatuss*
Anorexin*
Anorexin One-Span*
Apcohist Allergy*
Appedrine*
Appress

Atussin D.M.
  Expectorant*
Atussin Expectorant*
Ayds Weight
  Suppressant
Bayaminicol*
Bayaminic Extract*
Bayaminic Syrup*
Bayer Children's
  Cold*
Bayer Cough for
  Children*
Bayer Decongestant*
Bayhistine*
Bay-Ornade*
Bio Slim T*
Bowman Cold Tablets*
Breacol*
Brocon Chewable*
Brocon C.R.*
Bromphen*
Cafamine T.D.*
Caramiphen Edisylate*
Cenadex
Cheracol Plus*
Chexit*
Children's Hold 4
  Hour Cough
  Suppressant*
Childrens Co Tylenol*
Chlor-Rest*
Codimal Expectorant*
Codrin L.A*
Coffee, Tea & A New
  Me
Coffee Break Cubes
  Weight Reduction
  Plan
Coldecon
Comtrex*
Conex*
Conex with Codeine*
Conex DA*
Conex Plus*
Contac*
Contac Jr. Childrens'
  Cold Medicine*
Control
Cophene*
Coricidin "D"*
Coricidin
  Antitussive*
Corsym*
Coryban-D*
Covanamine*
Covangesic*
Cremacoat 3*
Cremacoat 4*
Dalca*
Daycare*
Deconade*
Deconex*
Decongestabs*
Deproist*
Dexatrim
Dextrotussin*
Dex-A-Diet II
Diadax
Dietac*
Dietac Drops
Dietac Maximum
  Strength
Diet Gard
Diet-Trim*
Dimalix*
Dimetane
  Expectorant*
Dimetane
  Expectorant-DC*
Dimetapp with
  Codeine*
Dimetapp Elixir*
Dimetapp Extentabs*
Dorcol Pediatric*
Drinophen*
Dristan Advanced
  Formula*
Drize*
D-Sinus*
Efed II*
Endecon*
Entex*
Entex LA*
Extendac*
Fernhist*
Fiogesic*
Fluidex Plus
Formula 44-D*
Ginsopan*
Grapefruit Diet Plan
  with Diadax

Grapefruit Diet Plan with Diadax Chewable Extra Strength
Grapefruit Diet Plan with Diadax Extra Strength Vitamin Fortified Continuous Action
Grapefruit Diet Plan with Diadax Vitamin Fortified Continuous Action
Halls*
Headway*
Head & Chest Cold Medicine*
Histabid Duracap*
Histalet Forte*
Histatapp Elixir*
Histatapp T.D.*
Hista-Vadrin*
Histosal*
Hold Liquid Cough Suppressant*
Hungrex Plus*
Hycomine*
Kleer Comp*
Kophane Cough & Cold Formula*
Korigesic*
Kronohist Kronocaps*
Lanatuss*
Lanatuss Expectorant*
Midatane Expectorant*
Midatap*
MSC Triaminic*
Naldecon*
Naldecon-CX*
Naldecon-Ex Pediatric*
Naldelate*
Naldetuss*
Napril Plateau Caps*
Nasahist*
Nazac Timed-Disintegration Decongestant*
Neophiban*
Neorhiban*
Nilcol*
Nobese
Nolamine*
Noraminic Syrup*
Norel Plus*
Norel Plus Injection*
Normatane*
Normatane Expectorant*
Novahistine*
Novahistine DH*
Novahistine Elixir*
Novahistine Expectorant*
Novamor*
Obestat
Odrinex*
Omex*
Orahist*
Ornacol*
Ornade*
Ornade 2 Liquid for Children*
Ornex*
Panadyl*
Permathene-12*
Phenatapp Extend*
Phenate*
Phenhist Elixir*
Phen APAP*
Phen-Lets
Poly-Histine-D*
Poly-Histine-D Elixir*
Poly-Histine Expectorant with Codeine*
Poly-Histine Expectorant Plain*
Probacon*
Probacon II*
Prolamine
Propadrine
Prothazine Expectorant*
Pro-Dax
Purebrom*
Puretapp Elixir*
Puretapp PA*

P.V.M. Appetite Control
P.V.M. Appetite Suppressant
Quadra-Hist*
Relemine*
Reletuss*
Resaid T.D.*
Resolution Half Strength
Resolution I
Resolution II
Respinol L.A.*
Rhindecon
Rhinex D-Lay*
Rhinidrin*
Rhinocaps*
Rhinolar*
Rhinolar-Ex*
Robitussin-CF*
Romilar III*
Rotane Expectorant*
Rotapp*
Ru-Tuss*
Ru-Tuss II*
Rymed-TR*
Ryna-Tussadine Expectorant*
Saleto-D*
Sinapils*
Sinarest*
Sine-Aid*
Sine-Off*
Sine-Off-Aspirin Formula*
Sine-Off Aspirin-Free Extra Strength*
Sine-Off Extra Strength - No Drowsiness*
Sinocon*
Sinubid*
Sinugen*
Sinulin*
Sinurex*
Sinustat*
Sinutab*
Sinutab Extra Strength*
Sinutab II*
Sinutrex*
Sinu-Lets*
Slim One*
Soltice*
Spantac*
Spantrol*
Spec-T Sore Throat/ Decongestant*
S.T. Decongest*
S-T Forte*
St. Joseph Cold for Children*
Super Odrinex*
Syracol*
Tagatap*
Tamine*
Tavist-D*
Timed Cold*
Tossecol*
T.P.I.*
Triaminic*
Triaminicin*
Triaminicin Allergy*
Triaminicin Chewables*
Triaminicin Nasal Spray*
Triaminicol*
Triaminicol Decongestant Cough*
Triaminic Allergy*
Triaminic-DM Cough Formula*
Triaminic Expectorant*
Triaminic Expectorant with Codeine*
Tricodene Forte*
Tricodene NN*
Tricodene Pediatric*
Trihista-Phen*
Tri-Medex*
Triminicol Cough Syrup*
Trind*
Trind DM*
Tri-Nefrin*

Tri-Phen*
Triphenyl
Expectorant*
Tri-Phen-Chlor*
Tudecon*
Tussagesic*
Tussaminic*
Tussanil Syrup*
Tuss-Ade*
Tuss Allergine*
Tuss-Ornade*
Tus-Oraminic*
Unitrol
Ursinus*
Vasominic TD*
Veltap*
Vicks Formula 44D
Decongestant Cough
Mixture*
Vita-Slim
Voxin-PG*
Westapp*
Westrim LA
4-Way*

PHENYLSALICYLATE
Dolsed*
UAA*

PHENYLSEMICARBAZIDE
Phenygenine

PHENYLTOLOXAMINE
Aceta-Gesic*
Amaril D*
Argesic*
Arthrogesic*
Bristamin
Conex DA*
Conex Plus*
Decongestabs*
Dilone*
Euphenex*
Histionex
Hyptran*
Kutrase*
Meadache*
Medache*
Mobigesic*
Momentum*
Myocalm*
Myocalm Revised II*
Naldecon*
Naldelate*
Naldetuss*
Neophiban*
Neorhiban*
Norel Plus*
Percogesic*
Phenylgesic*
Poly-Histine-D*
Poly-Histine-D
Elixir*
Quadra-Hist*
Rhinidrin*
Sinocon*
Sinubid*
Sinugen*
Sinustat*
Sinutab*
Sinutrex*
Sinu-Lets*
Tri-Phen-Chlor*
Tudecon*
Tussionex*
Volaxin*

PHENYRAMIDOL
Analexin

PHENYTOIN
Dantoin
Dilantin
Diphenylan
Ditan
Epanutin
Eptoin
Mebroin*

PHOLCODINE
Codylin
Ethnine
Ethnine Simplex

PHOSPHO-SODA
Fleet Prep Kit*
Fleet Prep Kit 2*
Fleet Prep Kit 3*
Kit 1*

PHOSPHORATED
CARBOHYDRATE
Calm-X
Eazol
Especol
Nausetrol

PHOSPHORUS
Neutra-Phos*

Neutra-Phos-K*
PHTHALYLSULFATHIAZOLE
Sulfathalidine
Thalazol
PHYSOSTIGMINE
Antilirium
Eserine Sulfate
Isopto Eserine
PHYTATE SODIUM
Rencal
PHYTONADIONE
Aquamephyton
Konakion
Mephyton
Mono-Kay
PILOCARPINE
Adsorbocarpine
Akarpine
Almocarpine*
E-Carpine*
E-Pilo*
E-Pilo-1
E-Pilo-2
Isopto Carpine
Miocarpine
Mistura P
Mi-Pilo
Ocusert
Ocusert Pilo
Optopilo
Pilocar*
Pilocel Oph
Pilomiotin
Piloptic
Pilovisc
P.V. Carpine
P1E1*
P2E1*
P3E1*
P4E1*
P6E1*
PIMINODINE
Alvodine
Cimadon
PIMOZIDE
Orap
PINAVERIUM
Dicetel
PINDOLOL
Visken
PINE TAR
Packer's Pine Tar
Polytar*
PIPAZETHATE
Selvigon
Theratuss
PIPENZOLATE
Piptal
Piptel
PIPERACETAZINE
Actazine
Quide
PIPERACILLIN
Pipracil
PIPERAZINE
Ancazine
Antepar
Bryrel
Entacyl
Multifuge
Oxucide
Parazine
Perin
Pincets
Pinsirup
Vermisol
Vermizine
Verm-X
Veroxil
PIPERIDOLATE
Dactil
PIPERILATE
Sycotrol
PIPEROCAINE
Metycaine
PIPERONYL BUTOXIDE
A-200 Pyrinate*
A-200 Pyrinated Liquid, Gel*
Rid*
RID Liquid Pediculicide*
PIPOBROMAN
Vercyte
PIPRADROL
Meratran
PIPRINHYDRINATE
Kolton
Mepedyl
Sea Legs

PIRACETAM
  Nootropil
PIRENZEPINE
  Gastrozepin
  Gastrozepine
PIROXICAM
  Feldene
PITUITARY, POSTERIOR
  Pituitrin
PIZOTYLINE
  Litec
  Mosegor
  Sandomigran
PLANTAGO SEED
  Casyllium*
  Effersyllium
  Hi-Fibran
  Hydrocil
  Hydrocil Fortified*
  Hydrocil Instant
  Hydrocil Plain
  Instant Mix
    Metamucil*
  Konsyl
  L. A. Formula*
  Metamucil
  Modane*
  Modane Bulk
  Mucillium
  Mucilose
  Naturacil
  Novo-Mucilax
  Perdiem*
  Perdiem Plain
  Petro-Syllium No. 1
    Plain*
  Petro-Syllium No. 2
    with
    Phenolphthalein*
  Plova*
  Prodiem*
  Prodiem Plain
  Prompt*
  Regacilium
  Reguloid
  Saraka
  Senokot with
    Plantago Seed*
  Serutan
  Siblin
  Sof-Lax Wafers*
  Syllact
  Syllact*
  Syllamalt*
  Syllamalt
    Effervescent*
  Tablucyl
  V-Lax
PNEUMOCOCCAL VACCINE
  Pnu-Imune 23
PODOPHYLLUM RESIN
  Podoben
POISON IVY EXTRACT
  Aqua Ivy
  Rhus Tox Antigen
POLDINE
  Nactate
  Nacton
POLIOVIRUS VACCINE,
    LIVE ORAL
  Orimune
  OPV
POLOXAMER
  Alaxin
POLOXAMER 188
  Magcyl
  Polykol
POLYCARBOPHIL
  Mitrolan
POLYESTRADIOL
  Estradurin
POLYFEROSE
  Jefron
POLYMYXIN B
  Aerosporin
  Alba-3 Ointment*
  BPN Ointment*
  Chloromyxin*
  Clinicydin*
  Cortisporin Cream*
  Cortisporin Ointment*
  Cortisporin Ointment
    Ophthalmic*
  Cortisporin
    Ophthalmic
    Suspension*
  Cortisporin Otic
    Solution*
  Cortisporin Otic
    Suspension*

Epimycin "A"*
Lidosporin Otic
Solution*
Mity-Mycin*
Mycitracin*
N.B.P.*
Neomixin*
Neosporin*
Neosporin-G Cream*
Neosporin G.U.
Irrigant*
Neotal*
Neo-Hydro*
Neo-Polycin*
Neo-Thrycex*
Novantrone*
Ophthocort*
Ortega Otic M*
Otocort Ear Drops*
Otoreid-HC*
Poly-Pred Drops*
Polyspectrin
Ophthalmic*
Polysporin*
Polysporin
Ophthalmic*
Pyocidin*
Pyocidin-Otic*
Relespor*
Septal*
Statrol Ophthalmic*
Terramycin with
Polymyxin B*
Terramycin Ointment*
Terramycin
Ophthalmic*
Terramycin
Ophthalmic
Ointment*
Terramycin Otic
Ointment*
Terramycin Topical
Ointment*
Terramycin Vaginal*
Terra-Cortril Spray
with Polymyxin B*
Triple Antibiotic*

POLYSACCHARIDE-IRON
COMPLEX
Hytinic
Niferex
Niferex with
Vitamin C*

POLYTHIAZIDE
Drenusil
Lotense
Minizide*
Nephril
Renese
Renese-R*

POLYVALENT
PNEUMOCOCCAL
VACCINE
Pneumovax
Pneumovax 23
Pnu-Imune

POLYVINYL ALCOHOL
Akwa Tears*
Aqua-Flow*
Contique Artificial
Tears
Contique Dual Wet*
Hy-flow*
Lens-Mate*
Lens-Wet*
Liquifilm Tears
Liquifilm Wetting*
Pre-sert*
Prolens*
Soquette*
Tears Plus*
Visalens Wetting*
Wet-N-Soak*
Wetting Solution*

POSION IVY EXTRACT
Rhus-All Antigen*

POTASSIUM
Neutra-Phos*
Neutra-Phos-K*

POTASSIUM ACETATE
Potassium Triplex*

POTASSIUM ACID
PHOSPHATE
K-Phos M.F.*
K-Phos Neutral*
K-Phos No.2*
K-Phos Original

POTASSIUM AMINOBENZOATE
Pabak
Pabalate-SF*

Potaba
POTASSIUM BICARBONATE
Alka-Seltzer Effervescent Antacid*
Kaochlor Eff*
Keff*
Klorvess Effervescent Granules*
Klorvess 10%*
K-Lyte
K-Lyte Cl*
K-Lyte Cl 50*
K-Lyte DS*
Potassium Triplex*
POTASSIUM BITARTRATE
Ceo-Two Suppositories*
Col-Evac*
POTASSIUM CARBONATE
Keff*
POTASSIUM CHLORIDE
Aqua-Flow*
BC*
Co-Salt*
Emplets
Kaochlor
Kaochlor Concentrate
Kaochlor Eff*
Kaochlor S-F
Kaochlor 10%
Kaochlor 20%
Kaon-Cl
Kaon Cl-10
Kato Powder
Kay Ciel
Keff*
K-Forte Potassium Supplement with Vitamin C Chewable*
K-LOR
Klor
Klor-Con
Klor-Con/25
Klorvess Effervescent Granules*
Klorvess 10%*
Klotrix
K-Lyte Cl*
K-Lyte Cl 50*
K-Lyte DS*
Kolyum Liquid/ Powder*
K-Tab
K-10
Micro-K
Pan-Cloride
Pfiklor
Potage
Roychlor
Slow-K
Slo-Pot
Slo-Pot 600
POTASSIUM CITRATE
Bicitra
Citrolith
Polycitra*
Polycitra-K*
Polycitra-LC--Sugar-Free*
Potassium Triplex*
Seltz K
Twin-K*
POTASSIUM GLUCONATE
Kaon
Kao-Nor
Kaylixir
Kolyum Liquid/ Powder*
Potassium Rougier
Royonate
Twin-K*
POTASSIUM GUAIACOLSULFONATE
Cerose*
Cerose DM*
Cetro-Cirose*
Codimal DM*
Codimal Expectorant*
Codimal PH*
DM-4 Children's Cough Control*
DM-8*
Efricon*
Kiddies Pediatric*
N-N Cough*
Noratuss*
Pinex
Poly-Histine Expectorant with Codeine*

Poly-Histine Expectorant Plain*
Prothazine Expectorant*
Thiocol

POTASSIUM IODIDE
Iodo-Niacin*
Isogen Compound*
Isogen Compound Elixir*
Isuprel Compound Elixir*
KIE*
Lugol's Solution*
Mudrane*
Mudrane-2*
Pediacof*
Pima
Quadrinal*
Rum-K
SSKI
Theodrin Pediatric Suspension*

POTASSIUM NITRATE
Dewitt's Pills for Backache & Joint Pain*

POTASSIUM OXYQUINOLINE SULFATE
Uroset

POTASSIUM PERCHLORATE
Perchloracap
Peroidin

POTASSIUM PHOSPHATE
Thiacide*
Uro-KP-Neutral*

POTASSIUM SALICYLATE
Neocylate*
Pabalate-SF*
Zarumin*

POTASSIUM TARTRATE
K-Med
Nati-K Nativelle
Wel-K

POTASSIUM THIOCYANATE
Rhocya

POVIDONE
Adapettes*
Fluress*
Subtosan
Tears Plus*

POVIDONE-IODINE
Acu-Dyne
Aerodine
Anbesol Antiseptic Anesthetic*
Betadine
Bridine
BPS
Efodine
Femidine
Final Step
Frepp Antiseptic
Isodine
Mallisol
Operand
Operand Douche
Pacadyne
Pharmadine
Polydine
Proviodine
PVP-Iodine
Sepp Antiseptic
Surgi-Sep

PRALIDOXIME
Protopam
2-Pam

PRAMOXINE
Dermarex*
Dureze Otic Drops*
F-E-P Creme*
Fungotic*
Otall Ear Drops*
Otic-HC Ear Drops*
Perifoam*
Proctofoam/Non-Steroid
Steramine Otic*
Stera-Form*
Tronolane
Tronothane
Viopramosone*
Vio Hydrosone*

PRAZEPAM
Centrax
Verstran

PRAZIQUANTEL
Biltricide

PRAZOSIN
Hypovase
Minipress
Minizide*

PREDNISOLONE
- Ataraxoid*
- Blephamide Liquifilm*
- Blephamide Ointment*
- Blephamide Ophthalmic*
- Blephamide S.O.P.*
- Cetapred*
- Delta-Cortef
- Econopred
- Fernisolone-P
- Hydeltra
- Hydeltrasol
- Hydeltra-T.B.A.
- Inflamase
- Isopto Cetapred*
- Meticortelone
- Metimyd*
- Meti-Derm
- Metreton
- Mydrapred Ophthalmic*
- Neo-Delta-Cortef*
- Neo-Hydeltrasol*
- Nova-Pred
- Optimyd*
- Paracortol
- Poly-Pred Drops*
- Predate-L.A.S.A.
- Predate-100
- Predne-Dome
- Prednicon
- Prednis
- Predoxine
- Predulose
- Pred Forte
- Pred Mild
- PSI-IV
- Sodasone
- Sterane
- Sterolone
- Ulacort

PREDNISONE
- Colisone
- Cortan
- Decortancyl
- Deltasone
- Delta-Dome
- Fernisone
- Listacort
- Meticorten
- Orasone
- Paracort
- Servisone
- SK-Prednisone
- Sterapred Uni-Pak
- Winpred
- Zenadrin

PREGNENOLONE
- Formula 405

PRENYLAMINE
- Hostaginan
- Sedolatan
- Segontin
- Synadrin

PRILOCAINE
- Citanest
- Xylonest

PRIMAQUINE
- Aralen*

PRIMIDONE
- Myidone
- Mylepsine
- Mysoline
- Primoline
- Ro-Primidone
- Sertan

PROBENECID
- Ampicin-PRB*
- Benemid
- Benuryl
- ColBenemid*
- Polycillin-PRB*
- Principen with Probenecid*
- Probalan
- Probampacin*
- Probenicillin*
- Pro-Biosan 500 Kit*
- Ro-Benecid
- SK-Probenecid
- Uricosid
- Wycillin and Probenecid*

PROBUCOL
- Lorelco

PROCAINAMIDE
- Novocamid
- Procan SR

Pronestyl
Pronestyl SR
Sub-Quin
PROCAINE
Anduracaine
Anuject
Durathesia
Glukor Injection*
Neocaine
Procolin*
PROCARBAZINE
Matulane
Natulan
PROCHLORPERAZINE
Combid*
Combid Spansule*
Compazine
Compazine Spansules
Eskatrol*
Isopro T.D.*
Iso-Perazine TR*
Prochlor-Iso*
Pro-Iso*
Stemetil
Tementil
PROCYCLIDINE
Kemadrin
Procyclid
PRODILIDINE
Cogesic
PROGESTERONE
Colprosterone
Femotrone
Gesterol
Lingusorbs
Lipo-Lutin
Lucorteum
Luteinol
Lutocylin
Lutromone
Membrettes
Nalutron
Profac-O
Progelan
Progestaject-50
Progestasert
Progesterol
Progestilin
Progestin
Proluton
Syngesterone
Syngestrets
PROLASE
Tri-Cone*
PROMAZINE
Atarzine
Intrazine
Norazine
Norzine
Promabec
Promanyl
Promazettes
Promwill
Protactyl
Prozine
Pro-Tan
Sparine
Verophen
PROMETHAZINE
Anergen 25
Atosil
Baymethazine
Fellozine
Ganphen
Histantil
Maxigesic*
Mepergan*
Phencen
Phenergan
Phenergan D*
Phenoject-50
Promatussin DM*
Prometh 25
Prorex
Prothazine
Provigan
Remsed
Synalgos*
Synalgos-DC*
V-Gan-25
ZiPan-25 & -50
PROPANIDID
Epontol
PROPANTHELINE
Banlin
Giquel
Norpanth
Novopropanthil
Propanthel
Pro-Banthine

Pro-Banthine with
Phenobarbital*
Robantaline
Ropanth
PROPARACAINE
Ak-Taine
Alcaine
Ophthaine
Ophthetic
PROPIOMAZINE
Largon
PROPIONIC ACID
Verdefam Cream*
Verdefam Solution*
PROPOXYCAINE
Neo-Cobefrin
Novocain
Ravocaine
PROPOXYPHENE
Algafan
Algodex
Darvocet-N*
Darvocet-N 100*
Darvon
Darvon with A.S.A.*
Darvon Compound-65*
Darvon-N
Darvon-N Compound*
Darvon-N With ASA*
Depronal
Develin Retard
Dolacet*
Dolene
Dolene-AP-65*
Dolene Compound-65*
Doloxene
Erantin
Femadol
Levadol
Neo-Mal
Novopropoxyn
Novopropoxyn
Compound*
Pargesic 65
Progesic
Proxagesic
Pro-65
SK 65
SK-65 APAP*
SK-65 Compound*
S-Painacet*
S-Pain-65
Unigesic-A*
Wygesic*
642
692*
PROPRANOLOL
Avlocardyl
Inderal
Inderal-LA
Inderide*
Novo-Pranol
PROPYLENE GLYCOL
Barsed Thera-Spray*
Buf Foot-Care
Lotion*
Cetaphil*
Decubitex*
Dureze Otic Drops*
Kerid Ear Drop*
Ortega Otic M*
Rhinocyn-DM*
Rhinocyn-PD*
Rhinosyn*
Tarlene*
Ultra derm*
PROPYLHEXEDRINE
Benzedrex
Dristan Inhaler
Eventin
PROPYLIODONE
Dionosil
PROPYLTHIOURACIL
Propacil
Propyl-Thyracil
PROTEASE
Bilezyme*
Converzyme*
Enzymacol*
Festal*
Festalan*
Kutrase*
Ku-Zyme*
Phazyme*
Phazyme-PB*
Phazyme-95*
Travase Ointment
PROTEINASE
Digolase*
PROTEOLYTIC ENZYMES

Ananase
PROTHIPENDYL
Timovan
Tolnate
PROTIRELIN
Relefact TRH
Thypinone
PROTOKYLOL
Caytine
Ventaire
PROTOVERATRINE A
Protalba
PROTRIPTYLINE
Concordin
Maximed
Triptil
Vivactil
PRUNE POWDER
Casyllium*
PSEUDOEPHEDRINE
Actacin*
Actagen*
Actamine*
Actifed*
Actifed with Codeine Cough Syrup*
Actifed-C*
Actifed Expectorant*
Actihist*
Acti-Prem*
Afrinol
Allerfrin*
Allerid-D.C.*
Ambenyl-D Decongestant Cough Formula*
Anafed*
Anamine*
Anamine T.D. Caps*
Baydec*
Benylin Decongestant*
Besan
Brexin*
Bromfed*
Broncholate*
Carbodec*
Cenafed
Chlorafed Timecelles*
Chlorated Adult Timecells*
Chlor-Trimeton Decongestant*
Codimal*
Codimal-L.A. Cenules*
Coldrine*
Congestac*
Congress Jr.*
Congress Sr.*
Contac Cough*
Contac Severe Cold Formula*
Contac Severe Cold Formula Night Strength*
Co-Pyronil*
Coryza Brengle*
Cosanyl Cough*
Cosanyl DM Improved Formula*
Cotrol-D*
Co Tylenol*
Co Tylenol Cold Formula for Children*
CoTylenol Liquid Cold Formula*
Deconamine*
Deconsmine*
D-Feda
Dimacol*
Disophrol*
Dristan Ultra*
Dristan Ultra Coughs Formula*
Drixoral*
Duo-hist*
Duralex*
Efedra P.A.*
Eltor
Emprazil*
Emprazil-C*
Fedahist*
Fedahist Expectorant*
Fedahist Syrup*
Fedrazil*
First Sign Nasal Decongestant
Guaifed*

Histalet*
Histalet DM*
Histarall*
Historal*
Hournaze*
Intensin*
Isoclor*
Kronofed-A
  Kronocaps*
Lo-Tussin*
Mor-Tussin P.E.*
Multi-Symptom*
Naldegesic*
Nasalspan*
Nasalspan
  Expectorant*
N.D. Clear T.D.*
Norafed*
Novafed
Novafed A*
Novahistine DMX*
Novahistine Sinus*
Nucofed*
Nucofed Pediatric
  Expectorant*
Phenergan D*
Polaramime
  Expectorant*
Poly-Histine-DX*
Promatussin DM*
Prothazine
  Expectorant*
Pseudodine*
Pseudofrin
Pseudo-Bid*
Pseudo-Hist*
Pseudo-Hist
  Expectorant*
Pseudo-Mal*
Respair-S.R.*
Rhinafed-Ex*
Rhinocyn-DM*
Rhinocyn-PD*
Rhinosyn*
Rhinosyn-X*
Robidrine
Robitussin DAC*
Robitussin-PE*
Rofed Syrup*
Rondec*
Rondec-DM*
Rondec-TR*
Ryna-Cx Liquid*
Ryna-C Liquid*
Ryna Liquid*
Sinacon*
Sine-Aid Extra
  Strength*
Sinufed
Sudadrine
Sudafed
Sudafed Cough*
Sudafed Plus*
Sudafed S.A.
Sudodrin
Sudo-60
Super Anahist*
Symptom 2
Tagafed*
Triacin*
Triafed*
Trifed*
Tri-Fed*
Triphed*
Tripodrine*
Triposed*
Tussend*
Tussend Expectorant*
Tylenol Maximum
  Strength Sinus
  Medication*
Viromed*
Zephrex*
Zephrex-La*

PYRANTEL PAMOATE
  Antiminth
  Combantrin
PYRAZINAMIDE
  Aldinamide
  Tebrazid
PYRETHRINS
  A-200 Pyrinate*
  A-200 Pyrinate
  A-200 Pyrinated
    Liquid, Gel*
  Barc
  Rid*
  RID Liquid
    Pediculicide*
PYRIDOSTIGMINE

Kalymin
Mestinon
Mestinon Bromide
Regonol
PYRIDOXINE
Alba-Lybe*
AVP Natal*
Beelith*
Beesix
Bendectin*
Cal-M*
Cerebro-Nicin*
Complement
Doxine*
Fortior-2B*
Gravidox
Hepp-Iron Drops*
Hexavibex
Hexa-Betalin
Hydoxin
Neuro B-12 Forte Injectable*
Thera-Combex H-P*
Vita-Metrazol*
PYRILAMINE
Albatussin*
Allerest*
Allertoc
Anthisan
Bayaminicol*
Bronitin*
Cardui*
Cenagesic*
Chexit*
Citra*
Codimal DM*
Codimal PH*
Compoz*
Copsamine
Covanamine*
Covangesic*
Dorantamin
Dormarex
Duadacin*
Duphrene*
Emeroid*
Endotussin-NN*
Enrumay
Excedrin P.M.*
Fernhist*
Fioaesic*
Ginsopan*
Histalet Forte*
Histan
Histosal*
Ivarest*
Kriptin
Kronohist Kronocaps*
Larylgan Throat Spray*
Maximum Cramp Relief*
MSC Triaminic*
Miles Nervine
Minihist
Napril Plateau Caps*
ND-Gesic*
Neo-Antergen
Pamprin*
Panadyl*
Paraminyl
Poly-Histine-D*
Poly-Histine-D Elixir*
Prefrin-A*
Premesyn PMS*
Primatene M*
Pyma
Pymafed
Pyramal
Pyra-Maleate
Quiet World*
Rectagene Balm*
Relemine*
Robitussin Night Relief*
Rynatan*
Ryna-Tussadine Expectorant*
Sleep-Eze
Stamine
Sunril*
Thylogen
Tossecol*
Triaminic*
Triaminicol*
Triaminicol Decongestant Cough*
Triaminic Expectorant*

Triaminic
Expectorant with
Codeine*
Tricodene C-V*
Trihista-Phen*
Triminicol Cough
Syrup*
Tussagesic*
Tussaminic*
Tussanil Syrup*
Ursinus*
Vasominic TD*
WANS*
Zem-Histine
4-Way Nasal Spray*
PYRIMETHAMINE
Daraprim
Fansidar*
PYRITHIONE ZINC
Danex
Dan-Gard
Donex
DHS Zinc
Hair Power
Head & Shoulders
Ionil
Vancide ZP
Zincon
Zincon Dandruff
Shampoo
Zinc Omadine
ZP 11 Medicated
Shampoo
PYRROBUTAMINE
Pyronil
PYRVINIUM PAMOATE
Molevac
Pamovin
Poquil
Povan
Pyr-Pam
Vanquin

Q

QUINACRINE
Atabrine
Tenicridine
QUINALDINE BLUE
Vernitest
QUINESTROL
Estrovis
QUINETHAZONE
Aquamox
Hydromox
QUINIDINE
Biquin Durules
Cardioquin
Cin-Quin
Duraquin
Kinidine
Quinaglute
Quinate
Quinicardine
Quinidex Extentabs
Quinora
Rhythmidine
SK-Quinidine
QUINIDINE
PHENYLETHYL-
BARBITURATE
Natisedine Nativelle
Quinobarb
QUININE
Coco-Quinine
Dentojel
Kinine
Quinamm
Quine
Quinite*
Quiphile
QM-260
Strema

R

RABIES IMMUNE GLOBULIN
RIG
RABIES IMMUNE GLOBULIN,
HUMAN
Hyperab
Imogam Rabies
RABIES VACCINE, HUMAN
Imovac Rabies
RACEMETHIONINE
A-D-R
Dequasine*
Meonine

Monile
Ninol
Pedameth
Uracid
Uranap
RANITIDINE
Zantac
RAUBASINE
Raubaserp
RAUWOLFIA SERPENTINA
Hywolfia
Raudixin
Raupena
Rauserfia
Rauserpa
Rauserpin
Rautina
Rauval
Rauverid
Rauzide*
Rawfola
Ru-Hy-T
Serfoliar
Wolfina
RESCINNAMINE
Anaprel-500
Cinnasil
Moderil
Raurescin
Rescisan
RESERPINE
Alkarau
Alserin
Butiserpazide*
Chloroserpine*
Demi-Regroton*
Diupres*
Diupres-250*
Diutensen-R*
Dralserp*
Ebserpine
Eskaserp
Exna-R*
Geneserp
Hiserpia
Hydrap-ES*
Hydropres*
Hydroserp*
Hydroserpine*
Hydrotensin*
Hygroton-Reserpine*
Hyser Plus*
Lemiserp
Liquapres*
Metatensin*
Naquival*
Neo-Serp
Rauloydin
Raurine
Rau-Sed
Regroton*
Releserp-5
Renese-R*
Resercen
Resercrine
Reserfia
Reserjen
Reserpanca
Reserpoid
R-HCTZ-H*
Ro-Chloro-Serp*
Rolserp
Ropres*
Roxinoid
Ruhexatal with Reserpine*
Salutensin*
Salutensin-Demi*
Sandril
Ser-Ap-Es*
Serfin
Serpalan
Serpanray
Serpasil
Serpasil-Apresoline*
Serpasil-Esidrix*
Serpate
SK-Reserpine
Thiaserp*
Triserp
Unipres*
Vioserp
Vio-Serpine
Zepine
RESORCIN
Neo-Castaderm*
RESORCINOL
Acne-Aid*
Acne-Dome Creme & Lotion*

Acnomel*
Acnycin*
Alphaone*
Bensulfoid*
Bicozene Creme*
Castellanis Paint*
Cenac*
Clearasil*
Clearasil Vanishing Formula*
Contrablem*
Euresol
Exzit*
Hill Cortac Lotion*
Lanacane Medicated Creme*
Mazon*
Microsyn*
PhisoAc*
Resulin*
Rezamid*
Rid-Itch Liquid*
Sulforcin*
Tar-Doak Lotion*

RH D IMMUNE GLOBULIN, HUMAN
Gamulin Rh
Hyp Rho-D
Rho Gam

RIBOFLAVIN
Alba-Lybe*
Cerebro-Nicin*
Geravite Elixir*
Thera-Combex H-P*
Vita-Metrazol*

RICINOLEIC ACID
Aci-Jel*

RIFAMPIN
Rifadin
Rifamate*
Rifomycin
Rimactane
Rimactane/INH Dual Pack*
Rofact

RISTOCETIN
Spontin

RITODRINE
Pre-Mar
Yutopar

ROLITETRACYCLINE
Lidociclina
Reverin
Syntetrex
Syntetrin
Tetrazotyl
Transcycline
Velacycline

ROSE PETAL AQUEOUS
Estrivin

ROSOXACIN
Eradacil
Roxadyl

ROTOXAMINE
Twiston
Twiston R-A

RUBELLA VIRUS VACCINE
Meruvax II
MR Vax II

RUTIN
Peridin-C*

S

SACCHARIN
Saxin
Sucaryl

SALICYCLIC ACID
Akne Drying*
Mazon*
Sebasorb*
Sebex*

SALICYLAMIDE
Akes-N-Pain*
Anodynos*
Anodynos Forte*
Arthralgen*
Bancap*
Bancap With Codeine*
Banesin*
BC Powder*
BC Tablets*
Cenagesic*
Citra*
Codalan*
Codimal*
Cortiforte*
Cystex*
Dapase

Dewitt's Pills for
  Backache & Joint
  Pain*
Dolomide
Dropsal
Duadacin*
Duoprin*
Duradyne-Forte*
Emagrin*
Emagrin Forte*
Fendol*
Hista-Compound No.5*
Kiddisan*
Kleer Comp*
Kolephrin*
Korigesic*
Maldex*
Meadache*
Medache*
Midran Decongestant*
Myocalm*
Os-Cal-Gesic*
Panodynes Analgesic*
Panritis*
Presaline*
Raspberin
Rhinex D-Lay*
Rhinogesic*
Rid-A-Pain*
S-A-C*
Salamide
Saleto-D*
Salimeph*
Salocol*
Salphenyl*
Salrin
Sedacane*
Sinexin*
Sino-Comp*
Sinulin*
Sinurex*
Sominex (USA)*
S.P.C.*
Stanback*
Super-Decon*
S45 Anti-Pain
  Compound*
Thru Penetrating
  Liquid*
Triaprin*
Twilight*
Volaxin*
Zarumin*
SALICYLANILIDE
  Salinidol
SALICYLATE
  Gaysal*
  Gaysal-S*
  Ivy-Chex*
  Mobidin
  Prosed*
  Urised*
  Vatronol Nose Drops*
  Vicks Sinex
    Decongestant Nasal
    Spray*
  Vicks Vatronol Nose
    Drops*
SALICYLIC ACID
  Acnaveen*
  Acne-Dome Medicated
    Cleanser*
  Acnesarb
  Acno*
  Acnotex*
  Alphaone*
  Barbseb*
  Barsed Thera-Spray*
  Bevill's Lotion
  Blis-To-Sol*
  Buf Acne-Cleansing
    Bar*
  Calicylic
  Clearasil Medicated
    Cleanser
  Compound W*
  Daliderm*
  Derma+Soft Creme
  Domerine*
  Dry and Clear Acne
    Cream*
  Dry and Clear Acne
    Medication
  Dry and Clear
    Cleanser
  Drytex
  Duofilm*
  Exzit Medicated
    Cleanser*
  Fomac Foam

Formac
Fostex Cake*
Fostex Cream*
Fostex Medicated
  Cleanser*
Freezone*
Gordofilm*
Hydrisalic
Keralyt
Klaron*
Komed*
Komed HC*
Listerex Golden
  Lotion
Listerex Herbal
  Lotion
Medicated Face
  Conditioner
Medicated Foot
  Powder*
Mediplast
Meted Shampoo*
Meted 2 Shampoo*
Microsyn*
Multiscrub*
NP-27 Cream*
NP-27 Liquid*
NP-27 Powder*
Off-Ezy
Oxipor VHC Lotion
  for Psoriasis*
Panscol*
Pernox*
Podiaspray*
Pragmatar*
P&S Shampoo*
Rid-Itch Liquid*
Salacid
Sal-Dex*
Saligel
Salonil
Sastid A1*
Sastid Plain*
Sastid Soap*
Sebaveen*
Sebucare
Sebulex*
Sebulex Scalp Care
  Lotion
Sebutone*
Solvex Ointment*
Solvex Powder*
Stri-Dex Medicated
  Pads
Tar-Doak Lotion*
Tarlene*
Tarsum*
Therac*
Theracort*
Therapads*
Tinver*
T-4-L*
Vanseb*
Vanseb-T*
Verdefam Cream*
Verdefam Solution*
Viranol*
Wart-Off
Whitfield's*
Whitsphill*
Xseb Shampoo
Xseb-T Shampoo*

SALINE SOLUTION
  Ayr

SALSALATE
  Arcylate
  Disalcid
  Duragesic*
  Momentum*
  Persistin*
  Saloxium

SARALASIN ACETATE
  Sarenin

SCARLET RED
  Decubitex*

SCOPOLAMINE
  Bellaphen*
  Bellastal*
  Butabell HMB*
  Comhist*
  Donnagel*
  Donnagel-PG*
  Donnamor Elixir*
  Donnazyme*
  Donphen*
  Hasp*
  Hybephen*
  Hyosophen*
  Isopto Hyoscine
  Kinesed*

Kwells
Malatal*
Neoquess Tablets*
Omnibel*
Palbar No. 2*
Panzyme*
Plexonal*
Pylora*
Quiagel*
Quiagel PG*
Relaxadon*
Ru-Tuss*
Seds*
Sidonna*
Spalix*
Spasaid*
Spaslin*
Spasmolin*
Spasmophen*
Spasmorel*
Spasquid*
Susano*
Transderm-SCOP
Triptone
Vanatal*
Vanodonnal*

SECOBARBITAL
Barbosec
Bi-Secogen*
Duo-Barb*
Hyptran*
Hyptrol
Novamo-Secobarb*
Secogen
Seconal
Secotabs
Sedonal Natrium
Seotal Sodium
Seral
Tuinal*
Tuinal Pulvules*
Tuisec
Tuo-Barb*

SELENIUM SULFIDE
Exsel
Lethopherol*
Losel 250
Sebusan
Selsun
Selsun Blue
Selsun Suspension
Sul-Blue

SENNA
Bekunis Herbal Tea
Black Draught
Casafru
Dr. Caldwell's Senna Laxative
Fletcher's Castoria
Gentlax
Gentlax B
Gentlax S*
Glysennid Norsenna
Mucinum-F
Norsena
Nytilax
Perdiem*
Prodiem*
Senexon
SenoKap DSS*
Senokot
Senokot with Plantago Seed*
Senokot-S*
Senolax
Swiss Kriss
X-Prep

SENNOSIDES A AND B
Castoria
Glysennid
Prompt*

SILVER IODIDE COLLOIDAL
Neo-Silvol

SILVER PROTEIN
Argyrol

SILVER SULFADIAZINE
Flamazine
Silvadene

SIMETHICONE
Amphojel 65*
Barriere
Chemgastric*
Di-Gel*
Diovol*
Flacid*
Gas-X
Gelusil*
Gelusil II*
Gelusil M*
Laxsil*

Maalox Plus*
Mygel*
Mylanta*
Mylanta II*
Mylanta-2 Extra Strength*
Mylicon
Mylicon 80
Ovol
Ovol 80
Phazyme*
Phazyme-PB*
Phazyme-95*
Riopan Plus*
Rioplus*
Sidonna*
Silain-Gel*
Simeco*
Tri-Cone*
Tri-Cone Plus*

SINCALIDE
Kinevac

SITOSTEROLS
Cytellin

SMALLPOX VACCINE
Dryvax

SODIUM ACETRIZOATE
Urokon Sodium

SODIUM ACID PHOSPHATE
K-Phos M.F.*
K-Phos Neutral*
K-Phos No.2*
Uro-Phosphate*

SODIUM ACID PYROPHOSPHATE
Phos-pHaid*
Vacuetts Adult*

SODIUM AMINOBENZOATE
Pabalate*

SODIUM ASCORBATE
Ascorbin
Cee-500
Ferancee*
Ferancee-HP*
Fero-Grad-500*
Liqui-Cee
Niferex with Vitamin C*

SODIUM BENZOATE
Caffeine And Sodium Benzoate*

SODIUM BICARBONATE
Algemol*
Alka-Seltzer Effervescent Antacid*
Alka-Seltzer Effervescent Pain Reliever and Antacid*
Antacid Powder*
Aqua-Flow*
Bell-Ans
BiSoDol*
Brioschi
Bromo-Seltzer*
Ceo-Two Suppositories*
Citrocarbonate*
Col-Evac*
Dewitt's Antacid Powder*
Diatrol*
Eno*
Gasticans*
Instant Mix Metamucil*
Lobana*
Neut
Ocean Mist
Sal Hepatica*
Sellymin
Soda Mint
Syllamalt Effervescent*
Vacuetts Adult*

SODIUM BIPHOSPHATE
Barium Enema Prep kit*
Fleet Enema*
Fleet Pediatric Enema*
Lavoptik Eye Wash*
Phos-pHaid*
Phospho-Soda*
Saf Tip Phosphate Enema*
Vacuetts Adult*

SODIUM BORATE
Antibiopto Ophthalmic*
Blinx*

Blistex*
Boil n Soak*
Trichotine
Unisol*
SODIUM CAPRYLATE
Larylgan Throat Spray*
Verdefam Cream*
Verdefam Solution*
SODIUM CELLULOSE
Calcisorb
SODIUM CELLULOSE PHOSPHATE
Calcibind
SODIUM CHLORIDE
Adsorbonac
Boil n Soak*
Efa Steri-Opt
Hyperopto
Hypersal Ophthalmic
Lauro*
Lavoptik Eye Wash*
Lensrins*
Muro-128
NaSal
Salinex
Unisol*
SODIUM CITRATE
Albatussin*
Bicitra-Sugar Free*
Citrocarbonate*
Eno*
Polycitra*
Polycitra-LC--Sugar-Free*
Sal Hepatica*
Vicks Formula 44 Cough Mixture*
SODIUM FLUORIDE
Adeflor Chewable*
Adeflor Drops*
Dentavite*
Florvite*
Flozenges
Flo-Tabs
Fluor-A-Day
Fluoretyl
Fluorident
Fluorinse
Fluoritab
Flura-Drops
Karidium
Les-Cav
Luride
Luride Lozi-Tabs
Novacebrin with Fluoride*
Oro-Naf
Pediaflur
Pedi-Dent
Phos-Flur
Phos-Flur Oral Rinse/Supplement
Point-Two Dental Rinse
Primadent
Solu-Flur
Thera-Flur
Vi-Daylin w/Fluoride Chewable*
Vi-Daylin/F + Iron*
Vi-Daylin/F ADC + Iron Drops*
Vi-Daylin/F ADC Drops*
Vi-Daylin/F Drops*
Vi-Penta F Chewables*
Vi-Penta F Infant Drops*
Vi-Penta F Multivitamin Drops*
SODIUM HYALURONATE
Healon
SODIUM HYPOCHLORITE
Hygeol
SODIUM IODIDE
Iodotope
Iodotope Therapeutic
SODIUM NITROPRUSSIDE
Nipride
Nitropress
SODIUM NITROPRUSSIDE REAGENT
Acetest
Ketostix
SODIUM OXYCHLOROSENE
Clorpactin WCS-90
SODIUM PHENOLATE
Cherry Chloraseptic*

Chloraseptic DM
Cough Control
Lozenges*
Chloraseptic Gel*
Chloraseptic
Lozenges*
Chloraseptic Spray*
SODIUM PHOSPHATE
Barium Enema Prep
kit*
Fleet Enema*
Fleet Pediatric
Enema*
K-Phos Neutral*
Lavoptik Eye Wash*
Phosphotape
Phospho-Soda*
Saf Tip Phosphate
Enema*
Uroqid-Acid*
Uroqid-Acid No.2*
Uro-KP-Neutral*
SODIUM POLYSTYRENE
SULFONATE
Kayexalate
SPS
SODIUM SALICYLAMIDE
Tisma*
SODIUM SALICYLATE
Alysine
Corlin Infant Drops*
Cystex*
Dodds Pills
Entrosalyl
Klev
Pabalate*
Parbocyl-Rev
PhisoDan*
Tranquil*
Uracel
SODIUM TARTRATE
Eno*
Limonade Asepta
Limonade Rodeca
SODIUM TETRABORATE
DECAHYDRATE
Komex
SODIUM TETRADECYL
SULFATE
Sotradecol
Trombovar
SODIUM THIOSALICYLATE
Arthrolate
Asproject
Jecto Sal
Nalate
Rexolate
Thiocyl
Thiodyne
Thiosal
Thisul
Tusal
TH Sal
SODIUM THIOSULFATE
Komed*
Komed HC*
Sulfactol
Tinver*
SOLASULFONE
Sulphetrone
SOMATROPIN
Asellacrin
SORBITOL
American Mcgaw
Travenol
SPARTEINE
Actospar
Spartocin
Tocine
Tocosamine
SPECTINOMYCIN
Trobicin
Trobicin Sterile
Powder
SPIRAMYCIN
Rovamycine
Selectomycin
SPIRITS OF TURPENTINE
Vicks Vaporub*
SPIRONOLACTONE
Aldactazide*
Aldactone
Novo-Spiroton
Sincomen
STANOLONE
Androlone
Neodrol
Protona
STANOZOLOL
Stromba
Winstrol
STIBOGLUCONATE

Pentostam
STIBOPHEN
Fuadin
STREPTODORNASE
Varidase*
STREPTOKINASE
Bistreptase
DornoKinase
KabiKinase
Streptase
Streptodornase
Varidase*
STREPTOMYCIN
Isoject-Streptomycin
Strepolin
Streptosol 25%
Strycin
STREPTONICOZID
Streptohydrazid
STREPTOZOCIN
Zanosar
STYRAMATE
Sinaxar
SUCCINYLCHOLINE
Anectine
Brevidil 'M'
Quelicin
Scoline
Sucostrin
Sux-Cert
SUCCINYLSULFATHIAZOLE
Cremosuxidine
Sulfasuxidine
SUCRALFATE
Carafate
Sulcrate
Ulcerban
SULFABENZAMIDE
Sultrin*
SULFACETAMIDE
Bleph
Blephamide Liquifilm*
Blephamide Ointment*
Blephamide Ophthalmic*
Blephamide S.O.P.*
Bleph-10 Liquifilm
Cetamide
Cetapred*
Isopto Cetamide
Isopto Cetapred*
Metimyd*
Ophthel-S
Op-Sulfa30
Optimyd*
Optosulfex
Sebizon
Sodium Sulamyd
Sulamyd Sodium
Sulfacel-15
Sulfacet-R Lotion*
Sulf-10
Sulf-30
Sultrin*
Vasosulf*
SULFACHLORPYRIDAZINE
Consulid
Cosulfa
Nefrosul
Sonilyn
SULFACYTINE
Renoquid
SULFADIAZINE
Codiazine
Coptin*
Cremodiazine
EsKadiazine
Microsulfon
Solu-Diazine
Sulfadets
Sulfonamides Duplex*
SULFADIMETHOXINE
Agribon
Albon
Levisul
Madribon
Neostreptal
SULFADOXINE
Fansidar*
SULFAETHIDOLE
Globucid
Sethadil
Sul-Spansion
SULFAMERAZINE
Sulfonamides Duplex*
SULFAMETER
Sulla
SULFAMETHAZINE
Cremomethazine
Diazil
Sulfadine
Vertolan

SULFAMETHIZOLE
- Azo-Sulfstat*
- Azotrex*
- Microsul
- Microsul-A*
- Proklar
- Signa Sul-A*
- Sulfstat Forte
- Thiosulfil
- Thiosulfil-A*
- Thiosulfil-A Forte*
- Thiosulfil Duo-Pak*
- Thiosulfil Forte
- Unisul
- Uremide*
- Urifon
- Uri-pak*
- Urolucosil
- Utrasul

SULFAMETHOXAZOLE
- Azo Gantanol*
- Gantanol
- Sinomin
- Urobak
- Uro-Gantanol*

SULFAMETHOXYPYRIDAZINE
- Kynex
- Midicel

SULFAMOXOLE
- Sulfuno

SULFANILAMIDE
- Amide-VC*
- AAS*
- AVC with Dienestrol*
- AVC Cream*
- AVC Suppositories*
- Benegyn*
- Cervex Vaginal Cream*
- DeHavac*
- Femguard*
- Nil*
- Par*
- Par-Vag*
- Prontylin
- Strepocide
- Sufamal*
- Vagacreme*
- Vagidine*
- Vagitrol Cream/ Suppositories*
- Vagi-Nil*

SULFAPHENAZOLE
- Orisul
- Sulfabid

SULFAPYRIDINE
- Dagenan

SULFASALAZINE
- Azopyrin
- Azulfidine
- Azulfidine En-Tabs
- Rorasul
- Salazopyrin
- SAS-500
- Sulfadyne

SULFATHIAZOLE
- Sulfadrin Nasal Suspension*
- Sulfamul
- Sultrin*

SULFINPYRAZONE
- Anturan
- Anturane
- Anturidin
- Enturen
- Zynol

SULFISOMIDINE
- Aristamid
- Elkosin
- Sulfamethin

SULFISOXAZOLE
- Azosul*
- Azo Gantrisin*
- Azo-Soxazole*
- Azo-Sulfisoxazole*
- Cantri Vaginal Cream*
- Entusul
- Gantrisin
- Gantrisin Cream
- Koro-Suff Vaginal Cream
- Lipo Gantrism
- Novosoxazole
- Pediazole*
- Rosoxol
- SK-Soxazole
- Suldiazo*
- Sulfalar
- Sulfizole
- Vagilia Cream/ Suppositories*

SULFISOXAZOLE ACETYL
  Lipo Gantrisin
SULFOBROMOPHTHALEIN
  Bromsulphalein
SULFOXONE
  Diasone
  Diasone Sodium
    Enterab
SULFUR
  Acnaveen*
  Acnederm Lotion*
  Acne-Aid*
  Acne-Dome Creme &
    Lotion*
  Acne-Dome Medicated
    Cleanser*
  Acno*
  Acnomel*
  Acnotex*
  Acnycin*
  Akne Drying*
  Bensulfoid*
  Boil-Ease*
  Cenac*
  Clearasil*
  Clearasil Vanishing
    Formula*
  Contrablem*
  Cuticura
  Dry and Clear Acne
    Cream*
  Epi-Clear*
  Exzit*
  Exzit Medicated
    Cleanser*
  Finac
  Fostex Cake*
  Fostex Cream*
  Fostex CM
  Fostex Medicated
    Cleanser*
  Fostril
  Hill Cortac Lotion*
  Klaron*
  Liquimat
  Lotio Alsulfa
  Medrol Acne Lotion*
  Meted Shampoo*
  Meted 2 Shampoo*
  Multiscrub*
  Pernox*
  PhisoAc*
  PhisoDan*
  Pisec
  Postacne Lotion
  Pragmatar*
  Resulin*
  Rezamid*
  Sastid Al*
  Sastid Plain*
  Sastid Soap*
  Seale's Lotion
  Sebaveen*
  Sebex*
  Sebulex*
  Sebutone*
  Solvex Powder*
  Sulfacet
  Sulfacet-R Lotion*
  Sulfoil
  Sulforcin*
  Sulfoxyl Lotion*
  Tar-Doak Lotion*
  Teenac
  Therac*
  Theracort*
  Thylox Medicated
    Soap
  Transact
  Vanseb*
  Vanseb-T*
  Xerac
  Zinc Sulfide
    Compound Lotion
SULINDAC
  Clinoril
SULISOBENZONE
  Screen-Tex
  Spectra-Sorb UV 284
  Sungard
  Uval
  Uvinol MS-40
SUMAC EXTRACT
  Rhus-All Antigen*
SURAMIN
  Antrypol
  Bayer 205
  Germanin
SUTILAINS
  Travase

SYROSINGOPINE
  Singoserp

T

TALBUTAL
  Lotusate
TAMOXIFEN
  Nolvadex
TANNIC ACID
  Amertan
  Dalidyne*
TEMAZEPAM
  Euhypnos Forte
  Restoril
TERBUTALINE
  Brethine
  Bricanyl
  Filair
TERFENADINE
  Seldane
TERPIN HYDRATE
  Broncho-Tussin*
  Chexit*
  Cotussis*
  Creo-Terpin*
  Mycinettes Sugar
    Free*
  Noratuss*
  Prunicodeine*
  Toclonol with
    Codeine*
  Toclonol
    Expectorant*
  Tricodene C-V*
  Tussagesic*
  Tussaminic*
TESTOLACTONE
  Fludestrin
  Teslac
TESTOSTERONE
  Android-T
  Andro-Cyp 100
  Andro-Cyp 200
  Andro 100
  Andrusol
  Anthatest
  Delatestryl
  Depo-Testadiol*
  Depo-Testosterone
  Di-Genik*
  Duogen*
  Everone
  Histerone 100
  Histerone 50
  Malogen
  Malogen Aquaspension
  Malogex
  Mertestate
  Orchisterone-P
  Oreton
  Oreton Buccal
  Oreton Pellets for
    Subcutaneous
    Implantation
  Oreton Propionate
  Perandren
  Synandrol F
  Testaqua
  Testate
  Testaval 90/4*
  Testex
  Testoject-E.P.
  Testoject-50
  Testone
  Testosteroid
  Testostroval P.A.
  Testrone
  Test-Estrin*
  Virosterone
TETANUS IMMUNE
    GLOBULIN
  TIG
TETANUS IMMUNE
    GLOBULIN, HUMAN
  Homo-Tet
  Hu-Tet
  Hyper-Tet
  Tet-Conn-G
TETANUS TOXOID
  Triogen*
  Tri-Immunol*
  Wyeth*
TETRACAINE
  Anacel
  Anethaine
  Cetacaine Topical
    Anesthetic*
  Medihaler-Tetracaine

Metraspray
Pontocaine
TETRACHLOROETHYLENE
Nema
TETRACYCLINE
Achromycin
Achromycin Ophthalmic
Achromycin V
Achrostatin V*
Azotrex*
Bio-Tetra
Bristacycline
Cantet
Cefracycline
Comycin*
Cycline-250
Cyclopar
Decycline
Deltamycin
Double-T
G-Mycin
GT-250
GT-500
Hosta 'P'
Hosta 500
Maytrex
Medicycline
Muracine
Mysteclin-F*
Neo-Tetrine
Nor-Tet
Novotetra
Paltet
Panmycin
Piracaps
Polycycline
Quidtet
Retet
Robitet
Ro-Cycline
SK-Tetracycline
Steclin
Sumycin
T-Caps
Tepicycline
Tetrabiotic
Tetracaps
Tetrachel
Tetracrine
Tetracyn
Tetralan-250
Tetralean
Tetram
Tetrastatin*
Tetra-C
Tetrex
Tetrosol
Topicycline
T-125
T-250
Wintracin
TETRAHYDRONAPHTHALENE
Cuprex*
TETRAHYDROZOLINE
Clear&Bright
Murine Plus
Murine 2
Ocusol Drops
Opt-Ease
Soothe Eye Drops
Tetracon
Tetrasine
Tyzine
Visine Eye Drops
THALIDOMIDE
Imidan
Kevadon
Talimol
THENALIDINE
Sandostene
THENYLDIAMINE
Neo-Synephrine Compound*
Thenfadil
THEOBROMINE
Diuretin
Theocalcin
Thesodate
THEOBROMINE MAGNESIUM OLEATE
Athemol
Athemol-N*
THEOPHYLLINE
Accurbron*
Acet-Am Expectorant*
Aerolate III
Aerolate Jr.
Aerolate Liquid
Aerolate Sr.
Aqualin Suprettes

THEOPHYLLINE

Aquaphyllin
Asbron G Inlay*
Asmalix
Asma-Lief*
Asminorl Improved*
Asminyl*
Asthmagyl*
Asthmophylline
Azma Aid*
Bronchial Capsules*
Bronitin*
Bronkaid*
Bronkodyl
Bronkodyl S-R
Bronkolixir*
Bronkotabs*
Chemfedral*
Constant-T
Co-Xan*
Dicurin Procaine*
Dorsaphyllin
Duraphyl
Elixicon Suspension
Elixophyllin
Elixophyllin-GG Oral Liquid
Elixophyllin SR
Entair*
Glycerol-T*
Guiaphed Elixir*
Hydromax Syrup*
Hydrophed Tabs*
Hylate-tabs*
Isogen Compound*
Isogen Compound Elixir*
Isotil Tabs*
Isuprel Compound Elixir*
Labid
Lanophyllin
Lanophylline-GG Capsules*
Lardet Expectorant Tabs*
Lardet Tabs*
Liquophylline
Lixolin
Lodrane
Marax*
Mudrane GG Elixir*
Phedral*
Physpan
Primatene M*
Primatene P*
Quadrinal*
Quibron*
Quibron Plus*
Respid
Respirol*
Slo-Bid
Slo-Phyllin Gyrocaps,
Slo-Phyllin GG*
Slo-Phyllin 80
Somophyllin-CRT
Somophyllin-T
Sustaire
Synophylate
Synophylate-GG*
Tedral*
Tedral Elixir*
Tedral Expectorant*
Tedral SA*
Tedral-25*
T.E.P.*
Thalfed*
Thecord*
Theobid Durcap
Theobid Jr. Durcaps
Theobron SR
Theocap
Theoclear
Theoclear L.A.
Theocyne
Theodrin Pediatric Suspension*
Theofedral*
Theolair
Theolair-Plus 250*
Theolixir
Theon
Theophedrizine*
Theophenyllin*
Theophyl Chewable
Theophyl-SR
Theophyl-225
Theoral*
Theospan
Theospan SR
Theospan 80

Theostat
Theotabs*
Theovent Long-Acting
Theozine*
Theo-Dur
Theo-Dur Sprinkle
Theo-Guaia*
Theo-Organidin*
Theo-Sly-R*
Theo-24
Uniphyl
Uniphyl 400
Verequad*
Verquad*
Wesmatic Forte*

THIABENDAZOLE
Mintezol

THIALBARBITAL
Kemithal

THIAMINE
Alba-Lybe*
Becrinol
Betalin-S
Betaxin
Bewon
Cal-M*
Cenalene*
Cerebro-Nicin*
Fortior-2B*
Geravite Elixir*
Glukor Injection*
Hepp-Iron Drops*
Ironized Yeast*
Neuro B-12 Forte Injectable*
Neuro B-12 Injectable*
Thera-Combex H-P*
Tia-Doce Injectable Univial*
Trophite*
Troph-Iron*
Troph-Iron Liquid*
Vinothiam
Vita-Metrazol*

THIAMYLAL
Surital

THIETHYLPERAZINE
Torecan
Toresten

THIMEROSAL
Adapettes*
Boil n Soak*
Lensrins*
Lens-Wet*
Mersol
Merthiolate

THIOCYANATE
Scyan

THIOGUANINE
Lanvis
Tabloid Brand Thioguanine

THIOPENTAL
Pentothal

THIOPROPAZATE
Dartal

THIOPROPERAZINE
Majeptil
Mayeptil
Vontil

THIORIDAZINE
Mellaril
Mellaril-S
Novoridazine
Thioril

THIOTHIXENE
Navane
Orbinamon

THIPHENAMIL
Trocinate

THONZYLAMINE
Anahist
Neohetramine
Resistab

THROMBIN
Fibrindex
Thrombostat

THYME OIL
Dewitt's Oil for Ear Use*

THYMOL
Vicks Vaporub*

THYROGLOBULIN
Proloid
Thyractin
Thyroprotein

THYROID
Dathroid
Delcoid

S-P-T
Thyrar
Thyrocrine
Thyronol
Thyro-Teric
Tuloidin
Westhroid 1/4
THYROTROPIN
Thyrotron
Thytropar
THYROXINE
Armour Thyroid*
Thyroid Strong*
TIAPROFENIC ACID
Surgam
TICARCILLIN
Ticar
TICLOPIDINE
Ticlid
Ticlodix
Ticlodone
TICRYNAFEN
Selacryn
TIMOLOL
Betim
Blocadren
Temserin
Timcacor
Timolide*
Timoptic
Timoptol
TINCTURE OF BENZOIN
Vicks Vaposteam*
TINCTURE OF OPIUM
Dia-Quel Liquid*
TINIDAZOLE
Fasigyn
Simplotan
TIOCARLIDE
Isoxyl
TITANIUM DIOXIDE
A-Fil*
Buf Foot-Care Soap*
Meltex*
TOBRAMYCIN
Nebcin
Tobrex
TOCAINIDE
Tonocaid
Tonocard
Tonogard
TOLAZAMIDE
Diabewas
Norglycin
Tolinase
TOLAZOLINE
Priscoline
Tolzol
TOLBUTAMIDE
Dolipol
Mellitol
Mobenol
Neo-Dibetic
Novobutamide
Oramide
Orinase
Rastinon
SK-Tolbutamide
Tolbutone
TOLMETIN
Tolectin
Tolectin DS
TOLNAFTATE
Aftate
Pitrex
Sporiline
Tinactin
Tinaderm
Tonoftal
TOLONIUM
Blutene
TOLYL BIGUANIDE
Buf Foot-Care Soap*
TRANEXAMIC ACID
Cyklokapron
TRANYLCYPROMINE
Parnate
TRAZODONE
Desyrel
TRETINOIN
Aberel
Aquasol A Cream
Retin-A
Vitamin A Acid Gel
TRIACETIN
Enzactin
Fungacetin
Fungoid
Fungoid Tincture
Vanay
TRIAMCINOLONE
Aristform*

Aristform D*
Aristform R*
Aristocort
Aristoderm
Aristogel
Aristosol
Aristospan
Axmacort
Azmacort
Cinalone 40
Cinolone-T
Flutex
Flutone
Kenac
Kenacomb*
Kenacort
Kenalog
Kenalog in Orabase
Kenalog-E
Mycolog*
Myco Triacet Cream & Ointment*
Mytrex*
Nysolone*
SK-Triamcinolone
Spencort
Tracilon
Tramacin
Triacet Cream
Triaderm
Triamalone
Tricilone NNG*
Trimacort
Tri-Statin*
Trymex
Viaderm-TA

TRIAMTERENE
Apo-Triazide*
Dyazide*
Dyrenium
Dytac
Jatropur
Maxzide*
Novotriamzide*
Novo-Triamzide*

TRIAZOLAM
Halcion

TRICHLORMETHIAZIDE
Aquex
Diurese
Iperdiuren
Kirkrinal
Metahydrin
Metatensin*
Naqua
Naquival*
Ropres*
Trichlorex

TRICHLOROETHYLENE
Chlorylen
Trilene

TRICLOBISONIUM
Triburon

TRICLOFOS
Triclos

TRICLOSAN
Adasept Cleanser
Clearasil Medicated Soap
Irgasan DP 300
Promani
Rhulicaine*
Solvex Athlete's Foot Spray*
Tersaseptic
Zemo*

TRIDIHEXETHYL
Claviton
Mepro-Hex*
Milpath*
Pathibamate*
Pathilon

TRIETHANOLAMINE TROLAMINE SALICYLATE
Aspercreme

TRIFLUOPERAZINE
Chem-Flurazine
Clinazine
Jatroneural
Novoflurazine
Pentazine
Solazine
Stelazine
Terfluzine
Triazine
Triflurin
Tripazine

TRIFLUPROMAZINE
Psyquil 25
Siquil
Vesprin

TRIFLURIDINE
  Viroptic
TRIHEXYPHENIDYL
  Antitrem
  Aparkane
  Artane
  Hexyphen
  Novohexidyl
  Pipanol
  T.H.P.
  Tremin
  Trihexane
  Trihexidyl
  Trihexy-2
  Trixyl
TRILOSTANE
  Modrastane
TRIMEPRAZINE
  Panectyl
  Temaril
  Theralene
  Vallergan
TRIMETHADIONE
  Tridione
  Trimedone
TRIMETHAPHAN CAMSYLATE
  Arfonad
TRIMETHIDINIUM
    METHOSULFATE
  Ostensin
TRIMETHOBENZAMIDE
  Tegmide
  Tigan
  Xametina
TRIMETHOPRIM
  Bactrim
  Coptin*
  Proloprim
  SMZ-TMP
  Trimpex
TRIMIPRAMINE
  Stangyl
  Surmontil
TRIOXSALEN
  Trisoralen
TRIPARANOL
  Mer/29
TRIPELENNAMINE
  Benzoxal
  Di-Delamine*
  PBZ
  PBZ Expectorant
    w/Ephedrine*
  PBZ Lontabs
  PBZ-SR
  PBZ with ephedrine*
  Poly-Histine-D*
  Poly-Histine-D
    Elixir*
  Pyribenzamine
  Pyrizil
  Rhulihist*
  Ro-Hist
  Tri-Tumine
TRIPHENYLTETRAZOLIUM
  Uroscreen
TRIPROLIDINE
  Acridil
  Actacin*
  Actagen*
  Actamine*
  Actidil
  Actidilon
  Actifed*
  Actifed-C*
  Actifed with Codeine
    Cough Syrup*
  Actifed Expectorant*
  Actihist*
  Acti-Prem*
  Allerfrin*
  Norafed*
  Pro-Actidil
  Pseudodine*
  Rofed Syrup*
  Tagafed*
  Triacin*
  Triafed*
  Trifed*
  Triphed*
  Tripodrine*
  Triposed*
  Tri-Fed*
TRIZYME
  Arco-Lase*
  Arco-Lase Plus*
  Co-Gel Liquitabs*
TROLAMINE
  Buf Foot-Care
    Lotion*

Seratyl
TROLAMINE SALICYLATE
Exocaine Cream
Mobisyl Creme
Myoflex
Royflex
TROLEANDOMYCIN
Cyclamycin
Olicin
Tao
TROLNITRATE
Angitrit
Metamine
Nitretamine
Vasomed
TROMETHAMINE
Tris Amino
THAM
TROPICAMIDE
Mydriacyl
TRYPSIN
Biozyme*
Granulex*
Orenzyme*
Parenzyme
Parenzymol
Tryptar
TRYPTOPHAN
Trofan
Tryptacin
TUAMINOHEPTANE
Heptedrine
Heptin
Rhinosol
Tuamine
TUBERCULIN
Aplisol
Aplitest
Sclavo Test-PPD
Tubersol
TUBOCURARINE
Tubadil
Tubarine
TUBOCURARINE DIMETHYL ETHER
Mecostrin Chloride
TURPENTINE OIL
Sloan's Liniment*
TYBAMATE
Benvil
Effisax
Solacen
Tybatran
TYROPANOATE SODIUM
Bilopaque
TYROTHRICIN
Bactratycin
Hydrotricine
Soluthricin
Tyroderm

U

UNDECYLENIC ACID
Blis-To-Sol*
Desenex*
Desenex Liquid
Fungiderm
Merlenate*
Nuvola Medicated Shampoo
Podiaspray*
Quinsana Plus*
Quinsana Plus Medicated Foot Powder
Rid-Itch Cream*
Sal-Dex*
Solvex Athlete's Foot Spray*
Undoguent*
Verdefam Cream*
Verdefam Solution*
UREA
Akne Drying*
Amino-Cerv
Aquacare
Calmurid
Carmol
Carmol 10 Lotion
Elaqua XX
Kerid Ear Drop*
Lowila Cake*
Nutraplus
Panafil Ointment*
Panafil-White Ointment*
Ultra Mide
Ureaphil

Uremol
Uremol HC*
Uretex
Urisec
Velvelan
UROKINASE
Abbokinase
Abbokinase
Breokinase
Win-Kinase

V

VALETHAMATE
Epidosin
Murel
VALPROATE SODIUM
Depakote*
Epilim
VALPROIC ACID
Depakene
Depakote*
Ergenyl
Urekene
VANCOMYCIN
Vancocin
VASOPRESSIN
Insipidin
Pitressin
Pitressin Tannate in Oil
VERAPAMIL
Calan
Cordilox
Iproveratril
Isoptin
Vasolan
VIDARABINE
Ara-A
Vira-A
VILOXAZINE
Vivalan
VINBARBITAL
Delvinal
VINBLASTINE
Velban
Velbe
VINCRISTINE
Oncovin
VINDESINE
Eldisine
VINYL ETHER
Vinethene
VIOMYCIN
Vinactane-P
Viocin
VITAMIN A
A.C.N.*
Acon
Afaxin
Alphalin
Alphamettes*
Anatola
Andoin*
Aquasol A
Aquasol A & D*
Aret-A
Arovit
A-Sol
A-Vitan
AVP Natal*
Desitin Ointment*
Dispatabs
Formule A
Homagenets Aoral
Pedi-Vit A
Proctodon*
Scott's Emulsion*
Super A
Testavol S
Tri-Vi-Flor*
Tri-Vi-Flor w/Iron Drops*
Tri-Vi-Sol*
Tri-Vi-Sol with Iron*
Vio-A
Vi-Alpha
Vi-Daylin ADC Drops*
Vi-Daylin/F ADC + Iron Drops*
Vi-Daylin/F ADC Drops*
Vi-Daylin Plus Iron ADC Drops*
Vi-Zac*
VITAMIN B COMPLEX
Albafort Injectable*
Becotin

Becotin-T*
Becotin With Vitamin C*
Bejectal
Bejectal with Vitamin C*
Bejex*
Beplete
Berocca*
Berocca-C*
Betalin
Feraplex Liquid*
Heptuna Plus*
I.L.X. B12*
I.L.X. B12 Elixir*
L-Glutavite*
Mega-B
Solu-B with Ascorbic Acid Sterile Powder*
Solu-B Sterile
Thera-Complex H-P*
Thex Forte*
Vibelan
Zentrol Chewable*
Zentron Liquid*
Zintinic*

VITAMIN D
Caltrate 600 + D*

VITAMIN E
Aprisac*
Aquasol E
Cardialine
Dalfatol
Daltose
E-Ferol
Ephynal
Eprolin
Epsilan-M
Esorb
E-Toplex
Kell-E
Lan-E
Lethopherol*
Maxi-E
Natopherol
Novo E
Phytoferol
Super Cardialine
Tocopherex
Tofaxin
Tokols
TriHemic 600*
Vascuals
Vita-E
Vi-Zac*

VITAMINS, MULTIPLE
Abdec Baby Drops
Abdec Kapseal
Abdec Teens
Abdec Teens with Iron*
Abdol with Minerals*
About Face
Adabee
Adabee with Minerals*
Adeflor Chewable*
Adeflor Drops*
Allbee with C
Allbee-T
Al-Vite*
B-C-Bid
B Complex
B-Complex
B Complex with Vitamin C
Beminal Forte with Vitamin C
Beminal 500
Betacrest
Beta-Vite with Iron Liquid
Beta-Vite Liquid
Betonal Cap
Bewon Elixir
B Nutron
Brewer's Yeast
Calcicaps
Calcicaps with Iron*
Calciwafers
Calinate-FA
Cal-Prenal
Cardenz
Cari-Tab Softab*
C-B Vone
Cebefortis
Cebetinic
Cecon Solution
Ceebec

Cefol
Centrum
Cevi-Bid
Chenatal*
Cherri-B Liquid
Chew-E
Chew-Vite
Chocks
Chocks-Bugs Bunny
Chocks-Bugs Bunny Plus Iron*
Chocks Plus Iron*
Citrotein*
Clusivol
Clusivol 130
Cod Liver Oil with Vitamin C
Cod Liver Oil Concentrate
Combex Kapseals
Combex Kapseals with Vitamin C
Dayalets
Dayalets Plus Iron*
De-Cal
Dentavite*
Dical-D with Vitamin C
Duo-CVP
Dura-C 500 Graduals
Eldec Kapseals*
Eldercaps*
Eldertonic*
En-Cebrin*
En-Cebrin F*
Engran-HP
Feminaid
Feminins
Femiron with Vitamins*
Ferritrinsic
Ferrolip Plus
Filibon*
Flintstones
Flintstones Plus Iron*
Florvite*
Folbesyn
Fortespan
Fosfree*
Ganatrex
Geralix Liquid
Geriamic
Gerilets
Geriplex
Geriplex-FS Kapseals
Geriplex-FS Liquid
Geritinic
Geritol
Geritol Junior
Geritol Junior Liquid
Geritol Liquid
Gerix Elixir*
Gerizyme
Gevrabon
Gevral
Gevral Protein
Gevral T
Gevrite
Glutofac*
Glytinic*
Golden Bounty B Complex with Vitamin C
Golden Bounty Multivitamin Supplement with Iron
Hemocyte Plus Tabules*
Hemo-Vite*
Hi-Bee with C
Hyplex
Hyrex
Iberet
Iberet Oral Solution
Iberet-500
Iberet-500 Oral Solution
Iberol
Incremin with Iron*
Iodine Ration
Iromin-G*
Larobec
Lederplex
Lipoflavonoid
Lipotriad
Lipo-Nicin*
Liquid Geritonic

Livitamin
Lofenalac
Lonalac*
Lufa
Maltlevol*
Maltlevol-M*
Maltlevol 12*
Materna*
Megadose*
Methischol
Mevanin-C*
Minuteman
Mission Prenatal*
Mi-Cebrin*
Mi-Cebrin T*
Monster Vitamins
Monster Vitamins & Iron*
Mucoplex
Multicebrin
Mulvidren Softabs
Myadec
M.V.I.
M.V.I.-12
M.V.M. Liquid
Nap Tabs
Natabec
Natacomp-FA*
Natafort Filmseal*
Natalins
Natural Theratab
NaturSlim II*
Neofol B-12
Neo-Calglucon
Niferex-PN*
Norimex
Norimex-Plus
Norlac
Novacebrin with Fluoride*
Nu-Iron-V*
Obron-6
One-A-Day
One-A-Day Plus Iron*
One-A-Day Vitamins Plus Minerals*
Optilets-M-500
Optilets-500
Orexin Softabs
Ostrex Tonic
Os-Cal Forte*
Os-Cal Plus*
Paladac
Paladac with Minerals*
Pals
Pals with Iron
Peritinic
Poly-Vi-Flor*
Poly-Vi-Flor with Iron*
Poly-Vi-Sol
Poly-Vi-Sol with Iron*
Pramet FA*
Pramilet FA*
Probec-T
Ragus*
Ray-D
Roeribec
Rovite*
Sclerex*
Sigtab
Simron Plus
Solu-B-Forte(S-B-F) Sterile Powder
Spancap C
S.S.S. Tonic
Stresscaps
Stresstabs 600
Stresstabs 600 with Iron*
Stresstabs 600 with Zinc*
Stuartinic
Stuart Formula
Stuart Formula Liquid
Stuart Hematinic
Stuart Hematinic Liquid
Stuartnatal*
Stuart Prenatal*
Stuart Prenatal Formula
Stuart Therapeutic Multivitamin
Super Calcicaps
Super D Cod Liver Oil

Super D Perles
Super Hydramin
Super Plenamins
Surbex
Surbex-T
Surbex with C*
Surbex 750 with Iron*
Surbex 750 with Zinc*
Tabron Filmseal*
Taka-Combex Kapseals
Tega-C
Tega-E
Therabid
Theracebrin
Theragran
Theragran Liquid
Theragran-M*
Therapeutic Vitamins
Therapeutic Vitamins and Minerals*
Thera-Combex H-P Kapseals
Thera-Combex Kapseals
Thera-Spancap
Theron
Tonebec
Tri-Vi-Sol with Iron Drops*
Tri-Vi-Sol Chewable
Unicap
Unicap Chewable
Unicap M
Unicap Plus Iron*
Unicap Senior
Unicap T
Vastran
Venthera
VG*
Vi-Aqua
Vicon
Vicon-C*
Vicon Plus
Vi-Daylin w/Fluoride Chewable*
Vi-Daylin Chewable
Vi-Daylin Drops
Vi-Daylin/F + Iron*
Vi-Daylin/F Drops*
Vi-Daylin Liquid
Vi-Daylin Plus Iron*
Vigran
Vigran Chewable
Vigran Plus Iron*
Vi-Magna
Viopan-T*
Vio-Bec
Vio-Geric
Vi-Penta F Chewables*
Vi-Penta F Infant Drops*
Vi-Penta F Multivitamin Drops*
Vi-Penta Infant Drops
Vi-Penta Multivitamin Drops
VM Preparation
Vi-Syneral One-Caps
Vitacrest
Vitagett
Vita-Kaps
Vita-Kaps-M
Viterra
Viterra High Potency
Vi-Zac
Z-Bec
Zentinic*
Zincaps
Zymacap
Zymalixir
Zymasyrup

W

WARFARIN
- Athrombin-K
- Coufarin
- Coumadin
- Marevan
- Panwarfin
- Warcoumin
- Warfilone
- Warnerin

WITCH HAZEL
- Neutrogena Acne-Drying Gel*
- Optrex

Tucks Cream
Tucks Ointment
Tucks Pads*

X

XANTHINOL NIACINATE
Angioamin
Complamin
XIPAMIDE
Diurexan
XYLOMETAZOLINE
Dristamead Long
Duramist PM
Hydra-Spray
Neo-Synephrine II
Otrivin
Sine-Off Once-A-Day
Sinex-L.A.
Sinus Spray
Sinutab Long-lasting Decongestant Sinus Spray
Sinutab Nasal Spray
Vicks Sinex Long-Acting Decongestant Nasal Spray
4-Way Long Acting Nasal Spray

Z

ZINC
Dequasine*
Stresstabs 600 with Zinc*
Surbex 750 with Zinc*
Zn-Plus
ZINC CHLORIDE
Freezone*
ZINC OXIDE
Acnederm Lotion*
Akne Drying*
Allersone*
Calamatum*
Calamine*
Caldesene Medicated Ointment
Cal-ZO Dressing*
Decubitex*
Derma Medicone-HC Ointment*
Derma Medicone Ointment*
Desitin Ointment*
Dome-Paste Bandage*
Emeroid*
Herisan
Hill Cortac Lotion*
HTO Stainless Manzan Hemorrhoidal Tissue Ointment*
Rectagene Balm*
Saratoga*
Supertah*
Wyanoids Hemorrhoidal Suppositories*
Wyanoids HC Rectal Suppositories*
Zincofax
Ziradryl Lotion*
ZINC PHENOLSULFONATE
Amogel*
Corrective Mixture*
Corrective Mixture with Paregoric*
Infantol Pink*
Pabizol with Paregoric*
ZINC PHOSPHATE
Vi-Zac*
ZINC PYRITHIONE
Ionil-T
ZINC STEARATE
Blis-To-Sol*
Ting*
ZINC SULFATE
Acnederm Lotion*
Anusol*
Anusol-HC*
Anusol Ointment*
Anusol Suppositories*
Eyephrine*
Medizinc
Neozin*
Optised Ophthalmic*

Orazinc
Phenylzin*
Verazinc
Zincfrin-A*
Zinc-220
Z-Pro-C*

ZINC UNDECYLENATE
Cruex Medicated Cream
Daliderm*
Desenex*
Deso-Creme*
Devines Kool Foot
Fung-O-Spray*
NP-27 Spray Powder
Quinsana Plus*
Rid-Itch Cream*
Undoguent*

ZIRCONIUM OXIDE
Rhulicream*

ZOMEPIRAC
Zomax